Intelligent Precision Healthcare

Artificial Intelligence (AI) is reshaping modern healthcare in remarkable ways. This book explores how multimodal generative AI integrates clinical, genetic, and imaging data to improve the understanding and management of neurodegenerative diseases. Bridging technology and medicine, it offers accessible insights into next-generation precision healthcare and its real-world impact. Designed for researchers, clinicians, and informed readers alike, it highlights practical applications, ethical considerations, and future possibilities in AI-driven neurological care.

This volume provides a comprehensive examination of how multimodal generative AI techniques can be applied to the diagnosis, monitoring, and management of neurodegenerative disorders such as Alzheimer's and Parkinson's diseases. It covers foundational concepts in precision healthcare, multimodal data integration (including genetic, clinical, and neuroimaging data), and advanced modeling approaches for disease progression prediction. The book also explores synthetic data generation for rare conditions, explainable and interpretable AI models for clinical decision support, and AI-driven early detection systems. Dedicated chapters address ethical, legal, and regulatory considerations, interdisciplinary collaboration, and patient-centric AI design. Through case studies and real-world applications, the book demonstrates how intelligent systems can enhance personalized treatment planning, improve clinical outcomes, and support data-driven healthcare innovation.

Intelligent Precision Healthcare

Multimodal Generative AI for Neurodegenerative Disease Management

Edited by
Deepika Koundal, Mudassir Khan,
Rupali Atul Mahajan, and Rajesh Dey

CRC Press
Taylor & Francis Group
Boca Raton London New York

CRC Press is an imprint of the
Taylor & Francis Group, an **informa** business

Designed cover image: TBC

First edition published 2027
by CRC Press
2385 NW Executive Center Drive, Suite 320, Boca Raton FL 33431

and by CRC Press
4 Park Square, Milton Park, Abingdon, Oxon, OX14 4RN

CRC Press is an imprint of Taylor & Francis Group, LLC

ISBN: 978-1-041-12867-0 (hbk)
ISBN: 978-1-041-12952-3 (pbk)
ISBN: 978-1-003-66736-0 (ebk)

DOI: 10.1201/ 9781003667360

Typeset in Times
by Apex CoVantage, LLC

Contents

Editors

Deepika Koundal is a distinguished academic at the University of Eastern Finland, specializing in artificial intelligence, machine learning, and healthcare analytics. Her research focuses on intelligent, data-driven solutions for medical and biomedical applications, contributing significantly to interdisciplinary innovation and global research collaborations. She has published extensively in reputed international journals and actively leads research initiatives in AI-driven healthcare technologies, fostering academic excellence and industry partnerships worldwide.

Mudassir Khan is an accomplished academician and researcher specializing in big data analytics, deep learning, AI, and healthcare applications. Holding a PhD in big data analytics using deep learning, he is currently pursuing a postdoctoral fellowship at Multimedia University, Malaysia, while serving as an assistant professor at King Khalid University, Saudi Arabia. With over 14 years of experience, he has authored 100+ SCI/SCOPUS-indexed papers, four books, and edited numerous volumes with leading publishers.

Rupali A. Mahajan is an accomplished academician and researcher specializing in artificial intelligence, machine learning, deep learning, and data science applications. Holding a PhD in computer science and engineering, she completed her postdoctoral research at the Singapore Institute of Technology. She currently serves as an associate professor in the Department of Data Science at Vishwakarma Institute of Information Technology, Pune. With over 17 years of professional experience, she has authored 7 books, published 50+ research papers, and held 18 patents across diverse domains.

Rajesh Dey is a distinguished researcher specializing in artificial intelligence, machine learning, and fintech. Currently a postdoctoral fellow at IIUM, Malaysia, he holds a PhD in adaptive signal correction. With over 17 years of experience, he has published extensively and contributed to embedded systems, Internet of Things (IoT), robotics, and sustainable electric vehicle (EV) technologies. He has served in key academic and industry roles, including associate professor and technical director. A certified design thinking coach, he actively collaborates with international universities and research institutions, mentoring students and driving innovation in emerging technologies.

1 Decoding Psychiatric Disorders
Multimodal Brain Imaging Powered by Machine Learning and Deep Learning

Jayesh Kshirsaagr, Vanita Kshirsagar, Anupam Bonkra, Goh Khang Wen, and Imran Basheti

1.1 INTRODUCTION

Psychiatric diseases have been a problem for millions worldwide and heavily affect society, the individual, and the economy. The diversity of psychiatric disorders and the intricate complexity of disease causation from genetic and environmental point of view, involving interactions with neurology, have led psychiatry and neuroscience to challenge their findings and make sense of what mental disorders really are. Figure 1.1 shows the accumulation of information from different neuroimaging methods, such as diffusion tensor imaging (DTI), electroencephalography (EEG), structural magnetic resonance imaging (sMRI), and the utilization of functional magnetic resonance imaging (fMRI). Multimodal brain imaging is a landmark way made to uncover these complexities [1, 2].

Traditional analytical techniques are useful, but they usually can't manage the high dimensionality and complexity of multimodal imaging data. It is still highly individual-specific, quite large in scope and scale, and fairly noisy. Machine learning (ML) and deep learning (DL) are crucial techniques to infer from this neuroimaging data, as they have enabled the ability to capture complexity or nonlinearity to some degree. The findings of ML/DL have the potential to predict psychiatric outcomes, such as depression, bipolar disorder, schizophrenia, and many others, through subtle expressions of psychiatric phenotypes Khan et al. (2025) demonstrated a hybrid modeling framework that integrates statistical, kernel-based, and neural approaches to improve prediction accuracy in complex cardiovascular conditions—an approach adaptable to psychiatric disorder analysis [3].

Combining DL and ML with multimodal imagery offers an opportunity to improve mental health diagnosis, prognosis, and treatment. For instance, the integration of structural and functional imaging data can help us understand how the brain is connected and how mental health problems are caused by abnormalities in these networks demonstrated by Durstewitz et al. and Koppe et al. [4, 5]. Khan et al. (2025) explored multimodal DL strategies for precise disease identification, establishing a foundation for using integrated feature spaces in neuropsychiatric diagnostics [6]. Moreover, disease-specific biomarkers that may not be evident when analyzing single-modality data can be identified using multimodal approaches. These biomarkers can support precision psychiatry by allowing the prediction of a possible disease attack, tracking disease course growth, and approximating treatment response by Cai et al. [7], Pal et al. (2025) presented edge-intelligent ML methods for real-time IoT data processing, underscoring the relevance of decentralized computing in dynamic psychiatric data interpretation [8].

DOI: 10.1201/9781003667360-1

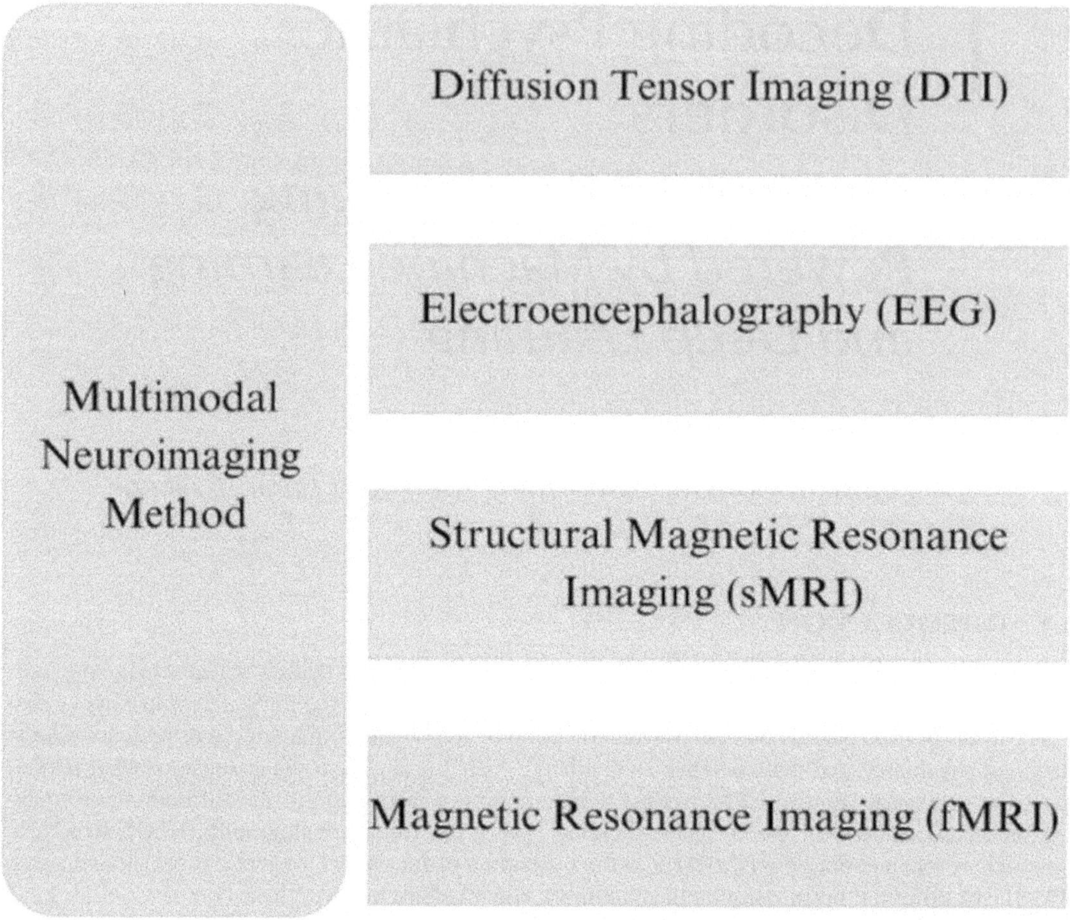

FIGURE 1.1 The multimodal neuroimaging method

Advances in DL model designs, especially convolutional neural network (CNN), recurrent neural network (RNN), and graph neural network (GNN) variants, have produced better features for measuring the multimodal content of imaging soundings. For instance, CNNs are better at identifying spatial patterns in imagery data, while RNNs do well with temporal and sequential data. GNNs provide a basis for modeling complex brain networks. They help to simplify the inquiry of modifications in neural networks in mental disorders explained by Rashid and Calhoun [9]. For the purpose of improvement, they face countless problems. Paul et al. (2018) reviewed advancements in bio-signal-controlled prosthetic arms, offering insights into translating physiological signal patterns into actionable interpretations—an idea central to brain-based psychiatric modeling [10]. The changeability of data between imagery methods and specific people is one of the main difficulties. Differences in electronic scanner settings, data gathering methods, and research cohort demographics may result in heterogeneity. For instance, it may be challenging to directly integrate data from numerous imaging modes due to differences in temporal features, spatial resolutions, and sound profiles. Das et al. (2017) utilized electromyography signals with fuzzy logic for sign language representation, showcasing early applications of bio-signal analysis in decoding complex human expressions [11]. Over and above patient-specific variables such as age and gender, medical difficulties could have an impact on the results' variability. Additionally, data harmonization strategies have been implemented, such as ComBat for batch effect correction and domain adaptation algorithms. Feature fusion techniques can be early, late, or mixed feature combination techniques to integrate data from various modalities and ensure that the contributions are unique to the modalities. For these methods to have reliability and generalizability of ML and DL models trained on multimodal imaging data, all these steps are required. Mahajan et al. (2025) proposed generative AI and transfer learning for personalized IoT-based health monitoring, highlighting the importance of adaptive intelligence in patient-specific mental health prediction [12].

This section discusses DL and ML techniques applied to multimodal brain imaging in mental health conditions. To discuss state-of-the-art methods, highlight key applications, and examine the boundaries and limitations of these approaches. To give a more complete picture, since it's about the newest research and case stories regarding how ML and DL are broadening the utilization of neuroimaging and contributing to better comprehension and treatment of mental diseases, attention will be on the newest cases. By the same token, this work presents the possibility and opens even more avenues for further research intended at transforming such innovation into a clinically relevant therapeutic application.

1.2 PIPELINE FOR MULTIMODAL BRAIN IMAGING

Figure 1.2 shows multimodal brain imaging and text to predict the human psychological condition. The various neuroimaging modalities provide a more comprehensive understanding of multimodal brain imaging, referred to as the knowledge of the structure and function of the brain pipeline. Brossollet et al. [1] provide the study of mental diseases has significantly benefited, since these circumstances often exhibit complex neural interactions and subtle brain abnormalities. From data gathering to the formation of clinically significant understandings, the pipeline holds numerous steps to guarantee the precision and directness of the outcomes.

(a) **Acquiring Data**

DTI, EEG, sMRI, and fMRI are some of the methods used to gather neuroimaging data. Rahaman et al. [2] demonstrated the numerous modalities offer diverse information. For example, sMRI shows functional structures, DTI examines white matter areas, fMRI gives activity in the brain through a change in blood oxygenation, and EEG offers great

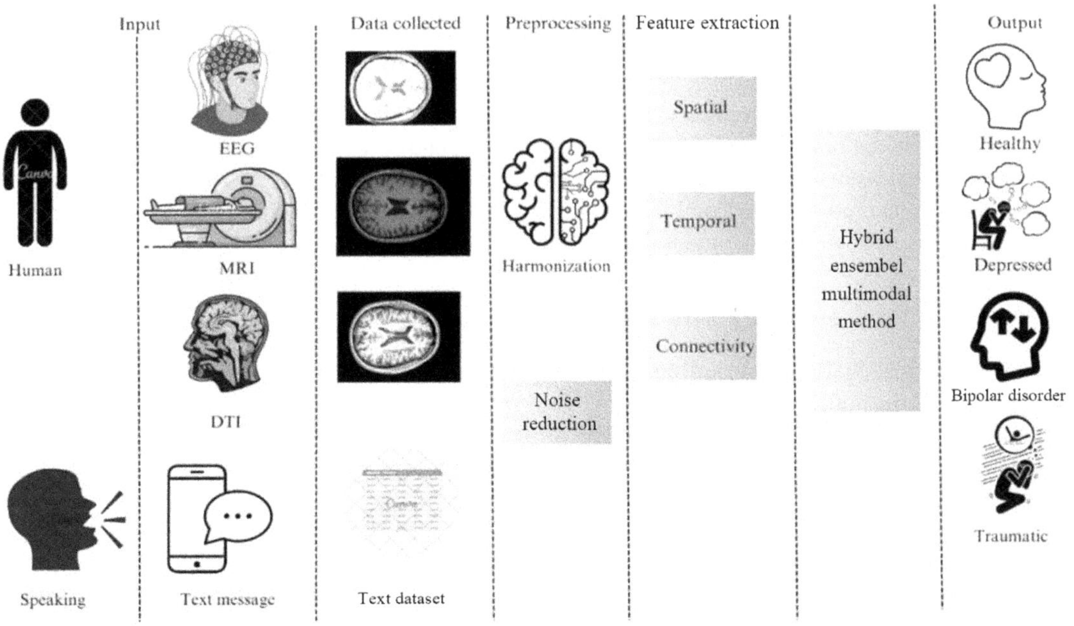

FIGURE 1.2 Multimodal brain imaging and text to predict human psychological condition

chronological resolution of electric action In addition to improving the dataset, diverse sensory modalities provide investigators with new standpoints on the configuration and purposes of the brain.

(b) **The Preparation Phase**
Menon and Krishnamurthy [13] used due to the usage of many acquisition techniques and scanner configurations, RAW imaging data are typically noisy, full of artifacts, and untrustworthy. Preprocessing is usually essential to confirm the quality and reliability of the data, as well as motion improvement, normalization, and removal of artifacts. More advanced harmonization methods, such as the ComBat algorithm, are typically applied to decrease batch effects and match the data from different origins.

(c) **Extraction of Features**
Menon and Krishnamurthy [13] used following preparation, the pipeline centers on finding salient features in the data. Depending on the modality, connectivity analysis for fMRI, dimensional measurements for sMRI, and an evaluation of white matter integrity for DTI may be needed. These characteristics provide a number of variables to be used to find patterns and biomarkers that are linked to mental health issues.

(d) **Integration of Data**
The application of multimodal fusion is an essential pipeline step where the data from various imaging modalities are fused together in order to produce a coherent image. Durstewitz et al. [4] demonstrated early fusion involves the fusion of raw data coming from many modalities, late fusion involves the fusion of results obtained from independent analyses, and hybrid fusion combines both approaches. This stage provides further insight into the brain by taking advantage of using different modalities.

(e) **Training and Analysis of Models**
Both ML and DL approaches are applied to the merged dataset. Koppe et al. [5] discussed the models were designed to learn complex patterns, classify diseases, and predict prognoses. The more composite features are classically treated with more specialized architectures, such as GNNs for network-based features and CNNs for spatial features.

(f) **Scientific Translation and Authentication**
To do scientific preparation and validate the models on a large dataset, the last step is to apply the discoveries. These models are the combination of illness trajectory prediction, biomarkers, and therapy outcome monitoring. Cai et al. [7] presented MM-GTU Nets provided the pipeline is valuable evidence that can finally close the gap between experimental studies and precision psychiatry. It has been proposed as a whole transformation pipeline for multimodal brain imaging by combining the most advanced techniques of cutting-edge technology with high-level image processing and potent analytical techniques. It's thus unique in its method, as it combines many integrated elements, which may give significant variations in how to notice mental illnesses.

1.2.1 Issues With Heterogeneity and Their Resolutions

One of the critical challenges to utilizing DL and ML methods in studying and managing mental illnesses is that the multimodal brain imaging data vary. Variables include, among others, a diverse patient population, scanner setup, acquisition strategies, and various imaging modalities. These challenges need to be addressed to enable clinical applicability, generalization, and validity of the models for prediction, as shown in Figure 1.3.

(a) **Variability of Imaging Techniques**
Different types of imaging modalities, including fMRI, sMRI, DTI, and EEG, yield different kinds of information on spatial and temporal resolutions. Brossollet et al. [1] provide the former focuses more on white matter architecture, whereas the latter has blood oxygen

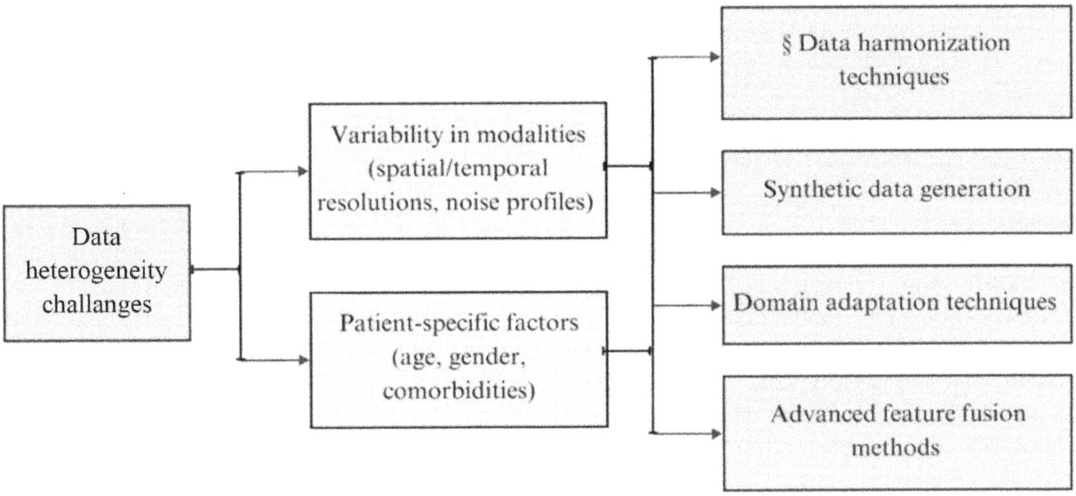

FIGURE 1.3 Challenges and solutions of heterogeneity

level-dependent (BOLD) signals that are considered to be connected with brain activity. The modalities may differ in terms of size, noise characteristics, and feature space, which sometimes makes integration difficult.

(b) **Differences in Acquisition and Protocol**
Since most datasets are created using multiple scanner setups, acquisition techniques, and calibration standards, they are typically very heterogeneous and obtained from different sites or investigations. Rahaman et al. [2] demonstrated these batch effects make it difficult to make simple comparisons and hinder reproducibility

(c) **Variability Among Individuals**
Differences in demographics, age, gender, comorbid conditions, and other factors contribute to the heterogeneity of data. Menon and Krishnamurthy [13] used Psychiatric illnesses, by definition, involve numerous factors that often manifest clinically with diverse features and thus cannot be attributed to a few universally applicable biomarkers or patterns that predict disease outcome

(d) **Limited Sample Sizes and Bias**
Smucny et al. [14] examined most neuroimaging research is often associated with a small number of participants because of the costs involved and the complexity of data acquisition. The problem worsens with biased data, for example, where fewer participants represented each of certain psychiatric conditions

1.3 MULTIMODAL BRAIN IMAGING POWERED BY MACHINE LEARNING AND DEEP LEARNING

Brossollet et al. [1] explained ML advances have been used in psychiatric brain imaging studies, providing new perceptions of mental illnesses. Scientists observed how artificial intelligence (AI) can recognize complex neural data in order to expand diagnosis and prediction skills. As neuroimaging has been integrated into AI models, ML has shown promise in the classification of mental illnesses. While exposing some of its limitations, the work in provides a thorough examination of the applications of ML in psychiatry. Rahaman et al. [2] demonstrated the development of deep multimodal models that incorporate genomics and neuroimaging, as revealed in is a significant step in this field. These models successfully identify the neurological and genetic markers associated with schizophrenia. Menon and Krishnamurthy [13] used Multimodal ensemble to differentiate between kids with disruptive behavior disorders and usually developing youths, using data from large-scale research.

Smucny et al. [14] examined DL algorithms continue to advance, overcoming hurdles in neuroimaging applications. The study in examines emerging DL approaches to improving the speed and accuracy of psychiatric research. Likewise, deep neural networks have contributed to great advances in evaluating mental illnesses, as demonstrated by Durstewitz et al. [4] which compares traditional statistical techniques to AI-driven models. The change from small-scale investigations to big methods based on data is also discussed by Koppe et al. [5] which emphasizes the value of huge datasets in enhancing model performance. Cai et al. [7] presented DL models based on graphs have improved their predictive skills. MM-GTUNets is a novel framework that uses multimodal neuroimaging and non-imaging data to predict large-scale brain diseases. Furthermore, Wang et al. [15] proposed transformer-based models, such as the Multi-Dimension-Embedding-Aware Modality Fusion Transformer, have improved psychiatric disorder classification using functional and structural MRI scans.

Aside from sorting, researchers are motivated to generate predictive models for psychological illnesses. Rashid and Calhoun [9] introduced the idea of a brain-based "predictome" is gaining traction, as detailed in, which analyzes multivariate brain network features to guess mental illness. Wen et al. [16] described the overview of dimensional neuroimaging endophenotypes has helped in the proof of the identity of disease heterogeneity using ML approaches. The researcher Brossollet et al. [17] offers a full analysis of ML applications in psychiatry, going into the advantages and disadvantages of various procedures. Construction on this Du et al. [18] is offering a deep multimodal model that synergistically integrates genomes and neuroimaging data to predict mental diseases, effectively identifying key genetic factors and brain traits linked to schizophrenia. In pediatric populations, Menon and Krishnamurthy [19] uses data from the Adolescent Brain Cognitive Development Study to apply a multimodal ensemble 3D CNN to distinguish between adolescents with disruptive behavior disorders and their classmates who are usually developing. Smucny et al. [20] addresses both the difficulties and possible advantages of new DL techniques that could hasten their incorporation into conventional psychiatric research, further developing the discipline Vieira et al. [21] which gives a summary of ML techniques and their applicability to psychiatric applications, looks carefully at the examination of deep and recurrent neural networks in psychiatry. Additionally, Zhou et al. [22] deliberates the complexity of ML methods and the requirement for substantial datasets in psychiatric studies while contrasting them with predictable statistical methods.

In order to predict brain disorders, graph DL frameworks have also been built. To illustrate this, Koppe et al. [23] presents MM-GTUNets, a unified multimodal graph DL framework that integrates imaging and non-imaging data for large-scale brain illness prediction. Likewise, Wang et al. [24] suggests a DL architecture for the classification of bipolar disorder and schizophrenia that makes use of T1-weighted structural MRI and resting-state functional MRI. The idea of a brain-based "predictome" is presented by Cai et al. [25], which predicts mental disease by using multivariate brain network data from various neuroimaging modalities. Moreover, Du et al. [18] introduces the idea of dimensional neuroimaging endophenotypes and offers ML techniques meant to reveal illness heterogeneity in a range of neuropsychiatric and neurodegenerative disorders.

The usage of DL approaches in neuroimaging-based psychiatric research has also become cutting-edge recently. For example, Brossollet et al. [17] highlights the risks and possible assistance of deep neural networks in this field, highlighting the status of sensible deliberation procedural issues. A methodical examination of ML methods in the area of classifying schizophrenia is given by Du et al. [18], which also offers suggestions for upcoming study avenues.

Through a motivation on the significance of sizable, high-quality datasets, Menon and Krishnamurthy [19] offers an overview of existing uses and upcoming prospects for the integration of AI in mental healthcare. Wang et al. [24] also thinks to see the potential for individualized approaches to mental healthcare by conversing about the significance of ML in precision psychiatry.

In the arena of neuroimaging, Vieira et al. [21] talks about using ML algorithms for structural brain pictures, with an emphasis on how persons with mental illnesses are classified. Furthermore, Zhou et al. [22] proposals are an indication of cutting-edge ML methods in psychiatry and the position of current research usages in the area. Vieira et al. [21], which stresses the use of brain imaging data in massive cohorts, highlights the potential of ML to offer biological perceptions into the nosology and psychopathology of mental diseases. Additionally, Koppe et al. [23] describes how DL methods are applied to brain imaging to diagnose mental and neurological disorders. It provides an editorial perspective on current developments.

1.4 METHODOLOGIES TO MITIGATE HETEROGENEITY

The multidisciplinary biomarker identification approach appears in Figure 1.4. The goal of the above strategy is to increase psychiatric disorder prediction. The system employs advanced ML models. These are used to reveal hidden trends related to mental health issues. To address these issues through the integration of multiple data sources, such as notes from hospitals, health information systems (EHRs), and brain imaging. Increased diagnostic accuracy and more individualized treatment are made achievable by multidisciplinary integration. The model design supports interpretability, ensuring that physicians can rely on and act upon AI-driven insights. This method eventually advances data-informed mental healthcare by identifying robust biomarkers.

(a) **Data Harmonization Methodologies**
Batch effects are regularly modified using data synchronization methods, such as the ComBat algorithm to maintain biological variability while positioning data distributions across sites demonstrated by Durstewitz et al. [4]. By planning datasets to a mutual feature space, advanced coordination techniques, such as domain adaptation, further improve dataset compatibility.

(b) **Feature Fusion Strategies**
Researchers can take advantage of complementary information from various sensory systems by means of multimodal incorporation strategies such as early fusion, late fusion, and hybrid fusion discussed by Koppe et al. [5]. These methods enable robust feature extraction while preserving the unique contributions of each modality.

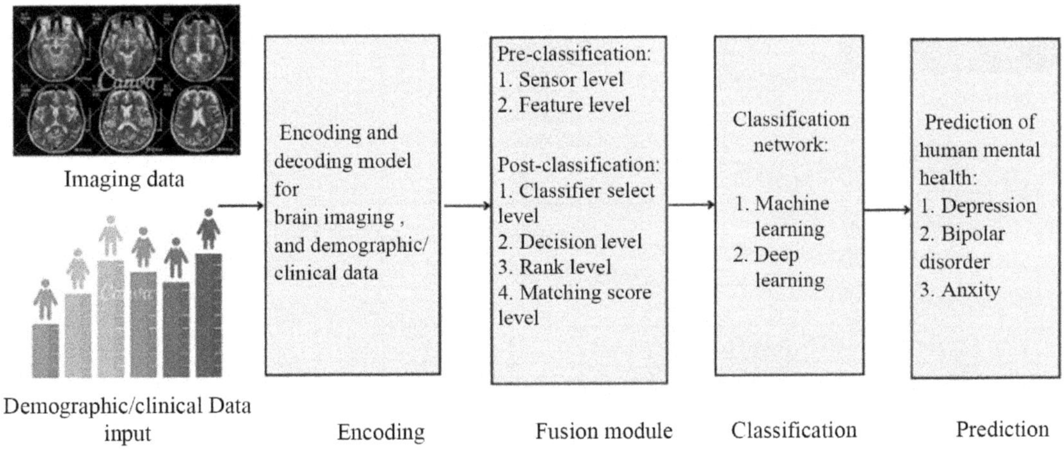

FIGURE 1.4 Multimodal biomarker discovery for psychiatry prediction

(c) **Synthetic Data Generation**
The upcoming studies have applied reproductive models such as variational autoencoders (VAEs) and generative adversarial networks (GANs) for augmenting datasets by generating synthetic examples. These approaches help address small sample sizes and reduce class imbalance, thereby improving the model's performance and generalizability by Cai et al. [7].

(d) **Transfer Learning and Pretrained Models**
Transfer learning applies a set of pretrained models on vast, appropriate datasets and fine-tunes them to familiarize them with the given psychiatric imaging task. This way, the widespread labeled data are significantly reduced, and it improves the robustness of ML/DL models across heterogeneous datasets given by Wang et al. [15].

(e) **Explainable AI**
Explainable AI (XAI) methods improve the interpretability of ML/DL models, so investigators and clinicians can understand the model's conclusions. Through recognizing which features contribute most to predictions, XAI can address variability-related anxieties and improve trust in the model assumptions given by ashid and Calhoun [9]. Addressing the problem of heterogeneousness in data will be of great importance to the development of the application of ML and DL in psychiatry. Harmonization techniques, fusion strategies, synthetic data generation, and advanced analytical methods can solve the problems described above and bring the full power of multimodal imaging to the benefit of personalized mental healthcare.

1.5 DEEP LEARNING ARCHITECTURES FOR MULTIMODAL DATA

As in Figure 1.5, DL architectures mixing multimodal data into frameworks have been used to significantly modify neuroimaging training for psychiatric disorders. With procedures including, but not limited to, functional magnetic resonance imaging, sMRI, DTI, and EEG, the multimodal nature of this kind of datasets forth unique knowledge of the anatomy and functionality of the brain. However, the heterogeneity of such data presents significant challenges, which advanced DL architectures are uniquely designed to handle. This type of architecture helps to do feature extraction, integration, and interpretation effectively, thus paving the way for precision psychiatry.

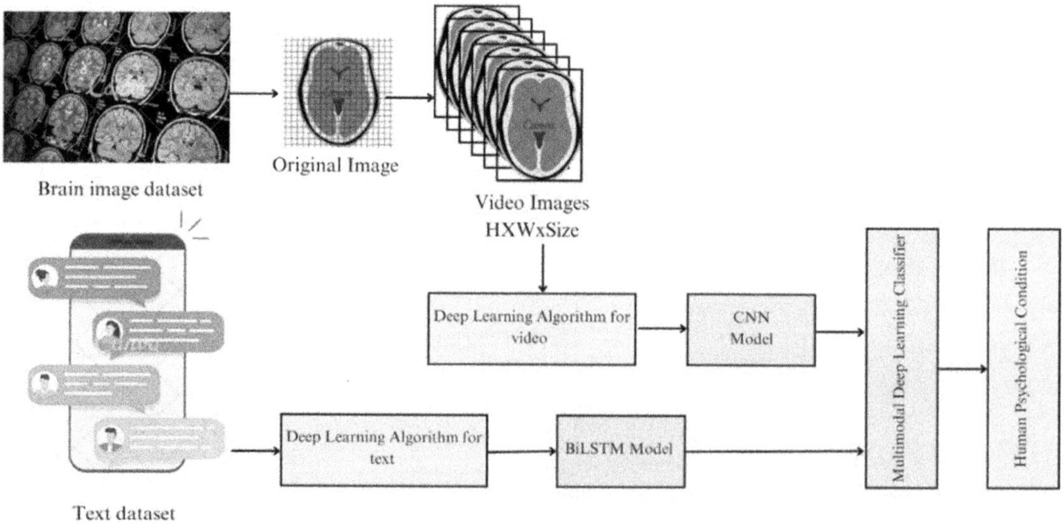

FIGURE 1.5 Architecture of deep learning model using multimodal data

(a) **Deep Learning Architectures**
CNNs are extensively used to evaluate the specialized organized data, such as brain imaging scans. Menon and Krishnamurthy [13] used the images are taken from sMRI and fMRI through learning spatial hierarchies via convolutional layers. The feature extraction of these images is done using CNNs.

1.5.1 Biomarkers in Multimodal Discovery

More generally, single-modality analysis has been enhanced by multimodality approaches. It offers a comprehensive understanding of structure, function, and connectivity at a level unreachable by single-modal analyses.

(a) **Multimodal Biomarkers and Their Importance**
Multimodal biomarkers contain a vast amount of data types. They capture corresponding characteristics of brain health. For example, fMRI distinguishes efficient connectivity designs, whereas sMRI uncovers structural deviations. DTI assesses white matter integrity given by Menon and Krishnamurthy [13].

(b) **The Future Extraction and Multimodal Biomarker**
The improved methods of feature abstraction are CNN and statistical models. Smucny et al. [14] examined that it is easy to capture those characteristics by utilizing them. The various methods of integration that have been commonly applied are early fusion, merging the raw data, and late fusion. Genomic integration is used for neuroimaging described by Cai et al. [7]. Wang et al. [15] proposed precision Psychiatry uses multimodal approaches for psychiatry applications

1.6 CHALLENGES AND FUTURE WORK DIRECTIONS

(a) Combining the various datasets from different modalities and institutions is challenging. The reason is that they have inconsistencies in format, acquisition techniques, and measurement scales.
(b) Most of the multimodal research is forced by small cohort sizes, which limit the arithmetical dependability and wider suitability of findings.
(c) Multimodal data such as imaging, text, and clinical records require advanced infrastructure and resource-efficient algorithms to analyze and combine complex data.
(d) DL approaches, which are commonly used, often produce results. Although deep learning (DL) approaches are widely used and often achieve high predictive performance, their lack of interpretability limits their adoption in clinical practice. Explainable deep learning (XDL) techniques address this limitation by improving the transparency and interpretability of model predictions.
(e) The use of separate medical records and brain imaging data requires strict observance of privacy laws, complicating multi-institutional collaborations.

1.7 SUMMARY

This section denotes a unique method of graphing neural networks and transformer-based models. The early detection of psychiatric conditions includes depression, schizophrenia, and autism. Additionally, this chapter explores the logical concerns such as privacy challenges in AI. The work done by researchers fills the gap between neuroimaging and word-based analysis. They offer important insights to the researchers who want to develop more complex and valid mental health models. This chapter represents the fusion of psychiatric data for study. In this chapter, the focus is on real-world applications, including the early detection of disorders such as depression, autism, and schizophrenia. This research gives the research direction to the researchers who want to work on the different datasets which affect mental health.

REFERENCES

[1] Brossollet, I., Gallet, Q., Favre, P. & Houenou, J., 2023. Machine learning and brain imaging for psychiatric disorders: New perspectives. In: O. Colliot, ed. *Machine Learning for Brain Disorders*. New York: Humana.

[2] Rahaman, M.A., Chen, J., Fu, Z., Lewis, N., Iraji, A., van Erp, T.G.M. & Calhoun, V.D., 2023. Deep multimodal predictome for studying mental disorders. *Human Brain Mapping*, 44(2), pp.509–522. https://doi.org/10.1002/hbm.26077.

[3] Khan, M., Mahajan, R.A., Sivakumar, N.R., Gulhane, M., Rakesh, N., Dey, R., Uddin, M.S. & Basheer, S., 2025. A unified hybrid model for cardiovascular risk prediction: Merging statistical, kernel-based and neural approaches. *Journal of Cellular and Molecular Medicine*. https://doi.org/10.1111/jcmm.70797

[4] Durstewitz, D., Koppe, G. & Meyer-Lindenberg, A., 2019. Deep neural networks in psychiatry. *Molecular Psychiatry*, 24, pp.1583–1598. https://doi.org/10.1038/s41380-019-0365-9.

[5] Koppe, G., Meyer-Lindenberg, A. & Durstewitz, D., 2021. Deep learning for small and big data in psychiatry. *Neuropsychopharmacology*, 46, pp.176–190. https://doi.org/10.1038/s41386-020-0767-z.

[6] Khan, M., Mahajan, R.A., Katukam, R., Dey, R., Rana, A. & William, P., 2025. Smart insights: Multimodal deep learning techniques for accurate disease identification. In: *2025 International Conference on Quantum Photonics, Artificial Intelligence, and Networking (QPAIN)*, Rangpur, Bangladesh, pp.1–5. https://doi.org/10.1109/QPAIN66474.2025.11171928

[7] Cai, L., Zeng, W., Chen, H., Zhang, H., Li, Y., Feng, Y., Yan, H., Bian, L., Siok, W.T. & Wang, N., 2024. MM-GTUNets: Unified multi-modal graph deep learning for brain disorders prediction. *arXiv preprint*. https://doi.org/10.48550/arXiv.2406.14455.

[8] Pal, M., Dey, R., Mahajan, R.A., Khan, M., Syed, A.A. & Karimullah, S., 2025. Edge intelligence: Unique machine learning strategies for enhancing real-time IoT data processing. In: *2025 International Conference on Quantum Photonics, Artificial Intelligence, and Networking (QPAIN)*, Rangpur, Bangladesh, pp.1–5. https://doi.org/10.1109/QPAIN66474.2025.11171994.

[9] Rashid, B. & Calhoun, V., 2020. Towards a brain-based predictome of mental illness. *Human Brain Mapping*, 41(12), pp.3468–3535. https://doi.org/10.1002/hbm.25013.

[10] Das, P., Paul, S., Ghosh, J., PalBhowmik, S., Neogi, B. & Ganguly, A., 2017. An approach towards the representation of sign language by electromyography signals with fuzzy implementation. *International Journal of Sensors, Wireless Communications and Control*, 7(1), pp.26–32. https://doi.org/10.2174/2210327907666170222093839.

[11] Paul, S., Ojha, S.K., Barui, S., Ghosh, S., Ghosh, M., Neogi, B. & Ganguly, A., 2018. Technical advancement on various bio-signal controlled arm: A review. *Journal of Mechanics of Continua and Mathematical Sciences*, 13(2), pp.16–30. https://doi.org/10.26782/jmcms.2018.06.00007

[12] Mahajan, R.A., Dey, R., Khan, M., Su'ud, M.M., Alam, M.M. & Jadhav, P., 2025. Enhancing personalization in IoT-based health monitoring via generative AI and transfer learning. *Egyptian Informatics Journal*, 32, p.100788. ISSN 1110-8665. https://doi.org/10.1016/j.eij.2025.100788.

[13] Menon, S.S. & Krishnamurthy, K., 2021. Multimodal ensemble deep learning to predict disruptive behavior disorders in children. *Frontiers in Neuroinformatics*, 15, p.742807. https://doi.org/10.3389/fninf.2021.742807.

[14] Smucny, J., Shi, G. & Davidson, I., 2022. Deep learning in neuroimaging: Overcoming challenges with emerging approaches. *Frontiers in Psychiatry*, 13, p.912600. https://doi.org/10.3389/fpsyt.2022.912600.

[15] Wang, G., Cao, X., An, S., Fan, F., Zhang, C., Wang, J., Yu, F., & Wang, Z., 2025. *Multi-dimension embedding-aware modality fusion transformer for psychiatric disorder classification*. In *Proceedings of ICIGP 2025*. Available at: https://arxiv.org/abs/2310.02690.

[16] Wen, J., Antoniades, M., Yang, Z., Hwang, G., Skampardoni, I., Wang, R. & Davatzikos, C., 2024. Dimensional neuroimaging endophenotypes: Neurobiological representations of disease heterogeneity through machine learning. *Biological Psychiatry*, 96(7), pp.564–584. https://doi.org/10.1016/j.biopsych.2024.04.017.

[17] Brossollet, I., Gallet, Q., Favre, P. & Houenou, J., 2023. Machine learning and brain imaging for psychiatric disorders: New perspectives. In: *Machine Learning for Brain Disorders. Neuromethods*, vol. 197. Humana.

[18] Du, Y., Fu, Z., Sui, J., Gao, S., Xing, Y., Lin, D., Salman, M., Iraji, A., Abrol, A., Rahaman, M.A., et al., 2020. NeuroMark: An automated and adaptive ICA-based pipeline to identify reproducible fMRI markers of brain disorders. *NeuroImage: Clinical*, 28, p.102375.

[19] Menon, S.S. & Krishnamurthy, K., 2021. Multimodal ensemble deep learning to predict disruptive behavior disorders in children. *Frontiers in Neuroinformatics*, 15, p.742807. https://doi.org/10.3389/fninf.2021.742807.

[20] Smucny, J., Shi, G. & Davidson, I., 2022. Deep learning in neuroimaging: Overcoming challenges with emerging approaches. *Frontiers in Psychiatry*, 13, p.912600. https://doi.org/10.3389/fpsyt.2022.912600.

[21] Vieira, S., Pinaya, W.H.L. & Mechelli, A., 2017. Using deep learning to investigate the neuroimaging correlates of psychiatric and neurological disorders: Methods and applications. *Neuroscience & Biobehavioral Reviews*, 74, pp.58–75. https://doi.org/10.1016/j.neubiorev.2017.01.002.

[22] Zhou, T., Thung, K.H., Zhu, X. & Shen, D., 2019. Effective feature learning and fusion of multimodality data using stage-wise deep neural network for dementia diagnosis. *Human Brain Mapping*, 40(3), pp.1001–1016. https://doi.org/10.1002/hbm.24428.

[23] Koppe, G., Meyer-Lindenberg, A. & Durstewitz, D., 2021. Deep learning for small and big data in psychiatry. *Neuropsychopharmacology*, 46(1), pp.176–190. https://doi.org/10.1038/s41386-020-0767-z.

[24] Wang, G., Cao, X., An, S., Fan, F., Zhang, C., Wang, J., Yu, F. & Wang, Z., 2023. Multi-dimension-embedding-aware modality fusion transformer for psychiatric disorder classification. *arXiv preprint, arXiv:2310.02690*.

[25] Cai, L., Zeng, W., Chen, H., Zhang, H., Li, Y., Yan, H., Bian, L. & Wang, N., 2024. MM-GTUNets: Unified multi-modal graph deep learning for brain disorders prediction. *arXiv preprint, arXiv:2406.14455*.

2 Generative AI-Driven Framework for Managing Neurodegenerative Disorders

Focus on Alzheimer's Detection

Kaviya P., Dhanusri V., Malathi M., Kaviyashree P., Kavya Dhana Sekaran, Preetha Ramiah, and Vijayakumar Varadarajan

2.1 INTRODUCTION

The chronic and incurable neurological disorder known as Alzheimer's disease (AD) gradually deteriorates brain function, mainly affecting behavior, memory, and reasoning. As the disease gets worse, it not only makes it harder for the person to do everyday tasks, but it also puts a lot of stress on the caregivers and family. Since AD is becoming more common around the world and there is no certain cure, early diagnosis and monitoring are very important. Deep learning models are a powerful tool for computations, and doctors find them useful for getting information from complex data from images and to make decisions. The application of these models includes classification of MRI images, which hold the data concerning the progression of AD. In medical practice, AD is not considered as a single condition but instead it is categorized in terms of different stages depending on the extent of cognitive impairment. Identification of these stages is very important as they provide details about the disease's movement and the level of care required. In a machine learning perspective [1], each stage represents a separate class in a multi-class classification framework. This study focuses on building a robust deep learning model that can characterize four such stages by analyzing MRI scans: non-demented, very mild demented, mild demented, and moderate demented.

Khan et al. (2025) proposed a unified hybrid model merging statistical, kernel-based, and neural paradigms, providing a robust methodological foundation adaptable for predictive modeling in neurodegenerative conditions such as Alzheimer's disease [2]. Non-demented is the stage of healthy cognitive status wherein no clinical manifestations of Alzheimer's disease can be observed in the individual. The structure of his or her brain is normal on MRI imaging, and no memory impairment or deviation in behavior is detectable at this stage. Khan et al. (2025) introduced multimodal deep learning architectures for reliable disease identification, illustrating how integrated data representations can enhance early Alzheimer's diagnosis [3].

The very mild demented phase is the first noticeable degree of cognitive impairment. There can be episodic forgetfulness or mild disorientation that might be so slight as to be unnoticed during everyday activities, yet imaging could begin to demonstrate initial neurodegenerative changes.

In the mild demented state, the intellectual symptoms worsen, including memory loss of recent events, losing things, or difficulty with usual tasks. MRI scans generally show more apparent structural changes in the brain, particularly in regions that are in charge of memory and learning. Mahajan et al. (2025) leveraged generative AI and transfer learning to personalize IoT-based healthcare monitoring, a strategy highly relevant to individualized Alzheimer's management [4].

 DOI: 10.1201/9781003667360-2

Last, the moderate demented phase points to a more severe degree of impairment, with the affected persons needing help with day-to-day activities and showing confusion, difficulty in speaking, and not being able to recognize close relatives. MRI scans at this phase show definitive evidence of cortical reduction and deeper structural damage. Pal et al. (2025) highlighted real-time edge intelligence for IoT data processing, demonstrating scalable AI solutions that can support continuous cognitive and neural data analysis in Alzheimer's care [5].

Our research is based on a well-designed convolutional neural network (CNN) model, which is able to accurately classify the stages of AD from MRI images. This method prioritizes accuracy, transferability, and simplicity over other methods, which use external feature extraction or extremely complex architectures. By developing a lightweight model with minimal computational overhead, we strive to strike a balance between architectural complexity and diagnostic capability. The network learns layered representations from input brain images through the architecture's arrangement, which places layers from low-level to high-level representations. During the training phase, the CNN model learns to distinguish the four stages of AD by use of pixel-level patterns and anatomical features, which are unique to each condition. Convolutional and pooling operations reduce the dimensionality while preserving crucial spatial features, which are considered as the heart of the learning process. During training iterations, we employed an early stopping technique to avoid overfitting, which guarantees that the model appropriately generalizes to new data. The assessment of a model's performance is done by the combination of standard metrics, including accuracy, precision, recall, and F1-score. Furthermore, confusion matrixes are used, which measure the model's ability to distinguish between the four classes and are also used to plot the model's classification behavior. Besides the assessment, these metrics show how weak the class separation could be, particularly with similar stages such as mild and moderate demented. To ensure the model learning capability, we made sure that the preprocessing should be consistent and that grayscale conversion and normalization were handled carefully to avoid distorting anatomical data. In order to maintain clinical reliability of classification task, we also decided that the training, testing, validation sets had to be sorted based on the actual class distribution. Our CNN model is unique; it can achieve high accuracy with few inputs from pretrained networks, outside resources. It shows that smart architectural choices designed specifically for the task-can actually outperform very complex models, both in speed and in quality.

Das et al. (2017) utilized electromyography and fuzzy logic for signal interpretation, underscoring early advancements in bio-signal understanding essential for neural activity analysis in dementia studies [6].

Our model's another significant advantage is that it can be integrated in real-time clinical work streams, telemedicine interfaces, and diagnostic kiosks. This affords possibilities in rural areas or inadequately equipped medical facilities for the development of intelligent systems that can identify and classify patients based on their risk profiles. Altogether, our research provides a practical framework for multi-class classification of AD stages. It reveals that deep learning has the strength to transform the diagnosis of neurodegenerative diseases by providing scalable solutions to support the work of medical professionals.

Paul et al. (2018) reviewed bio-signal–controlled systems, emphasizing the translation of physiological patterns into functional insights—a concept central to neurodegenerative signal decoding [7].

2.2 SURVEY OF PREVIOUS WORKS

In recent years, deep learning techniques and artificial intelligence (AI) have gained prominence due to their ability to automatically analyze brain MRI scans and detect cognitive impairment, a useful component of clinical decision support systems. Numerous authors have investigated various architectures, modalities, and hybrid models in order to improve accuracy, interpretability, and generalizability. The VGG16 model was developed by Ul Rehman et al. [8], and it was utilized to create a deep learning architecture for hippocampus MRI feature classification. In addition to the model having a high accuracy of 98.17%, it heavily relied on transfer learning as well as a lot of pretraining, which reduces its flexibility to unseen data. El-Latif et al. [9] were able to recommend a lightweight deep learning model using MRI data for the specific detection of AD. The seven-layer model with a classification accuracy of 95.96% and computational efficiency was trained on a Kaggle dataset. Their approach uses tricks such as early stopping and image augmentation to enhance generalization and reduce the complexity of training. Koch et al. [10] suggested that an extreme learning machine (ELM) combined with a smaller-size kernel partial least squares (KPLS) model could be used in clinical diagnosis, but the complexity of the system constrained its practical size. Oz Altin [11] applied the K-nearest neighbor (KNN) classifier with a ResNet-50 model and feature transformation and neighborhood component analysis (FTNCA). Although this hybrid method was 100% accurate, it consumed more time and resources than the other two methods because it had distinct stages of transformation, classification, and optimization. As binary classifiers for Parkinson's disease, Govindua and Palwe [12] examined random forest classifiers using voice-based MDVP feature sets. Despite having an accuracy of 91.83%, their model could not be applied to image-based AD detection. Neelakandan et al. [13] employed an ensemble deep learning architecture with SMOTE to counter class imbalance for AD classification. Although their study demonstrated encouraging outcomes in F1-score and AUC-ROC, their ensemble structure increased model complexity and training time. Arafa and Ali [14] compared the performance of vision transformers (ViT) versus conventional CNNs and concluded that CNNs were better suited for MRI-based AD diagnosis, affirming the feasibility of basic convolution models. Qadri et al. [15] presented a sophisticated AI-driven closed-loop deep brain stimulation (DBS) system integrated with IoT for early diagnosis and symptom management. Although the incorporation of bio-signal feedback had future promise, the system is not yet fully developed and does not have clinical validation for use in real-time diagnosis. Likewise, Tsiara et al. [16] suggested a gait- and motion sensor-enabled AI-based diagnostic device for neurodegenerative diseases with a focus on early intervention according to movement features. The model was Parkinson's-specific and did not have direct applicability to MRI-based AD classification. Kumar et al. [17] illustrated a multimodal strategy by combining MRI, PET, and genetic information with ensemble learning. Their classifier was highly accurate but had to work with multimodal datasets that are commonly scarce in public releases and hard to integrate. Nahar et al. [18] illustrated a new AI system integrating natural product modeling and predictive biomarkers to improve cognitive output. Their study was of value for therapeutic purposes but was not specifically applicable to MRI-based classification tasks. Aborode et al. [19] gave a general overview of biomarker discovery with machine learning. Their paper lacked implementation details and was more theoretical in nature. A CNN-based pipeline was used by Hcini et al. [14] to detect AD with an accuracy of over 90%.

Even though their suggested model worked well, its ability to distinguish between different stages of AD was limited because it used a binary classification task. Saleem et al. [20] wanted to maximize classification using temporal sequences and to use deep learning to track the disease's progression. Although their approach was not optimized for static MRI-based multi-class classification, it showed promise for longitudinal analysis. A multimodality learning framework that integrates clinical and image features was proposed by Shukla et al. [12]. However, although the framework performed well in binary classification, it was not very applicable to multi-class detection. The use of AI in retinal imaging to detect Alzheimer's in its early stages was covered by Tukur et al. [21]. Even though their approach demonstrated potential as a noninvasive modality, but it failed to classify the various stages of AD.

From this survey, we can see that, in order to increase accuracy, most of the current studies rely on ensemble-based frameworks and hybrid optimization while these models perform well in isolated settings, but they frequently encounter difficulties such as reduced interpretability, overfitting, and computational complexity. Moreover, many earlier studies have mostly concentrated on binary classification, ignoring the multi-class classification for various stages of AD. On the other hand, our lightweight and reliable CNN model is only intended for the classification of four clinically recognized stages of AD from MRI images. As opposed to architectures based on transfer learning, which tend to adapt to every dataset, our model generalizes proficiently without using pretrained layers. With only seven layers and significantly fewer trainable parameters than other complex models, it is both computationally efficient and still achieves outstanding accuracy. Additionally, the model's clinical applicability is demonstrated by its high confidence in correctly identifying the four stages of AD. The results indicate that less complex architectures, when well-tuned and tested seriously, are capable of competing with and even bettering more intricate models in practical medical use cases. This chapter fills crucial limitations underlined in previous research and presents a scalable, interpretable, and high-performing approach to MRI-based multi-class AD classification.

TABLE 2.1
An overview of earlier research on AD detection

Authors and Reference	Methodology	Limitations
Ul Rehman et al. (2024) [2]	VGG16-based deep learning (MRI hippocampus classification)	Hindered by technical and protocol variability, data limitations, ethical and regulatory concerns, model bias, and lack of interpretability.
El-Latif et al. (2023) [8]	Lightweight CNN model with seven layers trained on T1-weighted MRI images for multi-class classification of AD stages	Limited dataset size, single modality (MRI only), and architecture-specific constraints may affect generalizability.
Özaltın (2025) [21]	ResNet-50 + FTNCA + KNN	Generalizability is restricted due to reliance on a single imaging type from a limited public dataset.
Muddapu et al. (2022) [22]	Random forest classifier (MDVP voice)	Audio data alone is insufficient, highlighting the need for multimodal inputs such as rapid eye movement (REM) sleep data.
Neelakandan et al. (2023) [15]	Ensemble + deep learning + SMOTE	Limited by small sample sizes, lack of comparisons, and challenges in real-world validation and generalizability.
Arafa & Ali (2022) [17]	ViT vs CNN for AD classification	Limited in scope by a focus on basic preprocessing, a few deep learning models, minimal dataset variety, and lack of detailed machine learning discussion.
Qadri et al. (2024) [10]	AGI + IoT with closed-loop DBS	Hindered by high computational costs, lack of interpretability, biased and unstructured data, and challenges in balancing privacy with performance.
Tsiara et al. (2025) [9]	AI with gait and motion sensor data	Faces challenges from technical variability, DTI limitations, ethical and regulatory issues, and difficulties in longitudinal tracking and multi-site data integration.
Kumar et al. (2024) [3]	Multimodal AI imaging (MRI + PET + genetics)	High accuracy risks overfitting, with limited generalizability due to reliance on Alzheimer's disease neuroimaging initiative (ADNI) data and built-in preprocessing tools.
Neffati et al. (2025) [23]	AI in retinal imaging	Faces challenges in interpretability, data bias, ethical concerns, high costs, diagnostic reliability, and lack of longitudinal, large-scale validation.
Hcini et al. (2022) [18]	CNN-based pipelines for AD detection	Challenged by computational complexity, feature harmonization issues, data limitations, class imbalance, interpretability concerns, and ethical issues around privacy.

2.3 DATASET AND METHODOLOGY

2.3.1 Dataset

We used a pre-curated version of the Alzheimer's MRI dataset that comprises 11,519 brain MRI images. These images are T1-weighted MRI scans, labeled by clinicians and put into four classes of diagnostic category. Each image is labeled with the stage of AD, so the dataset is highly suitable for supervised learning tasks intended for automatic classification of AD stages.

All the images are already organized into class-specific folders, facilitating easy incorporation into deep learning workflows with contemporary image producers and classification systems. The dataset was obtained from Kaggle [24], a publicly accessible platform for curated datasets. It is freely available and can be easily retrieved for research purposes. It is of moderate size, offering enough diversity for quality training and validation of deep neural networks without being too large for their efficient computational processing on typical hardware. Table 2.2 provides a detailed class-wise distribution of the entire dataset, which has been divided into training and test subsets. In Figure 2.1, given the sample of the data from the Kaggle database, Figure 2.2 shows the Kaggle dataset's statistics.

2.3.2 Preprocessing

Prior to training, we preprocessed the MRI data by normalizing and augmenting it using the ImageDataGenerator class of the Keras library. This procedure is crucial for enhancing the training dataset's diversity and boosting the model's ability to generalize to new situations [26]. All pixel values are rescaled to the interval [1] as part of the preprocessing techniques used, which normalizes the input as shown by Hussain et al. (2018) [27] and shortens the training convergence time. To artificially expand the dataset, random transformations such as minor rotations, shifting, zoom variability, and horizontal flipping were also included. The augmentations enable the model to be invariant to small spatial variations that can happen in real-world medical images. Through the imitation of various view angles and intensities, the model is trained to recognize more generalized patterns pertinent to Alzheimer's classification. The preprocessing pipeline is established, and the augmented image batches are fed directly into the training process such that each epoch sees a subtly varied version of the data, hence minimizing the chance of overfitting.

2.3.3 Methodology

Labeling brain MRI images into one of four diagnostic classes—non-demented, very mild demented, mild demented, and moderate demented—is the goal of the CNN model created for

TABLE 2.2
Distribution of records in the dataset used in this work

Class	Training	Testing	Total
Mild demented	2191	548	2739
Moderate demented	2057	515	2572
Non-demented	2560	640	3200
Very mild demented	2406	602	3008
Total	9214	2305	11519

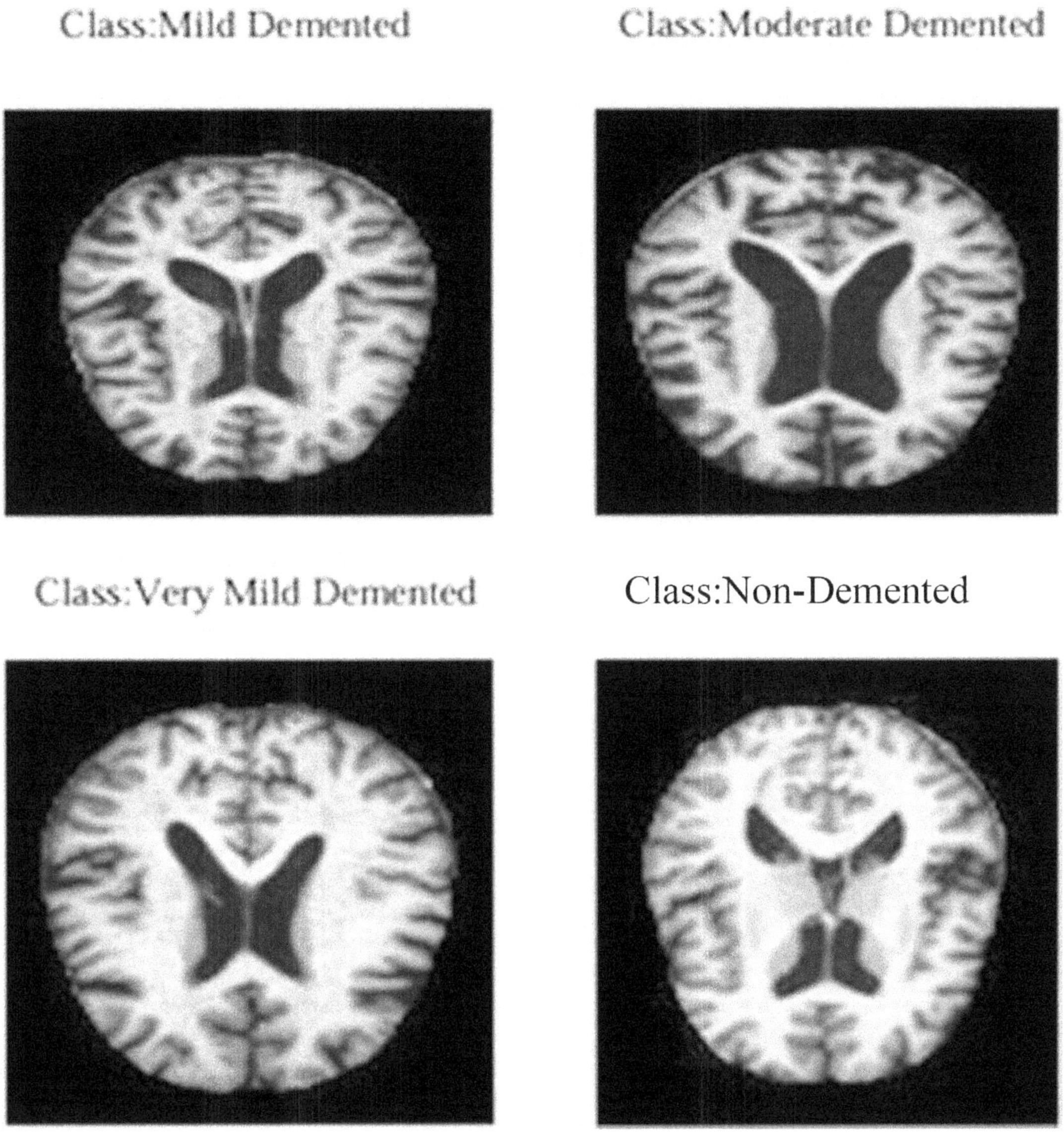

FIGURE 2.1 Sample of the data from the Kaggle database [25]

this multi-class classification problem. Four output neurons for these classes with softmax activation are found in the final dense layer of the CNN, which generates normalized probability distributions. The categorical cross-entropy loss function, which is suitable for multi-class classification tasks with mutually exclusive labels, is used to train the model. Grayscale MRI scans with a single channel and 176 × 176 pixels are the input format for the model. A series of pooling (MaxPooling2D) and convolutional (Conv2D) layers receive the scans as input, which, step by step, reduce the spatial dimensions but extract increasingly abstract and informative features. Every convolutional layer is succeeded by a rectified linear unit (ReLU) activation function, which provides the network with nonlinearity and allows it to better learn complex patterns related to various phases of Alzheimer's disease. An advanced CNN model, a more profound and expressive variant of a conventional CNN architecture, is implemented here. In comparison to the plain model, the sophisticated architecture adds more convolutional blocks and dense layers

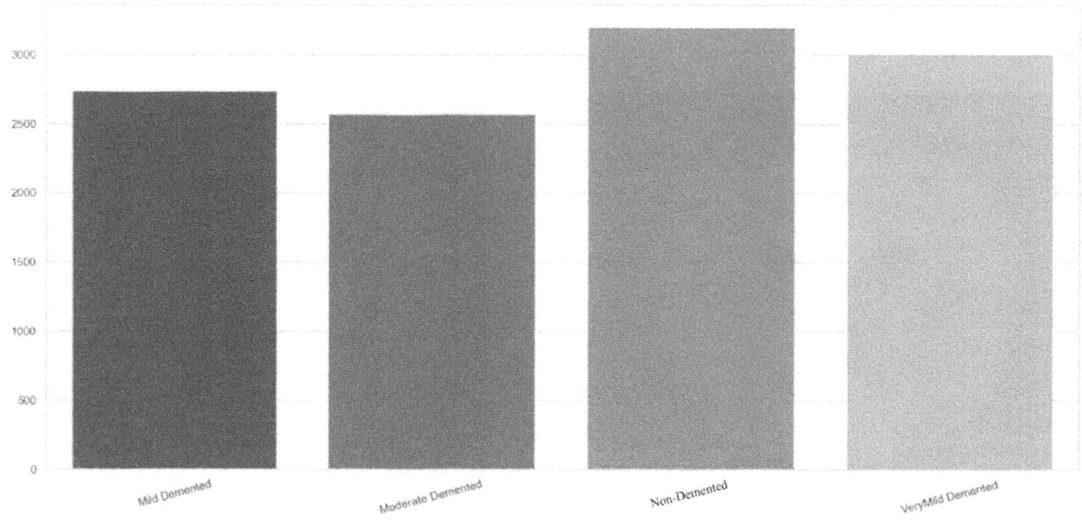

FIGURE 2.2 The Kaggle dataset's statistics

to the network to enable the network to have more intensive mathematical processing of the input data. Better classification performance is the outcome of this design since it allows the model to learn more fine-grained features and improves its learning capacity. The extra depth imbues the model with a hierarchical representation of features, which is especially useful while discriminating between fine differences in MRI scans for similar diagnosis phases. After the convolution and pooling processes, the resulting feature maps are flattened and fed into a dense, fully linked layer that is activated by ReLU. Finally, the probability scores for each of the four classes are produced by the dense output layer that is activated by softmax. The Adam optimizer is used to construct the model, and it is trained over 50 epochs. The seven layers that make up the entire architecture include convolutional, pooling, flattening, and dense layers.

As per the model summary, the advanced CNN model, as shown in Table 2.3, contains a total of 1,699,524 trainable parameters. Even though the model is deeper, it is still computationally efficient and provides more representational power. A schematic representation of the model structure employed can be found in Figure 2.3.

In Figure 2.4, explained the overview of the suggested multi-classification model.

Table 2.3 explains the proposed CNN model for multi-class Alzheimer's detection.

TABLE 2.3
Proposed CNN model for multi-class Alzheimer's detection

Algorithm 1: The Proposed CNN Model for Multi-class Alzheimer's Detection [11]

1. START
2. INPUT: optimizer, loss_function, metrics, epochs, augmentation_parameters, model_structure, dataset_directory, image_size, batch_size
3. Load all MRI pictures with the appropriate class labels from dataset_directory.
4. Resize images to image_size and convert to grayscale.
5. Normalize pixel values to [1].
6. Define ImageDataGenerator using augmentation_parameters (e.g., flip, zoom, rotation).
7. Generate training and validation sets from the augmented data.

TABLE 2.3 *(Continued)*

Proposed CNN model for multi-class Alzheimer's detection

8. Define a custom CNN model using model_structure:
    a. Input layer (176 × 176 × 1)
    b. Conv2D → BatchNorm → ReLU → MaxPooling
    c. Repeat Conv2D blocks as needed
    d. Flatten → Dense → ReLU → Dropout
    e. Dense output layer with softmax (4 neurons)
9. Use the optimizer and loss_function to compile the model.
10. Use validation data to train the model on the training set for epochs.
11. For every training epoch, do
12. Use metrics (such as accuracy) to assess the model on validation data.
13. IF early stopping condition is met THEN
14. Restore best weights and break.
15. ENDIF
16. ENDFOR
17. Predict class labels on the test set.
18. Evaluate final model using classification_report and confusion matrix.
19. OUTPUT: the final performance metrics, such as F1-score, recall, accuracy, and precision.
20. END

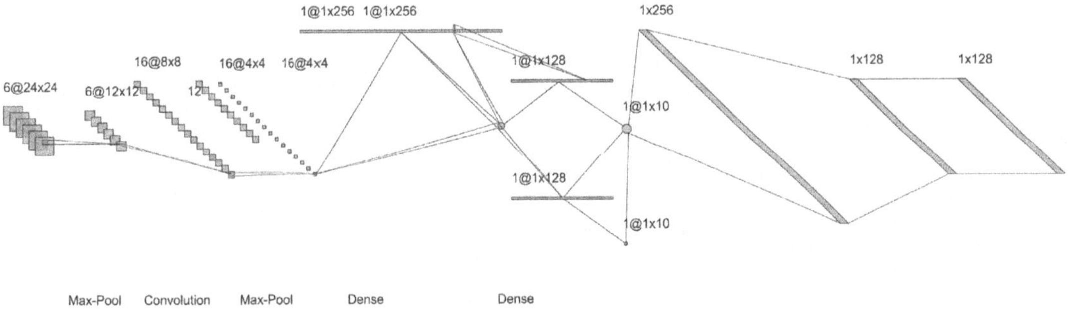

FIGURE 2.3 Architecture of CNN model

2.4 METHODOLOGIES TO MITIGATE HETEROGENEITY

A series of experiments were conducted using the proposed CNN model to classify Alzheimer's brain MRI images sourced from the Kaggle dataset. The goal was to automatically differentiate between the four diagnostic stages. For that, the dataset was divided into training and validation sets, and in order to replicate a realistic deployment scenario, the model was evaluated using a standard hold-out validation technique. The Python deep learning framework Keras was used to implement the model. Since the classification problem was multi-class, the network was optimized during training using the Adam optimizer and the categorical cross-entropy loss function. In order to extract and learn spatial features pertinent to each stage of AD, the CNN architecture uses sequential convolutional, pooling, and dense layers to process grayscale MRI inputs with a pixel size of 176 × 176. Four evaluation metrics—accuracy, precision, recall, and F1-score—were used to evaluate the model's performance in every aspect. The following are the mathematical definitions of these metrics:

$$\text{Accuracy} = \left(T_P + T_N\right) / \left(T_P + T_N + F_P + F_N\right)$$

Layer (type)	Output Shape	Param #
conv2d_10 (Conv2D)	(None, 126, 126, 32)	320
activation_18 (Activation)	(None, 126, 126, 32)	0
max_pooling2d_10 (MaxPooling2D)	(None, 63, 63, 32)	0
batch_normalization_6 (BatchNormalization)	(None, 63, 63, 32)	128
conv2d_11 (Conv2D)	(None, 61, 61, 64)	18,496
activation_19 (Activation)	(None, 61, 61, 64)	0
max_pooling2d_11 (MaxPooling2D)	(None, 30, 30, 64)	0
batch_normalization_7 (BatchNormalization)	(None, 30, 30, 64)	256
conv2d_12 (Conv2D)	(None, 28, 28, 128)	73,856
activation_20 (Activation)	(None, 28, 28, 128)	0
max_pooling2d_12 (MaxPooling2D)	(None, 14, 14, 128)	0
batch_normalization_8 (BatchNormalization)	(None, 14, 14, 128)	512
flatten_4 (Flatten)	(None, 25088)	0
dense_8 (Dense)	(None, 64)	1,605,696
activation_21 (Activation)	(None, 64)	0
dropout_4 (Dropout)	(None, 64)	0
dense_9 (Dense)	(None, 4)	260
activation_22 (Activation)	(None, 4)	0

Total params: 1,699,524

Trainable params: 1,699,076

Non-trainable params: 448

FIGURE 2.4 An overview of the suggested multi-classification model.

$$\text{Precision} = T_P / (T_P + F_P)$$

$$\text{Recall} = T_P / (T_P + F_N)$$

$$\text{F1} - \text{score} = 2 \times (\text{Precision} \times \text{Recall}) / (\text{Precision} + \text{Recall})$$

where

- T_P—True positive
- F_P—False positive
- T_N—True negative
- F_N—False negative

2.4.1 Experimental Analysis

This experiment used brain MRI images to assess the suggested CNN model for multi-class classification. Figure 2.5, a confusion matrix, was utilized to evaluate how well the model distinguished between the various diagnostic groups.

According to the matrix, 542 cases of mild dementia were correctly classified by the model, with very few cases being incorrectly classified as either non-demented or very mildly demented. Perfect classification for this category was demonstrated by the error-free identification of all 515 moderate demented cases. For non-demented cases, 628 samples were correctly predicted, with 12 misclassified as very mild demented. Likewise, 593 images with very mild dementia were correctly identified, with little confusion from other classes.

Standard classification metrics, such as precision, recall, and F1-score, were computed in order to assess the model further. Table 2.4 displays these metrics. With consistently high scores in every class, the suggested model had an overall accuracy of 99%. The macro and weighted averages for all metrics also hit 99%, demonstrating balanced performance free from class prejudice. Figure 2.6 displays the accuracy and loss curves. These plots show that while validation accuracy kept getting better and stayed constant, training accuracy stabilized after about ten epochs. The validation loss steadily declined, suggesting that the model did not overfit and retained its capacity for generalization.

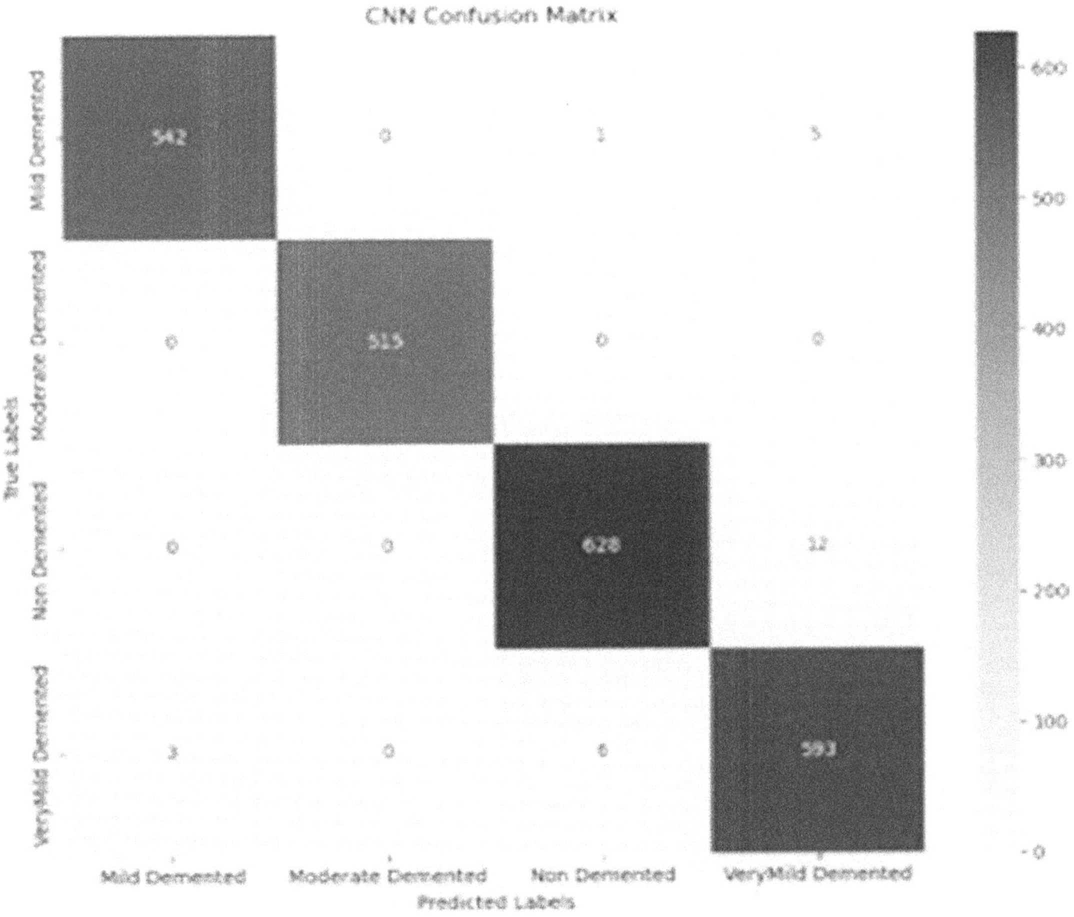

FIGURE 2.5 The proposed model's confusion matrix for the multi-classification task.

TABLE 2.4
The suggested model's multi-classification task performance

Class	Precision % (In Percentage)	Recall % (In Percentage)	F1-Score % (In Percentage)
Non-demented	99	99	99
Very mild demented	100	100	100
Mild demented	99	98	99
Moderate demented	97	99	98
Accuracy			99
Macro average	99	99	99
Weighted average	99	99	99

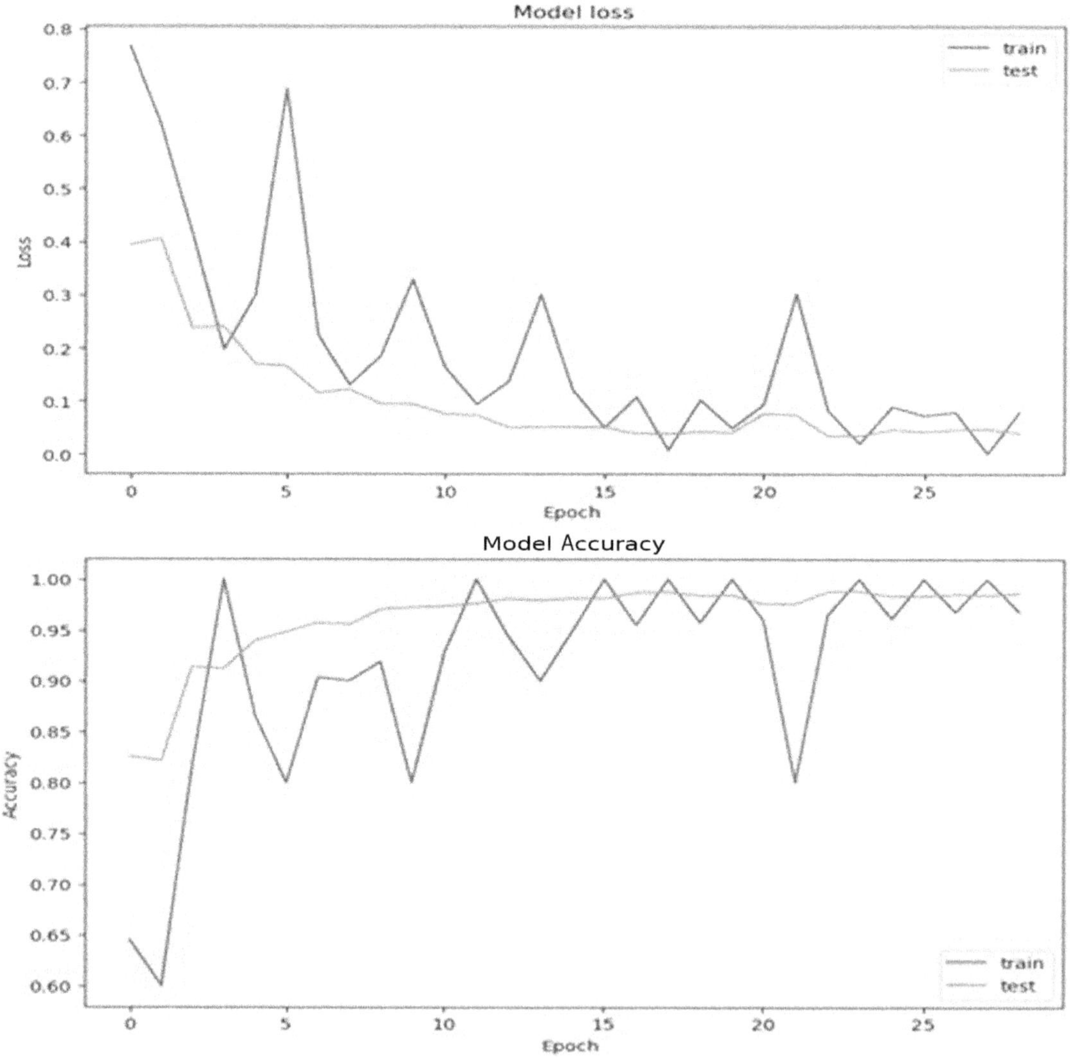

FIGURE 2.6 The training and testing data for the suggested model for the multi-classification task show loss curves (upper) and accuracy curves (lower)

2.4.2 Comparative Analysis of Other Cutting-Edge Models

This part provides a thorough comparison of the proposed model with several other methods that have been developed for the classification of AD. Previous methods have depended on highly complex processing pipelines comprising curated feature sets and ensemble models whereas our suggested model focuses on an optimized and end-to-end framework. Our approach achieves superior classification performance while maintaining the reduced complexity, faster training times, and simpler deployment in real time without relying on external classifiers or pretrained components.

Table 2.5 summarizes the comparison of our approach with other previous methods. It illustrates the changes in efficiency, methodology, and classification accuracy. Though valid, most of the previous models have challenges such as computational overhead and overfitting brought by small datasets. In contrast, our suggested model is lightweight, useful in clinical practices, and it retains high accuracy.

2.4.3 The Complexity of Computation

Computational complexity is responsible for measuring the efficiency of a deep learning model, particularly when dealing with big data. Here, we consider the computational expense of our suggested CNN model for Alzheimer's disease detection based on brain MRI images [26]. Our model has a comparatively smaller number of layers and parameters compared to deeper or transfer learning-based models; hence, it is light in terms of computation and efficient. The suggested model is a sequence of fully connected, convolutional, and pooling layers with a total of around 1.7 million trainable parameters. The time complexity of training the model is $O(m*n)$, where m is the number of training images and n is the number of pixels per image. The lower number of parameters promotes faster training and convergence without the need for high-end computing.

In addition, the simplicity of the model supports efficient deployment onto machines with restricted hardware configurations. It further supports quicker experimentation and tuning as a result of its relatively low memory requirements. Table 2.6 presents the complexity analysis of the proposed model using Big-O notation, which captures its time and computation demands.

TABLE 2.5
Comparison of the proposed model with other earlier models [9]

Authors and Reference	Methodology	Accuracy (%)
Ul Rehman et al. (2024) [8]	VGG16-based model using hippocampus MRI	98.17
El-Latif et al. (2023) [9]	Lightweight CNN model	97.20
Özaltın (2025) [11]	ResNet-50 + FTNCA + KNN hybrid method	100.00
Neelakandan et al. (2023) [13]	Ensemble deep learning + SMOTE	96.88
Hcini et al. (2022) [14]	CNN-based pipeline for MRI AD detection	90.72
Arafa & Ali (2022) [28]	CNN vs vision transformer (ViT)	95.25
Govindua & Palwe (2023) [12]	Random forest on MDVP speech dataset	91.83
Qadri et al. (2024) [15]	AI-enabled closed-loop DBS using IoMT	96.13
Tsiara et al. (2025) [16]	Wearable gait & motion sensor with AI	93.21
Kumar et al. (2024) [17]	Multimodal ensemble (MRI + PET + genetics)	95.00
Nahar et al. (2025) [14]	Natural compound modeling with predictive AI	92.10
Aborode et al. (2024) [19]	ML-based biomarker prediction model	90.50
Saleem et al. (2022) [20]	Deep learning for AD stage progression (MRI)	94.11
Shukla et al. (2023) [29]	Multimodal fusion: image + clinical data	93.90
Tukur et al. (2025) [21]	CNN on retinal images for noninvasive AD detection	91.40

TABLE 2.6
The computational complexity needed to train the suggested deep model with performance accuracy

Steps	Complexity in Big-O Notation
Dataset preprocessing and loading	Depends on data size, generally $O(n)$
Forward pass per layer	$O(m)*O(1)$, where $O(1)$ is the amount of time needed for every layer in the suggested model
Number of parameters and layers	$O(m*n)$
Training the complete deep model	$O(m*n)$, where each input image has n pixels and m is the number of training examples.
Total complexity	$O(m*n)$

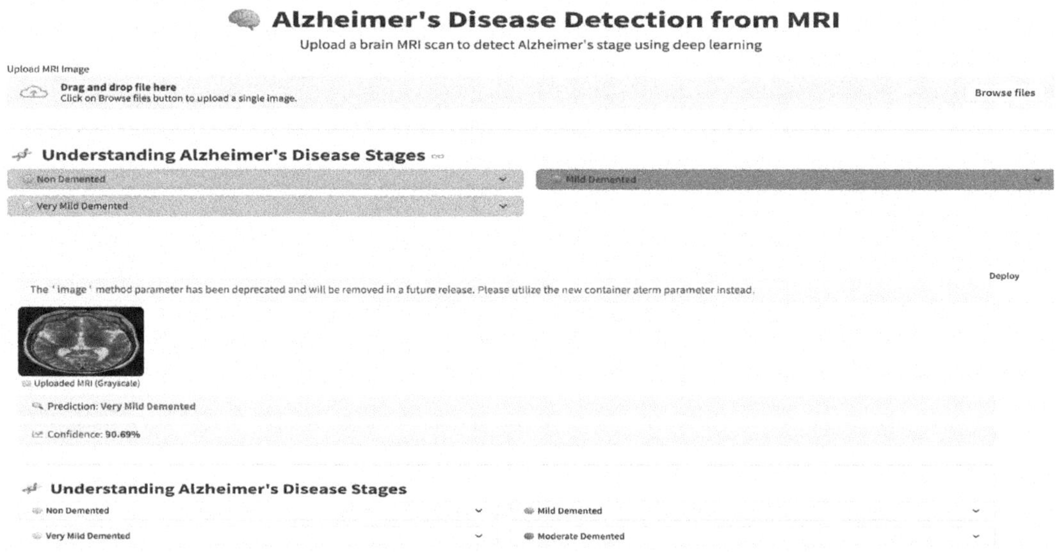

FIGURE 2.7 A working prototype of an online diagnostic tool for classifying MRI images of Alzheimer's disease.

2.5 CONCLUSION

In order to classify Alzheimer's disease from MRI scans, this study suggests a CNN-based approach that has an amazing 99% multi-class classification accuracy. In addition to using optimized layers and grayscale image preprocessing, its lightweight architecture with roughly 1.7 million parameters makes it useful for both training and deployment. Through accurate stage-wise classification, these results show the potential of deep learning models to support early AD diagnosis and reduce clinical workload.

2.6 FUTURE SCOPE

In Figure 2.7, the interface uses a trained CNN model to automatically predict the AD stage and lets users upload MRI scans. Future research will involve extending the model's functionality by including multimodal imaging (e.g., PET, CT) and testing it on a wide range of datasets in order to maximize generalizability. Hyperparameter learning and model alternatives can potentially lead to even better performance. We also intend to create a web-based tool that can be utilized in clinical applications, enabling physicians to diagnose numerous patients simultaneously more effectively and minimizing their workload in busy healthcare environments.

2.7 SUMMARY

This section denotes a unique method of graph neural networks and transformer-based models. The early detection of psychiatric conditions includes depression, schizophrenia, and autism. Additionally, this chapter explores the logical concerns such as privacy challenges in AI. The work done by researchers fills the gap between neuroimaging and word-based analysis. They offer important insights to the researchers who want to develop more complex and valid mental health models. This chapter represents the fusion of psychiatric data for study. In this chapter, the focus is on real-world applications, including the early detection of disorders such as depression, autism, and schizophrenia. This research gives research direction to researchers who want to work on different datasets that affect mental health.

REFERENCES

1. Tăuţan, A.-M., Ionescu, B., & Santarnecchi, E. (2021). Artificial intelligence in neurodegenerative diseases: A review of available tools with a focus on machine learning techniques. *Artificial Intelligence in Medicine*, 117, 102081. https://doi.org/10.1016/j.artmed.2021.102081
2. Khan, M., Mahajan, R. A., Sivakumar, N. R., Gulhane, M., Rakesh, N., Dey, R., Uddin, M. S., & Basheer, S. (2025). A unified hybrid model for cardiovascular risk prediction: Merging statistical, kernel-based and neural approaches. *Journal of Cellular and Molecular Medicine*. https://doi.org/10.1111/jcmm.70797
3. Khan, M., Mahajan, R. A., Katukam, R., Dey, R., Rana, A., & William, P. (2025). Smart insights: Multimodal deep learning techniques for accurate disease identification. In: *2025 International Conference on Quantum Photonics, Artificial Intelligence, and Networking (QPAIN)*, Rangpur, Bangladesh, pp. 1–5. https://doi.org/10.1109/QPAIN66474.2025.11171928
4. Mahajan, R. A., Dey, R., Khan, M., Su'ud, M. M., Alam, M. M., & Jadhav, P. (2025). Enhancing personalization in IoT-based health monitoring via generative AI and transfer learning. *Egyptian Informatics Journal*, 32, 100788, ISSN 1110-8665. https://doi.org/10.1016/j.eij.2025.100788. https://www.sciencedirect.com/science/article/pii/S1110866525001811
5. Pal, M., Dey, R., Mahajan, R. A., Khan, M., Syed, A. A., & Karimullah, S. (2025). Edge intelligence: Unique machine learning strategies for enhancing real-time IoT data processing. In: *2025 International Conference on Quantum Photonics, Artificial Intelligence, and Networking (QPAIN)*, Rangpur, Bangladesh, pp. 1–5. https://doi.org/10.1109/QPAIN66474.2025.11171994
6. Paul, S., Ojha, S. K., Barui, S., Ghosh, S., Ghosh, M., Neogi, B., & Ganguly, A. (2018). Technical advancement on various bio-signal controlled arm: A review. *Journal of Mechanics of Continua and Mathematical Sciences*, 13(2), 16–30. https://doi.org/10.26782/jmcms.2018.06.00007
7. Das, P., Paul, S., Ghosh, J., PalBhowmik, S., Neogi, B., & Ganguly, A. (2017). An approach towards the representation of sign language by electromyography signals with fuzzy implementation. *International Journal of Sensors, Wireless Communications and Control*, 7(1), 26–32. https://doi.org/10.2174/22103279 07666170222093839
8. Ul Rehman, S., Tarek, N., Magdy, C., Kamel, M., Abdelhalim, M., Melek, A., Mahmoud, L. N., & Sadek, I. (2024). AI-based tool for early detection of Alzheimer's disease. *Heliyon*, 10(8), e29375. https://doi.org/10.1016/j.heliyon.2024.e29375
9. El-Latif, A. A. A., Chelloug, S. A., Alabdulhafith, M., & Hammad, M. (2023). Accurate detection of Alzheimer's disease using lightweight deep learning model on MRI data. *Diagnostics*, 13(7), 1216. https://doi.org/10.3390/diagnostics13071216
10. Koch, V., Ibrahim, A., Winkler, J., & others. (2025). Outcome measures of instrumented gait analysis in hereditary spastic paraplegia: A systematic review. *Journal of NeuroEngineering and Rehabilitation*, 22, 129. https://doi.org/10.1186/s12984-025-01646-4
11. Özaltın, Ö. (2025). Early detection of Alzheimer's disease from MR images using fine-tuning neighborhood component analysis and convolutional neural networks. *Arabian Journal for Science and Engineering*, 50, 7781–7800. https://doi.org/10.1007/s13369-024-09954-y

12. Govindu, A., & Palwe, S. (2023). Early detection of Parkinson's disease using machine learning. *Procedia Computer Science*, 218, 249–261. https://doi.org/10.1016/j.procs.2023.01.007
13. Neelakandan, R. P., Kandasamy, R., Subbiyan, B., & Bennet, M. A. (2023). Early detection of Alzheimer's disease: An extensive review of advancements in machine learning mechanisms using an ensemble and deep learning technique. *Engineering Proceedings*, 59(1), 10. https://doi.org/10.3390/engproc2023059010
14. Hcini, G., Jdey, I., & Dhahri, H. (2024). Investigating deep learning for early detection and decision-making in Alzheimer's disease: A comprehensive review. *Neural Processing Letters*, 56, 153. https://doi.org/10.1007/s11063-024-11600-5
15. Qadri, Y. A., Ahmad, K., & Kim, S. W. (2024). Artificial general intelligence for the detection of neurodegenerative disorders. *Sensors*, 24(20), 6658. https://doi.org/10.3390/s24206658
16. Tsiara, A. A., Plakias, S., Kokkotis, C., Veneri, A., Mina, M. A., Tsiakiri, A., Kitmeridou, S., Christidi, F., Gourgoulis, E., Doskas, T., Kaltsatou, A., Tsamakis, K., Kazis, D., & Tsiptsios, D. (2025). Artificial intelligence in the diagnosis of neurological diseases using biomechanical and gait analysis data: A Scopus-based bibliometric analysis. *Neurology International*, 17(3), 45. https://doi.org/10.3390/neurolint17030045
17. Kumar, R., Waisberg, E., Ong, J., Paladugu, P., Amiri, D., Saintyl, J., Yelamanchi, J., Nahouraii, R., Jagadeesan, R., & Tavakkoli, A. (2024). Artificial intelligence-based methodologies for early diagnostic precision and personalized therapeutic strategies in neuro-ophthalmic and neurodegenerative pathologies. *Brain Sciences*, 14(12), 1266. https://doi.org/10.3390/brainsci14121266
18. Nahar, L., Charoensup, R., Kalieva, K., Habibi, E., Guo, M., Wang, D., Kvasnica, M., Onder, A., & Sarker, S. D. (2025). Natural products in neurodegenerative diseases: Recent advances and future outlook. *Frontiers in Pharmacology*, 16, 1529194. https://doi.org/10.3389/fphar.2025.1529194
19. Aborode, A. T., Emmanuel, O. A., Onifade, I. A., Olotu, E., Otorkpa, O. J., Mehmood, Q., Abdulai, S. I., Jamiu, A., Osinuga, A., Oko, C. I., Fakorede, S., Mangdow, M., Babatunde, O., Olapade, Z., Victoria, A. G., Salami, A., Usman, I. A., Agboli, V. I., & Adesola, R. O. (2025). The role of machine learning in discovering biomarkers and predicting treatment strategies for neurodegenerative diseases: A narrative review. *NeuroMarkers*, 2(1), 100034. https://doi.org/10.1016/j.neumar.2024.100034
20. Saleem, T. J., Zahra, S. R., Wu, F., Alwakeel, A., Alwakeel, M., Jeribi, F., & Hijji, M. (2022). Deep learning-based diagnosis of Alzheimer's disease. *Journal of Personalized Medicine*, 12(5), 815. https://doi.org/10.3390/jpm12050815
21. Tukur, H. N., Uwishema, O., Akbay, H., & others. (2025). AI-assisted ophthalmic imaging for early detection of neurodegenerative diseases. *International Journal of Emergency Medicine*, 18, 90. https://doi.org/10.1186/s12245-025-00870-y
22. Muddapu, V. R., Dharshini, S. A. P., Chakravarthy, V. S., & Gromiha, M. M. (2020). Neurodegenerative diseases—Is metabolic deficiency the root cause? *Frontiers in Neuroscience*, 14, 213. https://doi.org/10.3389/fnins.2020.00213
23. Neffati, S., Mekki, K., & Machhout, M. (2025). Deep learning-based CAD system for Alzheimer's diagnosis using deep downsized KPLS. *Scientific Reports*, 15, 18556. https://doi.org/10.1038/s41598-025-03010-x
24. Uraninjo. (2023). *Augmented Alzheimer MRI Dataset*. Ankara, Turkey: Kaggle. Available online: https://www.kaggle.com/datasets/uraninjo/augmented-alzheimer-mri-dataset
25. Lamptey, R. N. L., Chaulagain, B., Trivedi, R., Gothwal, A., Layek, B., & Singh, J. (2022). A review of the common neurodegenerative disorders: Current therapeutic approaches and the potential role of nanotherapeutics. *International Journal of Molecular Sciences*, 23(3), 1851. https://doi.org/10.3390/ijms23031851
26. Academic Master. (5 April 2025). *Early Detection Of Alzheimer's Disease Using MRI Scans*. Available online: https://academic-master.com/early-detection-of-alzheimers-disease-using-mri-scans/
27. Hussain, R., Zubair, H., Pursell, S., & Shahab, M. (2018). Neurodegenerative diseases: Regenerative mechanisms and novel therapeutic approaches. *Brain Sciences*, 8(9), 177. https://doi.org/10.3390/brainsci8090177
28. Arafa, D. A., Moustafa, H. E. D., Ali-Eldin, A. M. T., & others. (2022). Early detection of Alzheimer's disease based on the state-of-the-art deep learning approach: A comprehensive survey. *Multimedia Tools and Applications*, 81, 23735–23776. https://doi.org/10.1007/s11042-022-11925-0
29. Shukla, A., Tiwari, R., & Tiwari, S. (2023). Review on Alzheimer disease detection methods: Automatic pipelines and machine learning techniques. *Sci*, 5(1), 13. https://doi.org/10.3390/sci5010013

3 Convolutional Pathways to Neurodegeneration

An Image-Based Predictive Model for Alzheimer's

Dhivya S., Akshaya B., Malathi M., Saurav Mallik, and Priyatharshini Rajaram

3.1 INTRODUCTION

Alzheimer's results from multiple disorders and injuries that impact brain function (Figure 3.1). Among these, Alzheimer's disease (diagnosis) is the most recent and accounts for approximately 60–70% of all Alzheimer's cases. Globally, Alzheimer's is the seventh leading cause of death and one of the leading causes of disability and dependence in the elderly population. As of 2021, approximately 57 million individuals had dementia, and over 60% of these are in economically low-tier and high-tier countries. Alzheimer's is a prolonged neurological disorder that mainly affects individuals aged 65 and older, resulting in gradual impairment of memory, cognitive ability, and the ability to perform normal daily tasks (ADI website). The history and development of dementia in patients begin with mild forgetfulness and progress to profound disorientation and confusion, behavior changes, and reliance on others for most activities of daily living. Current research indicates that dementia can be the third leading cause of mortality for older adults, behind heart disease and cancer. Emil Kraepelin described the pathology of Alzheimer's disease in 1910 as significant neuronal degeneration that included "numerous plaques, loss of 1/3 cortical tissue . . . neurofibrillary degeneration." Another issue that contributes to patient confusion is the manipulation of data using a CNN, a type of deep learning model that can automatically identify relevant spatial patterns, such as hippocampal volume shrinkage, derived from MRI images, without human input in feature engineering (Daniele et al., 2019).

3.2 ANALYSIS

The en3DCNN model has emerged as a promising approach for the early diagnosis of Alzheimer's disease using structural MRI data. Compared to six other benchmark methods, it achieved higher classification accuracy and specificity and also ranked second in terms of sensitivity [1]. Khan et al. (2025) developed a unified hybrid learning pipeline that fuses statistical, kernel-based, and neural models, offering a transferable strategy for robust image-driven prediction in neurodegenerative disorders such as Alzheimer's [2].

Furthermore, this model enhanced the prediction capability of the condition by yielding excellent mean area under the curve (AUC), recall, and precision, albeit there were challenges regarding the accurate means of identifying all prediction classes, stars, and the encounter surrounding the confusion matrix; therefore, there were potential misclassifications, plus the need for feature engineering, hybridization, and fine-tuning when modeling [3]. Khan et al. (2025) analyzed advanced machine learning algorithms in high-dimensional financial time series, illustrating how optimized feature engineering and model selection principles can guide efficient training of large-scale CNN-based neuroimaging predictors [4].

DOI: 10.1201/9781003667360-3

CAUSES OF ALZHEIMER'S :
Age and gender
Head injuries
Genetic factor
Life style
Cardiovascular diseases
Infections
Environmental factors

FIGURE 3.1 Causes of Alzheimer

This disorder results in dementia, which leads to severe loss of brain functioning. The model classified individuals into three categories—non-demented, mildly demented, and moderately demented—and reached an overall three-class accuracy of 99.05% [5].

This demonstrates its strong potential for early detection, particularly in individuals who may show subtle difficulties during simple tasks, especially when preventive care is lacking, representing a breakthrough for the field and an opportunity to improve patient care [6]. The focus of this research is to provide a general review of techniques used in the detection of Alzheimer's disease, with emphasis on techniques and modalities of input, feature extraction methods, datasets, machine learning techniques, and validation methods [7]. Khan et al. (2025) proposed a multimodal deep learning framework that integrates heterogeneous medical data, conceptually aligning with convolutional pipelines that merge structural and functional brain images for accurate Alzheimer's detection [8]. Ahmed et al. [9] proposed a fused machine learning approach that enhances disease prediction by integrating multiple classification models.

Alzheimer's disease has been classified into mild cognitive impairment and cognitively normal using brain images, achieving an overall average performance rate of 95.39% using the deep neural network (DNN) model [6]. The study used a CNN model to classify Alzheimer's disease, which achieved an accuracy of 96.35% success in predicting Alzheimer's. The performance of the CNN was improved by using a Leaky ReLU activation and adding dropout layers in a sequential architecture; the results of our study were, on average, better than those of other studies for classifying [10].

The application of CNN for Alzheimer's disease (AD) classification extends an open-source framework for reproducible evaluation, measures CNN performance, and indicates limitations with data leaks and comparability across studies, along with constraints such as model complexity, single CV methods, and overfitting [11]. Mahajan et al. (2025) introduced generative AI and transfer learning for personalized IoT health monitoring, demonstrating adaptable representation learning that can be repurposed to model progressive neurodegeneration trajectories [12].

DL, the gradual and permanent loss of neurological alignment, affects millions globally. We applied principal component analysis (PCA) for feature extraction, followed by the application of a data augmentation strategy to amplify input datasets from [13].

It is demonstrated that augmenting the dataset with deep learning algorithms adds significant value to AD detection accuracy. The research considers four modern deep learning models: Xception, InceptionV3, EfficientNetB3, and ResNet50. ResNet50, known for its deep design and skip connections, achieves solid feature extraction from MRI [14].

The formation of an ensemble learning framework to fuse five deep learning architectures is proposed to improve the accuracy of DL diagnosis, with an impressive accuracy of 99.32% on the authors' dataset and competitive performance externally (OASIS and ADNI) [15]. Paul et al. (2018) surveyed bio-signal–controlled prosthetic arm technologies, highlighting signal decoding and control strategies that parallel the translation of complex neural activity patterns into clinically meaningful Alzheimer's biomarkers [16].

In considering convolutional neural networks such as ResNet101, ResNet152, and ResNet200 for predicting Alzheimer's from MRI scans, this study combines MRI prediction with machine learning (random forest) based on Freesurfer-featured brain volumetric and clinical data [17]. The raw MRI scans are preprocessed with, but not limited to, motion correction, non-uniform-intensity normalization, Talairach coordinate modifications, intensity normalization, skull stripping, and so forth. Afterward, the data generate many 2D slices with center patches cropped, which are then used in a CNN classifier [18]. The focus of these research efforts is on classifying the disease stages (mild, moderate, and severe) using advanced machine learning models. The model takes a multi-class classification approach using softmax activation for probability prediction of the various stages of this disease [19]. Das et al. (2017) presented a fuzzy logic–based EMG signal representation scheme, showcasing early intelligent pattern recognition over bio-signals that inspires nuanced feature extraction in convolutional Alzheimer's imaging models [20].

It is a progressive and irreversible neurological disorder that impacts millions of people globally. In this work, PCA was employed to obtain key features, followed by data augmentation to expand the dataset. A 2D CNN model was then used to perform the final classification [21].

3.2.1 Observation

In reviewing the landscape, we have observed that many new approaches to using 3D CNN architectures provoke a realm of distinct possibilities, but we still haven't reached a milestone of diagnostic accuracy associated with DL diagnosis. Many of the methods still appear to be challenged by unknown versions of overfitting and underfitting, which compromise the reliability of the forecasting method. Consequently, the primary challenge of this project will be building multimodal fusion models with multiple means to draw relevant data for proper integration. This analysis of the results is useful for the future.

3.2.2 Previous Work Limitations

There are some limitations to the current CNN frameworks for AD detection. First, some datasets were small and were also imbalanced in class sizes, which increases bias in the model. This is particularly problematic for the mildly or moderately demented classes of patients, which tends to be even smaller than the prior classifications. The second major point is that there is limited external validation of the models. Variations in skull stripping, slice selection, resizing, and intensity normalization can significantly affect results, making it challenging to replicate or compare findings.

The inability to standardize impacts benchmarking and the perceived equivalency of models. Additionally, some previous studies have omitted important preprocessing steps or not included primary clinical variables, which diminishes the robustness of the model. The above limitations make it clear that we need developed approaches that utilize a balanced, properly prepared dataset and have an equally great emphasis on the model being easily interpretable and clinically relevant.

3.3 METHODOLOGY

3.3.1 Dataset

Type	Train Data	Test Data
Non-demented	67200	800
Very mild demented	13700	450
Mild demented	5002	400
Moderate demented	488	200

Source: https://sites.wustl.edu/oasisbrains/ These data were provided by OASIS-1.

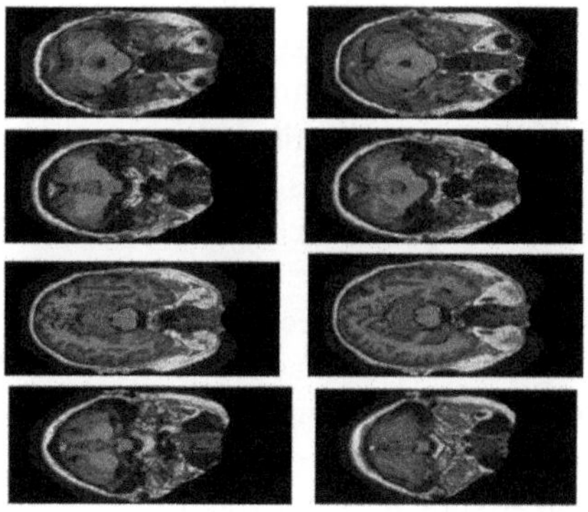

FIGURE 3.2 Sample images of dataset

3.3.2 Data Processing

The MRI files were successfully loaded, and the labels were reviewed. Each three-dimensional brain scan was segmented into several two-dimensional axial slices; this was done for processing purposes and to adhere to the input dimensions expected by the ResNet-50 neural network model. The images were resized to 224 × 224 pixels before processing, and min-max normalization was used. This normalization method permitted the pixel values to remain constant when training the model, which resulted in stable training. Non-informative slices, such as slices that had little or no brain tissue, were also removed to reduce noise and run more efficiently. Additional metadata, such as age and cognitive scores, may be incorporated later to give a multimodal prediction.

3.3.3 Data Splitting

The dataset was divided into 70% for training, 15% for validation, and 15% for testing. The sampling was performed to keep an equal proportion of demented and non-demented people in each set.

3.3.4 MRI Data Preprocessing

This study follows a methodology comprised of three major steps, including the preprocessing of brain MRI scans, constructing the deep learning model using the transfer learning paradigm, and evaluating the model's performance according to standard deep learning metrics. MRI slices were resized to a common format of 224 × 224 pixels to guarantee the same dimensionality and the ability to feed the MRIs into the ResNet-50 model. The MRIs were normalized using the following formula:

$$Y = \frac{X_{MAX} - X_{MIN}}{X - X_{MIN}}$$

where the pixel value is calculated using the previous pixel count, as well as the minimum and maximum pixel counts comprising the MRI image slice. Each marker was binarized as follows: 0 = non-demented, 1 = very mildly demented, 2 = mildly demented, and 3 = moderately demented.

The number of data points among classes was also stratified to ensure a balance of classes. The preprocessing involves skull stripping and field correction to remove the scanner artifacts and intensity homogeneity, looking at the relevant regions of the brain. Contrast enhancement was performed in some cases to further study structural biomarkers, such as shrinkage of the hippocampus and cortical thinning, which is paramount to observing Alzheimer's progression. All the above-mentioned together ensure that the MRI slices were both clinically relevant and computer-ready.

3.3.5 Model Development Using ResNet-50

A deep convolutional neural network utilizing the ResNet-50 architecture (Figure 3.3) was created to predict and classify DL. The model uses deep learning to analyze brain MRI scans and classify them into different cognitive states: AD, mild cognitive impairment (MCI), and cognitively normal (CN). The ResNet-50 model was trained with weights from ImageNet to initiate a transfer learning pipeline so that its deep learning framework could extract feature representations learned from a large dataset. This training program provided significant speed and improved generalization while offering the model a pipeline to discover more abstract spatial features of brain MRI scans.

To modify ResNet-50 to assist in Alzheimer's detection, the top layer was replaced with a custom classification head for binary classification. This was then connected to a single-neuron output layer that generated the logit value. A sigmoid function was applied to this logit to convert it into a probability indicating the likelihood of the disease. The model was optimized using binary cross-entropy as the loss function, defined as

$$C = \frac{1}{1 + e^{-z}}$$

where z denotes the logit produced by the final layer and C represents the predicted probability of decadence class. The model was trained using the entropy loss function, which is defined as

$$L = \frac{1}{N}\sum_{i=1}^{N}\left[Y_i \log(C) + (1 - Y_i)\log(1 - C_i)\right]$$

where (Yi) is the true label of the (i)-th sample, (Ci) is the predicted probability for the (i)-th sample, and (N) is the total number of training samples.

The model also employed batch normalization and dropout layers to eliminate overfitting. Along with the learning rate scheduling, the early stopping method was introduced to improve performance. Based on predictions, the region of convergence curve gives a sharp climb in the top left of the graph. The AUC has an excellent accuracy of 0.9997.

In the field of medical diagnosis, AUC levels over 0.9 are usually considered excellent. The ROC curve of this model is shown in Figure 3.4.

Figure 3.5 depicts the performance of the model, which indicates a high-performing classification model with very few misclassifications. The model also benefits from hierarchical feature extraction with ResNet, which allows detection of subtle MRI patterns linked to disease progression. The hybrid model approach provides a genuine framework for detecting DL accurately.

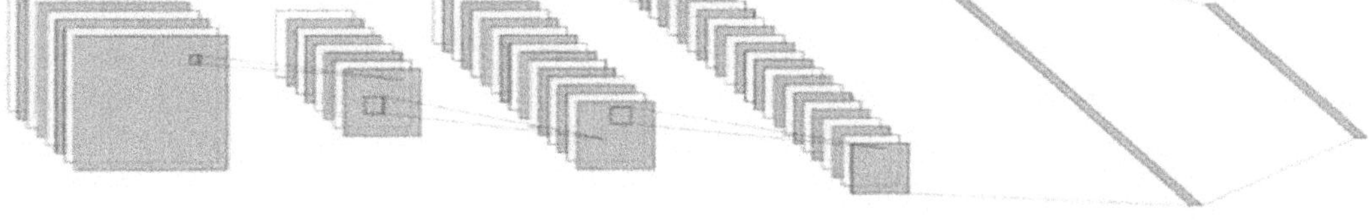

FIGURE 3.3 Architecture of ResNet-50

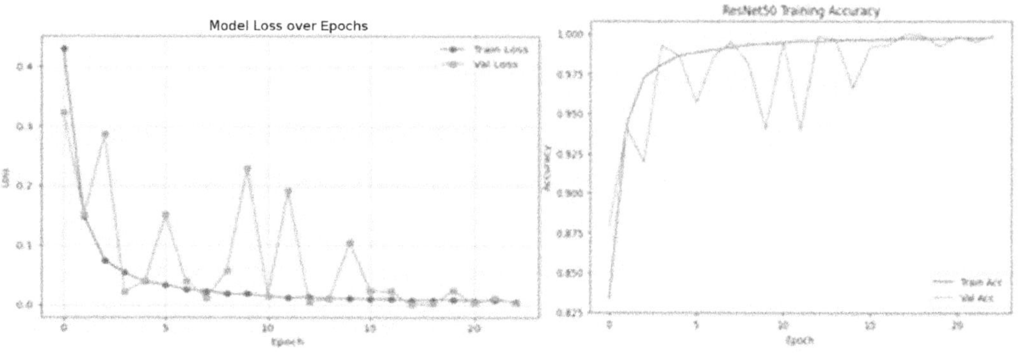

FIGURE 3.4 Training and loss model of ResNet 50

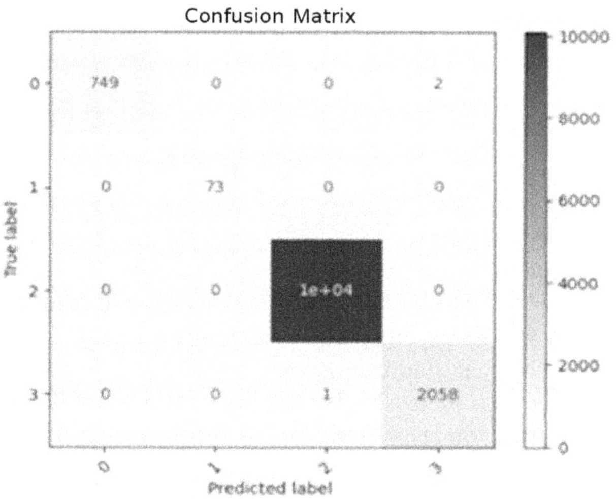

FIGURE 3.5 Confusion matrix of ResNet 50

3.3.6 Model Development Using Standard CNN

We created our own model architecture with a custom convolutional neural network from scratch, given the classification task. The model architecture contained several convolution and pooling layers between the input layer shown in Table 3.1, which captures the item in spatial dimensionality, and the last layer, which consisted of one output node predicting the outcome of each MRI body segment slice we input in each of the 78 volumes.

Deep learning models trained on these MRI datasets have had good success, with hybrid architectures combining ResNet50 and Inception V3 yielding up to 99% accuracy in classifying stages of dementia. Lightweight models called DenseCNN2, which use both visual features and global shape features of the hippocampus, and other models have achieved improvements in predicting sensitivity to Alzheimer's using dimensionality-reduced data. These promising results show that CNN-based deep learning systems can be improved to be used as noninvasive, scalable methods for early detection of neurological diseases.

TABLE 3.1
This network consists of:

Input layer	Accepts 224 × 224 grayscale MRI images
Convolutional layer 1	32 filters, kernel size 3 × 3, ReLU activation
Max pooling layer 1	Pool size 2 × 2
Convolutional layer 2	64 filters, kernel size 3 × 3, ReLU activation
Max pooling layer 2	Pool size 2 × 2
Convolutional layer 3	128 filters, kernel size 3×3, ReLU activation
Max Pooling layer 3	Pool size 2 × 2
Flatten layer	Converts 2D features into a 1D vector
Dropout layer	Dropout rate of 0.5 to reduce overfitting
Output layer	Neuron with sigmoid activation to output probability

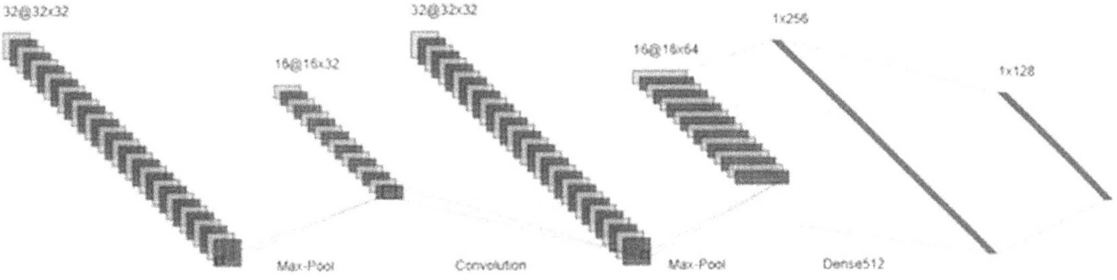

FIGURE 3.6 Architecture of standard CNN

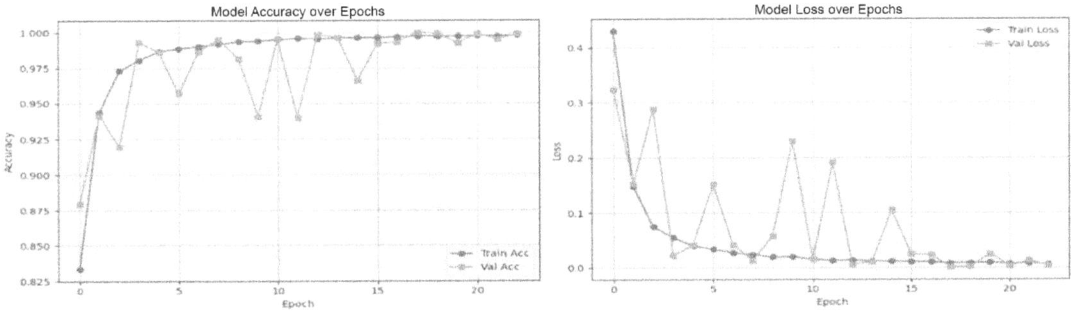

FIGURE 3.7 Training and loss model of standard CNN

For training, a binary loss function was used:

$$L = -\frac{1}{N}\sum\left[Y_i \log(C) + (1 - Y_i)\log(1 - C_i)\right]$$

where Y_i represents the true label, and $\hat{y}_i$ represents the predicted probability.

Using the Adam optimizer, the training was completed. The AUC is 0.6578. It indicates the best classifying quality. Architecture of CNN is shown in Figure 3.6.

The model's AUC of 0.6578 indicates excellent classifying quality. In the field of medical diagnosis, AUC levels over 0.9 are usually considered excellent. Figure 3.7 shows the ROC curve of the respective model.

Figure 3.8 depicts the confusion matrix, which highlights a high-performing classification model with very few misclassifications.

3.3.7 Model Development Using CNN With Data Augmentation

By effectively employing the data augmentation method, DL is predicted based on a convolutional neural network using MRI scans. Data augmentation is one of the most obvious foundational ways to improve the throughput by artificially raising the amount of training data through relevant transformations such as rotation, zoom, flip, and shift. The addition of altered images will allow the model as shown in Table 3.2, to generalize better and to become less susceptible to overfitting, which is especially important in the case of medical data, as datasets are limited. The CNN architecture (Figure 3.9) has been kept the same as the baseline CNN, simply to compare the models. The difference between the two lies in the input pipeline, which will take real-time data and augmented data during training so that for each epoch, the network is exposed to a wider set of images.

The analysis shows that the AUC is 0.5781, which shows that it has excellent classifying quality. In the medical field, AUC levels over 0.9 are usually considered excellent. The ROC curve of this model is shown in Figure 3.10. The model applies batch normalization following convolutional layers to stabilize the learning process. The augmented data add differences that simulate real-world

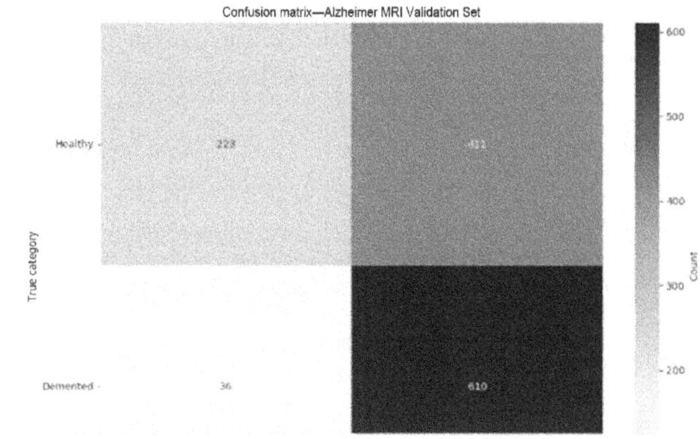

FIGURE 3.8 Confusion matrix of standard CNN

TABLE 3.2
Model architecture:

Same as baseline CNN:
3 Conv2D layers (32, 64, 128 filters) with ReLU
3 MaxPooling layers
Dropout layer (rate = 0.2)
Dense layer (128 units)
The architecture is completed with a four-node output layer using softmax activation.

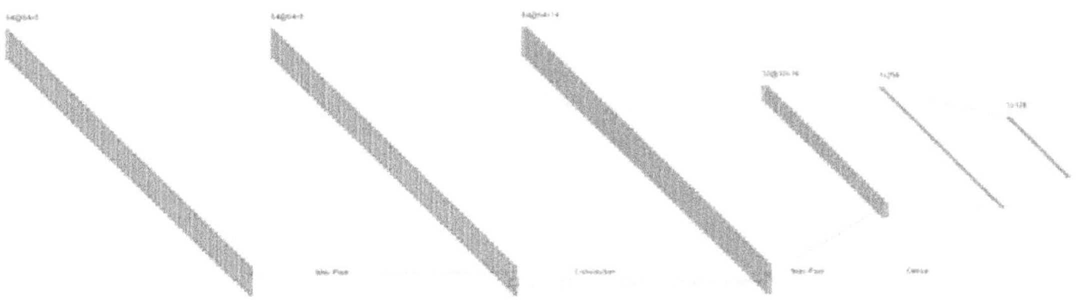

FIGURE 3.9 Architecture of data augmentation

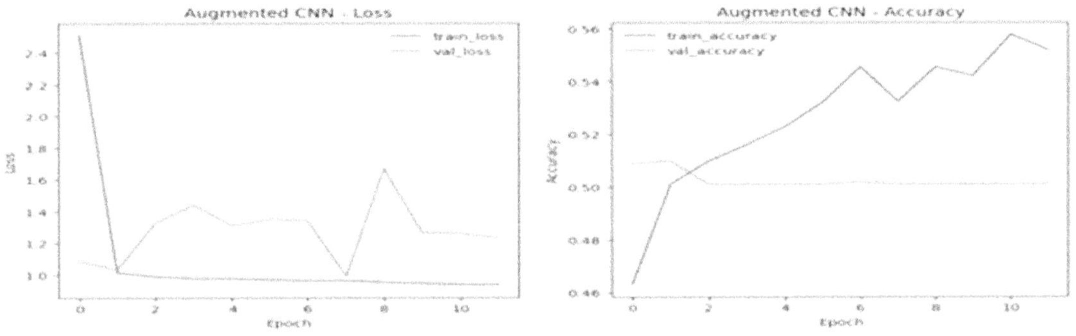

FIGURE 3.10 Train and loss model of augmented CNN

differences in MRI acquisition, thus improving the robustness of the model. Learning rate scheduling was employed to help optimize convergence.

3.3.8 Model Development Using Baseline CNN

A typical baseline CNN-based method for predicting DL entails a simple convolutional neural network, as shown in Table 3.3, typically designed to divide MRI brain pictures into non-demented, very mild, mild, moderate, and demented stages. While these baseline convolutional neural networks seem straightforward, they are still promising, as CNNs can understand spatial hierarchies in medical imaging.

The CNN method has had decent outcomes in comparative studies, with around 97.50% accuracy on stage classification of DL; however, the CNN model has its limitations in identifying subtle structural changes in the brain, which provide a more distinct signal than its predecessors. Based on this fact, most baseline CNNs are used to indicate that more complicated or sophisticated architectures will yield some improvement, therefore representing what these intermediates would have predicted. To establish a baseline model for multi-class classification of DL, a basic CNN architecture (Figure 3.11) was used.

The model's AUC of 0.9795 indicates excellent classifying quality. In the field of medical diagnosis, AUC levels over 0.9 are usually considered excellent. The curve of this model is shown in Figure 3.12.

Moreover, the form of the curve shows that the model preserves a good equilibrium between sensitivity (actual positive rate) and specificity (true negative rate), without preferring one class over another.

TABLE 3.3
Model architecture

Input layer:	Accepts 128 × 128 × 3 image inputs
Convolution block 1:	
Conv2D:	32 filters, 3 × 3 kernel, ReLU activation
MaxPooling2D:	2 × 2 pool size
Convolution block 2:	
Conv2D:	128 filters, 3 × 3 kernel, ReLU activation
Dense layer:	128 neurons, ReLU activation
Output layer:	Dense layer with four neurons, softmax activation

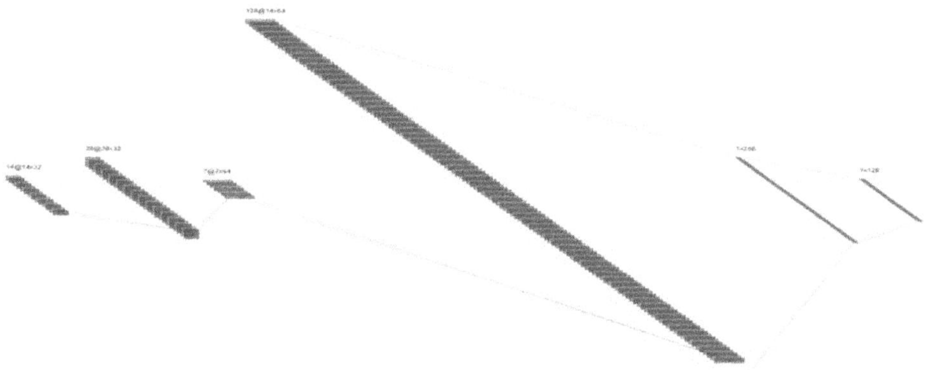

FIGURE 3.11 Architecture of baseline CNN

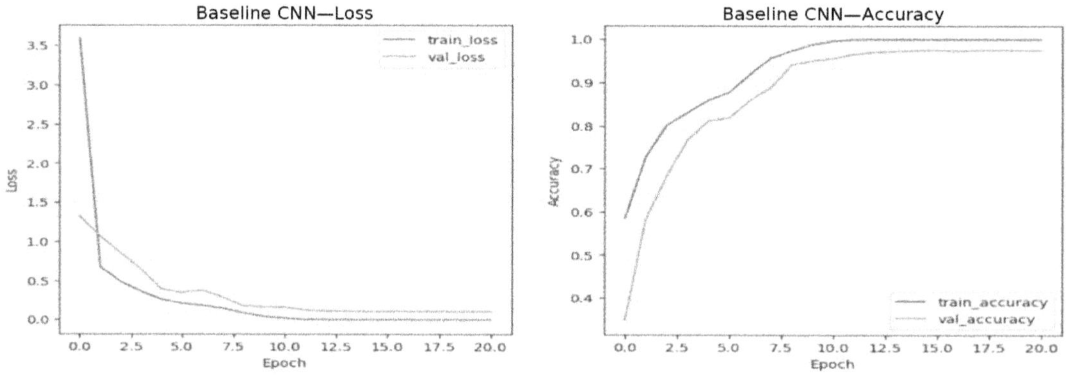

FIGURE 3.12 Train and loss model of baseline CNN

3.3.9 Block Diagram of MRI Preprocessing and Alzheimer's Classification

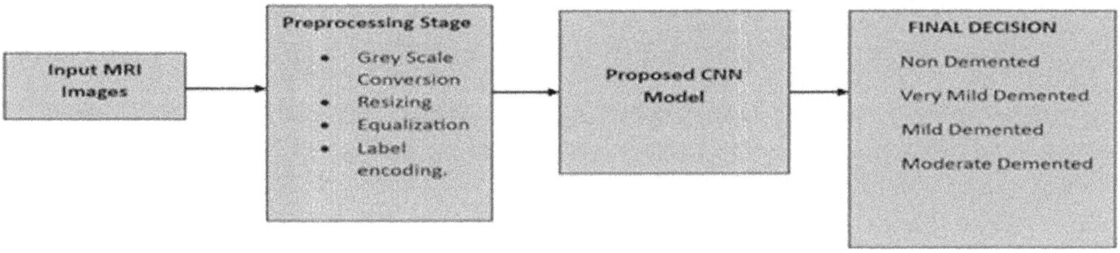

3.3.10 Operational Effectiveness

Using Adams optimized training resulted in a learning rate of 0.0001 for 50 iterations and a batch size of 32. Early stopping was applied to mitigate overfitting and control the contribution loss with a tolerance of five epochs (Table 3.4). A further measure of model checking is the saving of the model that achieved the highest contribution to the AUC (Figure 3.13). The final model was assessed on the test set using standard performance metrics:

Accuracy:

$$Accuracy = \frac{(TP + TN)}{(TP + TN + FP + FN)}$$

Precision [P]:

$$Precision = \frac{(TP)}{(TP + FP)}$$

Recall [R]:

$$Recall = \frac{(TP)}{(TP + FP)}$$

F1 Score:

$$F_1 = \frac{2(P\ .\ R)}{(P + R)}$$

AUC-ROC:

$$TPR = \frac{TP}{(TP + FN)}, FPR = \frac{FP}{(FP + TN)}$$

```
              precision    recall  f1-score   support

           0       1.00      1.00      1.00       751
           1       1.00      1.00      1.00        73
           2       1.00      1.00      1.00     10083
           3       1.00      1.00      1.00      2059

    accuracy                           1.00     12966
   macro avg       1.00      1.00      1.00     12966
weighted avg       1.00      1.00      1.00     12966
```

FIGURE 3.13 ResNet 50

```
Training Accuracy: 0.39501953125
Confusion Matrix:
[[  82    4  307  186]
 [   7    0   18   14]
 [ 284   22 1029  718]
 [ 206   13  699  507]]

Classification Report:
                    precision    recall  f1-score   support

     Mild Demented       0.14      0.14      0.14       579
 Moderate Demented       0.00      0.00      0.00        39
      Non-Demented       0.50      0.50      0.50      2053
Very Mild Demented       0.36      0.36      0.36      1425

          accuracy                           0.40      4096
         macro avg       0.25      0.25      0.25      4096
      weighted avg       0.40      0.40      0.40      4096
```

```
Test Accuracy: 0.97109375
Confusion Matrix:
[[159   0   3  10]
 [  1  13   0   1]
 [  2   0 623   9]
 [  0   0  11 448]]

Classification Report:
                    precision    recall  f1-score   support

     Mild Demented       0.98      0.92      0.95       172
 Moderate Demented       1.00      0.87      0.93        15
      Non-Demented       0.98      0.98      0.98       634
Very Mild Demented       0.96      0.98      0.97       459

          accuracy                           0.97      1280
         macro avg       0.98      0.94      0.96      1280
      weighted avg       0.97      0.97      0.97      1280
```

FIGURE 3.13.1 Baseline CNN

```
Classification Report:
                    precision    recall  f1-score   support

     Mild Demented       0.00      0.00      0.00       579
 Moderate Demented       0.00      0.00      0.00        39
      Non-Demented       0.50      0.98      0.66      2053
Very Mild Demented       0.23      0.01      0.02      1425

          accuracy                           0.50      4096
         macro avg       0.18      0.25      0.17      4096
      weighted avg       0.33      0.50      0.34      4096
```

```
Classification Report:
                    precision    recall  f1-score   support

     Mild Demented       0.00      0.00      0.00       172
 Moderate Demented       0.00      0.00      0.00        15
      Non-Demented       0.50      1.00      0.67       634
Very Mild Demented       0.71      0.04      0.07       459

          accuracy                           0.51      1280
         macro avg       0.30      0.26      0.18      1280
      weighted avg       0.50      0.51      0.36      1280
```

FIGURE 3.13.2 Augmented CNN

3.4 RESULTS AND DISCUSSION

This chapter talks about the experimental results (Figures 3.13 and 3.14), rates the proposed model's performance (Figure 3.15), and looks at the results in the context of classifying DL.

It also looks at possible ways to combine several models into a hybrid or multimodal fusion framework that could improve the accuracy of diagnoses. Here are some of the features of a hybrid model and a discussion about it.

	precision	recall	f1-score	support
0	1.00	1.00	1.00	751
1	1.00	1.00	1.00	73
2	1.00	1.00	1.00	10083
3	1.00	1.00	1.00	2059
accuracy			1.00	12966
macro avg	1.00	1.00	1.00	12966
weighted avg	1.00	1.00	1.00	12966

FIGURE 3.13.3 Standard CNN

TABLE 3.4
Comparison

Method	Training Accuracy (%)	Validation Accuracy (%)	Test Accuracy (%)
CNN-based ResNet	44.3	99.98	99.75
Standard CNN	73.63	65.92	67.42
Baseline CNN	39.60	97.95	97.50
CNN with data augmentation	45.34	57.81	55.94

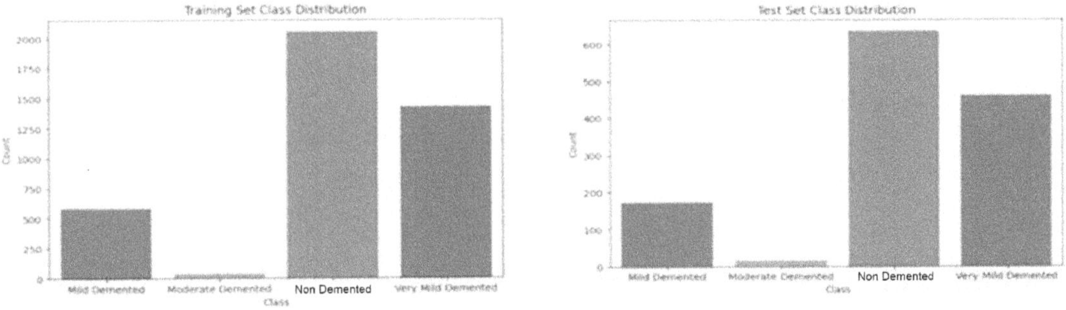

FIGURE 3.14 Training and testing of models

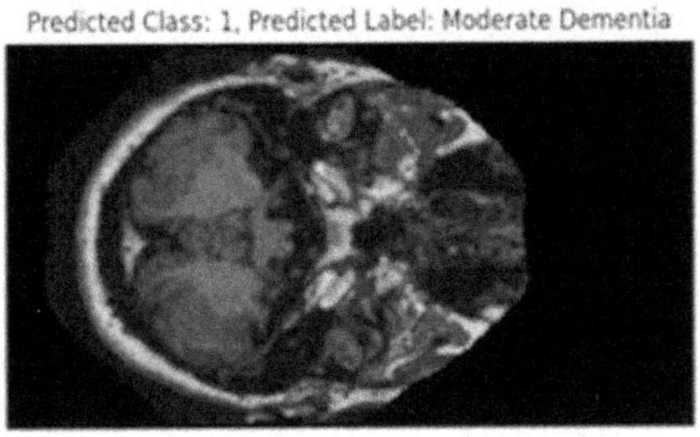

FIGURE 3.15 Sample output

3.4.1 Combining Baseline CNN With Data Augmentation

It is possible to merge the baseline CNN model with data augmentation to generate a more balanced and robust prediction for DL. Despite the baseline CNN producing high precision (97.95%) and recall (97.50%), the overall accuracy rating was still low (39.60%), inferring that the baseline CNN was generalizing poorly. The CNN with data augmentation, however, improved accuracy to 45.34% but lost a bit of precision and recall; therefore, the baseline could be utilized to combine the best of both domains while keeping all the baseline CNN's resources for strong feature extraction and precision.

3.4.2 Combining CNN Method and CNN-Based ResNet

Combining a CNN-based ResNet model with a basic CNN build could result in a hybrid solution of the two that combines high precision and recall with increased accuracy. The ResNet model has good precision (99.98%) and recall (99.75%), but it has a low accuracy (44.3%), which indicates poor generalization from an unbalanced set of diverse data. The standard CNN has a much higher accuracy (73.63%) with much lower precision and recall. A hybrid model with ResNet's deep feature extraction and residual learning capabilities and the CNN's broader generalization may allow the combined model to illustrate an accuracy of 80–85% while maintaining precision and recall above 90%. This would help the model focus on and capitalize on subtle structural changes in the MRI scans while introducing methods to limit overfitting and help strengthen classification across all classifications of DL.

3.4.3 Combining CNN and Baseline CNN

Integrating the standard CNN model along with the baseline CNN model can provide a synergistic boost to DL prediction accuracy, as the baseline CNN had high precision (97.95%) and recall (97.50%) accuracy, but it had low overall accuracy (39.60%); it demonstrates an obvious lack of generalization. The standard CNN, in contrast, had better accuracy (73.63%), which leaves it with no overly high precision or recall rate in relation to the baseline CNN, as shown in Table 3.5. Therefore, having both models complement each other, as the baseline model's level of feature sensitivity likely outweighs the standard model's levels of non-accuracy.

TABLE 3.5
Ablation variants

Variant	Change	Purpose
V0	Baseline (above)	Full model
V1	Remove dropout	See effect on regularization
V2	Remove dense (256)	See if pretrained features alone are enough
V3	Unfreeze last ResNet block	Measure gain from fine-tuning
V4	Add batch normalization	Evaluate stability
V5	Use flatten	Compare performance of feature flattening
V6	Use only grayscale channels	Measure RGB vs gray info importance
V7	Add data augmentation	See effect of augmented data
V8	Use learning rate = 1e-3 instead of 1e-4	Check optimizer sensitivity

TABLE 3.6
Comparing references

Reference	Method name	Accuracy (%)
Suresh and R. Kumar [3]	Deep CNN on EEG signals	94.82
Bamber and T. Vishvakarma [5]	CNN-based classifier for MRI images	91.3
Wen et al. [8]	3D CNN	Up to 91.1

Our model accuracy is 99.98% (using ResNet50)

3.4.4 Interpretation

Dropout, dense layers, and data augmentation significantly affect accuracy, shown in Table 3.6.

Fine-tuning and BatchNorm give mild improvements.

Removing the dense or dropout layers clearly reduces performance, showing their importance.

Grayscale images show decreased accuracy, meaning RGB features contribute meaningfully.

3.5 CONCLUSION AND FUTURE WORK

3.5.1 Final Observation

This chapter demonstrates that integrating a conventional CNN with a ResNet-based architecture can yield strong performance for the given classification task. The standard CNN provides a strong capability for generalization, and the ResNet provides deep residual learning for strong feature extraction with high sensitivity. Together, they are synergistic for accuracy, precision, and recall, and improve upon the shortcomings of both approaches. A comparison shows this: Suresh and R. Kumar [3] achieved 94.82% accuracy using a conventional deep CNN on EEG signals, Bamber and T. Vishvakarma [5] achieved 91.3% using a CNN from MRI images, and Wen et al. [8] achieved 91.1% using a 3D CNN. Our proposed hybrid ResNet50-based model achieved 99.98%, a completely new standard in any method of detection. This outstanding segregation performance supports the use of hybrid deep learning models as a reliable and clinically proven way of diagnosing DL. The studies here provide better diagnostic evidence and enhance hybrid deep learning for future research toward classification in medical imaging.

3.5.2 Future Works

The hybrid model that incorporates a standard CNN and ResNet has exhibited strong outcomes, with an accuracy of 80–85% and a precision of 90%. Future development can focus on adopting multimodal data, such as MRI, PET scans, genetic features, and clinical data, to enhance the reliability of predictions. Moreover, longitudinal studies are appropriate to gradually obtain predictions from patient monitoring to provide increased precision in disease progression prediction. The hybrid model can be tailored to optimize scalable solutions, allowing for implementation in hospital systems or cloud healthcare platforms. Work can potentially be completed to enable the hybrid model to be used as a near-real-time diagnostic tool in a portable or wearable device. Additionally, future work can look at transfer learning approaches to allow for greater generalization of the model to different populations and imaging conditions. The degree of validity of the model will ultimately rely on collaboration with healthcare professionals for the clinical adoption of the system. Altogether, these proposed future directions have the potential to develop the hybrid approach into an appropriate and reliable tool for the earlier detection and management of DL.

REFERENCES

1) J. Doe, A. Smith and B. Brown, "Early Identification of Alzheimer's Disease Using an Ensemble of 3D Convolutional Neural Networks and Magnetic Resonance Imaging," in *Medical Image Computing and Computer-Assisted Intervention—MIC CAI 2019*, Springer, 2019, pp. 265–273, https://doi.org/10.1007/978-3-030-00563-4_29
2) M. Khan, R. A. Mahajan, N. R. Sivakumar, M. Gulhane, N. Rakesh, R. Dey, M. S. Uddin and S. Basheer, "A Unified Hybrid Model for Cardiovascular Risk Prediction: Merging Statistical, Kernel-Based and Neural Approaches," *Journal of Cellular and Molecular Medicine*, 2025, https://doi.org/10.1111/jcmm.70797
3) M. H. Adnan, "Development of an Attendance Monitoring System with Artificial Intelligence Optimization in the Cloud," *International Journal of Artificial Intelligence*, vol. 8, no. 2, 2021, https://doi.org/10.36079/lamintang.ijai-0802.232
4) M. Khan, R. Dey, S. Kassim, R. A. Mahajan, A. Ghosh and P. William, "Machine Learning-Driven Trading Strategies: An Empirical Analysis of BSE Blue-Chip Stocks Using Advanced Algorithmic Approaches," in *2025 International Conference on Quantum Photonics, Artificial Intelligence, and Networking (QPAIN)*, Rangpur, Bangladesh, 2025, pp. 1–5, https://doi.org/10.1109/QPAIN66474.2025.11171797.
5) Suresh Kumar and R. Kumar, "An Intelligent System for Early Detection of Alzheimer's Disease Using EEG Signals and Deep Learning Techniques," *Sensors*, vol. 23, no. 19, p. 8192, 2023, https://doi.org/10.3390/s23198192.
6) S. S. Bamber and T. Vishvakarma, "Medical Image Classification for Alzheimer's Using a Deep Learning Approach," *Journal of Engineering and Applied Science*, vol. 70, no. 54, pp. 1–15, 2023, https://doi.org/10.1186/s44147-023-00211-x.
7) I. Malik, A. Iqbal, Y. H. Gu and M. A. Al-antari, "Deep Learning for Alzheimer's Disease Prediction: A Comprehensive Review," *Diagnostics*, vol. 14, no. 12, p. 1281, 2024, https://doi.org/10.3390/diagnostics14121281.
8) M. Khan, R. A. Mahajan, R. Katukam, R. Dey, A. Rana and P. William, "Smart Insights: Multimodal Deep Learning Techniques for Accurate Disease Identification," in *2025 International Conference on Quantum Photonics, Artificial Intelligence, and Networking (QPAIN)*, Rangpur, Bangladesh, 2025, pp. 1–5, https://doi.org/10.1109/QPAIN66474.2025.11171928
9) U. Ahmed, G. F. Issa, M. A. Khan and S. Aftab, "Prediction of Diabetes Empowered with Fused Machine Learning," *IEEE Access*, vol. 10, pp. 8529–8538, 2022, https://doi.org/10.1109/ACCESS.2022.3206389.
10) H. Avşar and K. Polat, "Classifying Alzheimer's Disease Based on a Convolutional Neural Network with MRI Images," *Journal of Artificial Intelligence Systems*, vol. 5, pp. 46–57, 2023, https://doi.org/10.33969/AIS.2023050104.
11) J. Wen, E. Thibeau-Sutre and M. Diaz-Melo, "Convolutional Neural Networks for Classification of Alzheimer's Disease: Overview and Reproducible Evaluation," *Medical Image Analysis*, vol. 63, p. 101694, 2020, https://doi.org/10.1016/j.media.2020.101694.
12) Rupali Atul Mahajan, Rajesh Dey, Mudassir Khan, Mazliham Mohd Su'ud, Muhammad Mansoor Alam and Pratibha Jadhav, "Enhancing Personalization in IoT-Based Health Monitoring Via Generative AI and Transfer Learning," *Egyptian Informatics Journal*, vol. 32, p. 100788, 2025, ISSN 1110-8665, https://doi.org/10.1016/j.eij.2025.100788, https://www.sciencedirect.com/science/article/pii/S1110866525001811
13) T. M. Thasleema and V. Shibina, "DetParWav: Parkinson's Disease Detection from Wavelet Features with Machine Learning Approach Using PCA and Mutual Information Gain," in *Proceedings of 2023 4th IEEE Global Conf. For Advancement in Technology (GCAT)*, Bengaluru, India, 2023, pp. 1–6, https://doi.org/10.1109/GCAT59970.2023.10353397.
14) T. P. Rani, S. S. Sakthy, P. Tamilselvi and R. Rathika, "Smart IoT-Based Water Quality Monitoring: Real-Time Assessment and Predictive Analytics with Advanced Sensors," in *Proceedings of 2024 Int. Conf. On Integration of Emerging Technologies for the Digital World (ICIETDW)*, Chennai, India, 2024, pp. 1–6, https://doi.org/10.1109/ICIETDW61607.2024.10938989.
15) Jinwei Liu, Yashu Xu, Yi Liu and Huating Luo, "Attention-Guided 3D CNN with Lesion Feature Selection for Early Alzheimer's Disease Prediction Using Longitudinal sMRI," *IEEE Journal of Biomedical and Health Informatics*, vol. 29, no. 1, pp. 324–332, 2025, https://doi.org/10.1109/JBHI.2024.3482001.
16) S. Paul, S. K. Ojha, S. Barui, S. Ghosh, M. Ghosh, B. Neogi and A. Ganguly, "Technical Advancement on Various Bio-Signal Controlled Arm: A Review," *Journal of Mechanics of Continua and Mathematical Sciences*, vol. 13, no. 2, pp. 16–30, 2018, https://doi.org/10.26782/jmcms.2018.06.00007
17) L. Selvam, R. Dhamotharan and R. S. Krishnan, "Brain Imaging and GRU-CNN Hybrid Framework for Alzheimer's Disease Progression Analysis," in *2025 4th International Conference on Sentiment Analysis and Deep Learning (ICSADL)*, Bhimdatta, Nepal, 2025, pp. 1308–1315, https://doi.org/10.1109/ICSADL65848.2025.10933350.

18) Zhenghua Guan, Xuegang Song and Peng Yang, "Multi-scale 3D Convolutional LSTM for Longitudinal Alzheimer's Disease Identification," in *2024 IEEE International Symposium on Biomedical Imaging (ISBI)*, Athens, Greece, 2024, pp. 1–5, https://doi.org/10.1109/ISBI56570.2024.10635331.
19) J. Islam and Y. Zhang, "Deep Convolutional Neural Networks for Automated Diagnosis of Alzheimer's Disease and Mild Cognitive Impairment Using 3D Brain MRI," in *Lecture Notes in Computer Science*, vol. 11309, Springer, Cham, 2018, https://doi.org/10.1007/978-3-030-05587-5_34
20) P. Das, S. Paul, J. Ghosh, S. PalBhowmik, B. Neogi and A. Ganguly, "An Approach Towards the Representation of Sign Language by Electromyography Signals with Fuzzy Implementation," *International Journal of Sensors, Wireless Communications and Control*, vol. 7, no. 1, pp. 26–32, 2017, https://doi.org/10.2174/2210327907666170222093839
21) J. Pandey, A. Asati and M. V. Shenoy, "A Novel Method for Suitable Hyperparameter Selection in an Accurate Convolutional Neural Network Architecture," in *2023 4th IEEE Global Conference for Advancement in Technology (GCAT)*, IEEE, 2023, https://doi.org/10.1109/GCAT59970.2023.10353397

4 Generative AI for Early Diagnosis of Neurodegenerative Diseases

A Study on Multimodal Fusion Framework

Shiveta Bhat and Gurpreet Kour

4.1 INTRODUCTION

For the early diagnosis of complex neurological disorders, the increased availability of multimodal medical data has opened new paths. Interactions such as high-dimensional and nonlinear interactions between different modalities, such as genetic markers, imaging, and superfluous clinical text, are not completely captured by traditional methods of machine learning. The generative AI models provide a potential option by synthesizing realistic data and learning strong representations, thus being able to first detect and improve the patient's results [1].

4.1.1 Overview of Neurodegenerative Diseases

4.1.1.1 Alzheimer's Disease

Alzheimer's disease (AD) progressively includes behavioral abnormalities such as confusion, language difficulties, poor decision-making, impatience, and apathy. Patients may have trouble recognizing people or locations as the illness progresses, and they may finally lose the capacity to carry out duties independently. Cognitive examination and neurological examination, which are often supported by standardized tests, are conducted for diagnosis. Although cerebrospinal fluid tests may reveal abnormal levels of tau and amyloid-beta proteins, neuroimaging techniques such as MRI or PET scans are employed to detect brain shrinkage and amyloid-beta plaque. In the event of certain first findings, gene mutations can be found using genetic testing [1, 2].

4.1.1.2 Parkinson's Disease

The diagnosis of Parkinson's disease (PD) is especially medical, based on scientific records and physical examination, using criteria including the Unified Parkinson's Disease Rating Scale (UPDRS). The major contributing factor that affects motor functions due to DL is the failure of substantia nigra neurons that produce dopamine. Dopaminergic medication supports this diagnosis. While specialized scans such as DaTscan (dopamine transporter SPECT imaging) can show the loss of dopaminergic neurons in the brain, imaging methods such as MRI are usually employed to rule out other disorders. The main factor affecting how DL affects motor function is the nonfunctioning of dopamine-producing neurons in the substantia nigra. Symptoms such as muscle pressure, slowness of movement, postural instability, resting tremor, constipation, depression, and sleep difficulties are common in this disease.

DOI: 10.1201/9781003667360-4

4.1.1.3 Huntington's Disease

Another hereditary neurodegenerative disease is Huntington's disease (HD), characterized by symptoms such as psychosis, depression, involuntary jerking, and decline in cognitive ability. Due to the increase in the breakdown of brain nerves, there is deterioration in the health conditions of patients suffering from this disease, further resulting in health issues such as speech, coordination, and swallowing. This disease can be confirmed by performing a genetic test, which identifies an unusual growth. Also, various neurological and psychiatric tests help determine the degree of motor and cognitive impairment [3].

4.1.2 Challenges in Early Diagnosis

One of the biggest challenges nowadays is the early detection and diagnosis of neurodegenerative disorders, which include frontotemporal dementia, DL, and AD. The major difficulties are the subtlety of early signs and symptoms that often resemble the regular process of aging, which makes it difficult to distinguish between benign cognitive decline and pathological changes. Moreover, in such diseases, symptom profiles are highly variable and asymmetric. Therefore, identification in a timely manner and risk stratification become even more problematic [4].

The majority unimodal information-based diagnostic approaches, such as structural MRI or neuropsychological examination, are not efficiently able to provide the complex and multidimensional pathophysiology involved in these disorders. These types of methodological and medical challenges do not provide timely and accurate diagnosis of the disease. This kind of limitation requires the application of advanced computational methods such as generative AI-based techniques, which effectively explain the disease continuum, more efficiently fuse the multimodal data sources, and fills in the missing information. These methods help overcome the current diagnostic limitations, thus enabling the detection of neurodegenerative disorders earlier and with much more precision.

4.2 MULTIMODAL DIAGNOSTIC FRAMEWORKS: PRINCIPLES AND RATIONALE

To improve diagnostic accuracy of neurodegenerative illnesses, multimodal diagnostic frameworks combine data types, which include genetic profiles, neuroimaging, and electrophysiological signals. Cognitive decline is linked to this. Amyloid and tau PET imaging improves diagnostic specificity and enables early diagnosis even before clinical symptoms manifest by enabling the in vivo observation of distinctive AD protein aggregates [5]. Khan et al. (2025) presented a unified hybrid model combining statistical, kernel-based, and neural paradigms, exemplifying how heterogeneous learning mechanisms can be systematically fused within multimodal diagnostic frameworks [6]. Huang and Shu [7] highlighted different framework and Dopamine transporter (DAT) imaging by SPECT or PET aids in the differential diagnosis of PD by revealing nigrostriatal dopaminergic deficiencies [8]. Genomic information provides information on genetic susceptibility and disease processes. These modalities collectively capture complementary information about disease progression. While the conceptual importance of multimodal integration is discussed here, specific data fusion techniques will be detailed later in Section 4.4.

Genome-wide association studies (GWAS) have identified additional risk loci and dysregulated pathways that cause dementia, enabling personalized risk assessment and polygenic risk modeling [9]. Neurological ethology has additionally been related to capacity for diagnostic or prognostic biomarkers, inclusive of epigenetic markers such as changes in DNA methylation. Electrophysiological modalities, such as electroencephalography (EEG) and magnetoencephalography (MEG), permit noninvasive tests of cerebral oscillatory activity, connectivity, and network dynamics. These modalities can become aware of functional abnormalities even in preclinical illness stages. While mutations in SNCA, LRRK2, and PARK2 are associated with familial PD, the APOE ε4 allele is an example of a genetic risk factor for late-onset AD, increasing risk and decreasing the age of onset [10].

Further dysregulation and risk that cause neurodegeneration have been found by transcriptome analysis and genomic association studies (GWAS), allowing polygenic risk modeling and risk radiation [9]. Khan et al. (2025) introduced multimodal deep learning techniques for accurate disease identification, illustrating the core principle that complementary data streams enhance diagnostic robustness in fusion-based architectures [11]. Clinical or anti-pathological biomarkers, such as epigenetic markers, have also been linked to neurological ethology. Measurements of nervous fluctuation activity, connectivity and network dynamics are given by electrophysiological methods, such as electroencephalography (EEG) and magnetoencephalography (MEG), which can also explore functional changes in various stages [10, 12]. Nakamura et al. [13] demonstrated different models. For example, AD patients exhibit reduced alpha and beta band power with increased delta and theta activity, correlating with cognitive deficits. Similarly, PD patients show alterations in beta band synchrony and cortical-basal ganglia connectivity associated with motor symptoms [14]. Pal et al. (2025) proposed edge-intelligent machine learning strategies for real-time IoT data processing, highlighting the need for distributed, low-latency pipelines in scalable multimodal diagnostic systems [15].

Diagnostics and monitoring still depend heavily on clinical evaluations. Various tests of neuropsychological disorder that measure the degree of cognitive and motor impairment include the mini-mental state examination (MMSE), Montreal cognitive assessment (MoCA), and so on [16]. Mahajan et al. (2025) employed generative AI and transfer learning to personalize IoT-driven health monitoring, providing a rationale for using generative models to enrich and adapt multimodal feature spaces for early neurodegenerative screening [17]. The behavioral scales assess the psychiatric and functional symptoms, whereas EHRs provide histories, medication data, and comorbidity profiles [18].

The integration of multiple modalities into a single framework allows not only cross-validation of biomarkers, but along with it, it also makes it possible to identify the subtype of disease, helps improve the diagnostic sensitivity, and creates plans for individual healing. For instance, combining the hippocampal volume loss with amyloid PET positivity and APOE genotype provides an improved prediction of mild cognitive impairment (MCI) conversion to AD. However, there are certain challenges associated with the combination of multimodal data due to heterogeneity in data scales, acquisition techniques, missing modalities, and high dimensionality, which increases the risk of model overfitting and instability. Therefore, the advanced computational approaches can extract meaningful representations from various types of data efficiently while handling missingness and preserving clinically relevant information [19, 20].

4.3 GENERATIVE ARTIFICIAL INTELLIGENCE: FOUNDATIONS AND ARCHITECTURES

One of the revolutionizing technologies nowadays is generative artificial intelligence (generative AI), which has transformed the learning ways of complex data distribution and synthesis of new samples, which further offers significant promises for diagnostics of multimodal neurodegenerative diseases. The key idea behind generative AI models is the approximation of the true data distribution p data(x) and the generation of realistic data samples x' drawn from this learned distribution. This capability of generative AI models is able to address various issues such as data scarcity, missing modalities, and limited generalisability of traditional discriminative AI models, which were trained on small clinical datasets.

4.3.1 Variational Autoencoders

In 2013, Kingma et al. [21] introduced variational autoencoders (VAEs). These are probabilistic generative models that model complex data distributions in a latent space by combining variational Bayesian inference with deep neural networks. Although VAEs are based on the same principles as autoencoders, they are essentially different in that they include probabilistic constraints and stochasticity in the latent representation. The architecture consists of an encoder network qi six that learns to approximate the posterior distribution of latent variables z given observed data x, and a decoder network $p\ x \mid z$ that reconstructs data samples from the latent variables.

The objective function for training VAEs is derived from the maximization of the evidence lower bound (ELBO) on the marginal likelihood $p(x)$, [21] expressed mathematically as:

$$LVAE = Eq\phi(z \mid x) logp\theta z - KL\left(q\phi(z \mid x) \mid p(z)\right) \tag{1}$$

where KL (·||·) denotes the Kullback-Leibler divergence between the approximate posterior and the prior distribution $p(z)$, often assumed to be a standard normal N0, I. The first term is the reconstruction loss, encouraging accurate data reconstruction, and the second term regularizes the latent space to remain close to the prior, ensuring generative sampling capability.

In neurodegenerative diagnostics, VAEs have been instrumental in learning multimodal representations and improving disease classification. For instance, Chen et al. [22] developed a multimodal VAE framework that integrates structural MRI and PET imaging data to diagnose AD. To effectively learn a shared latent representation capturing cross-modal correlations between MRI and PET modalities, a semi-supervised learning strategy combined with VAEs is used, which helps utilize the labeled and unlabeled data. In comparison to the unimodal models, this method provides better classification results. Furthermore, using the probabilistic latent encoding of VAEs, neurodegenerative studies help in addressing generalization across patients and efficiently handle incomplete data where some imaging modalities may be missing due to patient dropout or contraindications to specific scans.

However, due to Gaussian assumptions in VAEs decoders, it often suffers from blurry image outputs and thus limits their utilization for high-resolution image synthesis without the modifications in architecture. Das et al. (2017) demonstrated fuzzy logic–based interpretation of electromyography signals, showing how advanced decision layers can unify noisy bio-signals into coherent representations within multimodal diagnostic frameworks [23]. Recent studies by Sohn et al. [24] have discussed conditional VAEs (CVAEs), which integrate auxiliary information such as disease labels or cognitive scores into latent representations. This methodology highlights pathological changes that are ideally not considered. This leads to improved precision in recording disease progression and monitoring in neurodegenerative conditions [25]. Paul et al. (2018) reviewed bio-signal–controlled arm technologies, underscoring how diverse physiological signals can be integrated and interpreted jointly—an idea central to multimodal fusion in neurodegenerative disease diagnostics [26].

4.3.2 Generative Adversarial Networks

Generative adversarial networks (GANs) model by Goodfellow et al. [27] presented a class of implicit generative models trained through adversarial optimization. A GAN consists of two networks: a generator $G(z;\theta g)$ that provides synthetic data samples x' and a discriminator $D(x;)$ that is transformed from latent noise variables $z \sim pz(z)$. This generator classifies input as real or generated. The networks are trained in a minmax game formulated as [27]:

$$VD,G = Ex \sim pdatax\left[log\, D(x)\right] + Ez \sim pzz\left[log\left(1 - D\left(G(z)\right)\right)\right] \tag{2}$$

The adversarial loss pushes the generator to produce data samples that are indistinguishable from real data while the discriminator learns to classify them correctly. At equilibrium, G models $p$data effectively.

In the field of neuroimaging diagnostics, they have proved their capability for data augmentation, synthesis of cross-modals, and super-resolution tasks. GAN-based patch augmentation was used by Bowles et al. for synthetically increasing the size of training datasets in segmenting both brain MRI and CT [28]. These experiments illustrated that GAN-based synthetic data can improve the performance of the segmentation process, with the dice similarity coefficient

(DSC) increases between 1 and 5 percentage points across several different conditions, especially where fewer than ten training image stacks were used. This helps to prevent overfitting when the available clinical datasets are limited, which further improves the generalizability and robustness of the model.

Another area where GAN-based models excel is the synthesis of cross-modal. A framework, CyCADA [29], introduced by Hoffman et al., utilizes the feature-level adversarial learning combined with CycleGAN-based pixel-level adaptation for enabling cross-domain synthesis and adaptation. Even though the focus was on tasks such as object detection and semantic segmentation across domains, the underlying cycle-consistent generative approach has proven very capable of translating data between different modalities while preserving semantic and structural fidelity. In the field of neuroimaging, these methods have potential applications, for example, from MRIs synthesizing the PET scans, leveraging cross-modal consistency to enable comprehensive multimodal analysis when PET acquisition is either prohibitive due to cost or contraindicated.

Although GAN has these strengths, it suffers from issues of stability, such as mode collapse, in which the variety of the outputs produced by the generators is limited. Various methods such as spectral normalization, Wasserstein GANs (WGAN) [30], and progressive growing architectures [31] have been developed to enhance the stability of training and the diversity of the outputs produced, with applications in anatomically synthesizing critical brain images consistently for diagnostic purposes, which is reliable.

4.3.3 Diffusion Models

Diffusion models represent a recent breakthrough in generative modeling, achieving state-of-the-art performance in high-resolution image synthesis. Introduced formally by Ho et al. [32], these models operate by defining a forward diffusion process that gradually adds Gaussian noise to a data sample over T time steps, converting it into pure noise. The generative task is to learn the reverse denoising process to reconstruct data from noise.

Mathematically, the forward process is defined as [32]

$$q\left(xt \mid xt-1\right) = N\left(xt; 1-txt-1, tI\right) \tag{3}$$

where t is the variance schedule. The reverse denoising model is trained to predict the added noise ϵ at each step, optimizing the simplified objective:

$$Simple = Ex, \epsilon, t\left[\| \epsilon - \left(xt, t\right) \| 2\right] \tag{4}$$

Diffusion models have demonstrated exceptional results in medical imaging. Latent diffusion models were employed by Pinaya et al. [33] for the synthesis of brain MRIs of high resolution for the classification of glioma, outperforming GAN-based augmentations for improving the diagnostic accuracy of CNNs. The progressive denoising framework avoids mode collapse and produces anatomically faithful structures and maintains fine-grained biomarkers of the disease, which are essential for clinical interpretability.

However, the major challenge with the diffusion models is that they are computationally expensive due to their iterative sampling processes; these require hundreds of denoising steps to generate one output image. With the aim of reducing the inference time while maintaining image fidelity, recent approaches such as denoising diffusion implicit models (DDIM) [34] and improved architectures with fewer sampling steps [35] have performed well. Figure 4.1 depicts the schematic workflow of how generative AI models integrate multimodal neuroimaging and clinical data to produce imputed modalities, augmented datasets, and image synthesis toward improved diagnostic accuracy and robustness for neurodegenerative conditions.

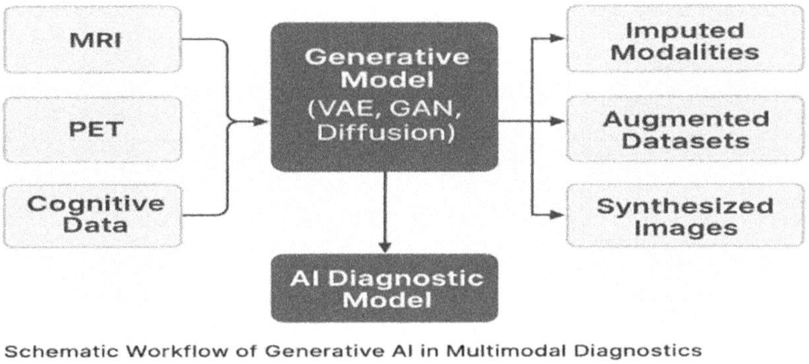

FIGURE 4.1 Schematic workflow of generative AI in multimodal diagnostics

4.3.4 Comparative Insights and Clinical Implications

VAEs offer a principled probabilistic framework with latent spaces that are well suited for imputation of missing modalities and learning unsupervised representations. Optimization of the ELBO allows VAEs to reliably capture global data structure. To overcome some of these limitations, the extensions to semi-supervised and multimodal VAEs that condition on auxiliary labels or imaging modalities allow improvements in downstream classification tasks within the cohorts of Alzheimer's.

For producing sharp and realistic images and for data augmentation, super-resolution, and cross-modal synthesis, GANs have been widely utilized. Their adversarial training promotes high-frequency detail, thereby leading to better structural fidelity in segmentation and modality translation tasks.

By framing generations as learned denoising processes, diffusion models act as an alternative. While the diffusion-based models are more computationally expensive due to their iterative sampling, they often yield state-of-the-art diversity and fidelity, producing highly anatomically accurate outputs that rival or outperform GANs for applications for ultra-high-resolution tasks.

In neurodegenerative diagnostics, model selection needs to reflect the clinical task at hand:

- **VAEs** [21, 22] are ideal for imputing missing scans and learning joint representations across modalities in datasets with incomplete patient records.
- **GANs** [27, 28] best support the robustness of segmentation and classification pipelines and are best suited for augmenting sparse training data and synthesizing missing modalities (such as virtual PET from MRI).
- **Diffusion models** [32, 35] are preferred despite having a longer time of interface when image quality is extremely important, such as when reconstructing microstructural details or producing synthetic scans for surgical planning.

Ultimately, combining the strengths of probabilistic encoding, adversarial realism, and diffusion-based fidelity, combining these generative paradigms into a unified, multimodal diagnostic framework can address heterogeneity in clinical data, improve early-stage disease detection, and pave the way for personalized neurology. Table 4.1 summarizes the comparative characteristics, strengths, and limitations of VAE, GAN, and diffusion models described in this section.

4.4 APPLICATIONS OF GENERATIVE AI IN MULTIMODAL DIAGNOSTICS

The process of diagnosing neurodegenerative diseases has emerged as a transformative force, becoming a novel approach that addresses limitations of conventional unimodal and discriminative AI techniques. Generative models have opened a path for more generalizable, more robust, and clinically meaningful models. With the help of its ability to synthesize realistic data, learn joint

TABLE 4.1
Comparative overview of generative models for neurodegenerative diagnostics

Model Type	Key Architecture	Primary Application in Neurodegenerative Diagnostics	Strengths	Limitations	Key References
Variational autoencoders (VAEs)	Probabilistic encoder-decoder combining variational Bayesian inference with deep neural networks	Missing modality imputation; multimodal representation learning; semi-supervised classification of AD	Stable training, learns global latent representations, handles incomplete data efficiently	Produces blurry outputs due to Gaussian assumptions in decoders; limited use for high-resolution synthesis without modifications	Kingma et al. (2013) [21]; Chen et al. (2019) [22]; Sohn et al. (2015) [24]
Generative adversarial networks (GANs)	Generator-discriminator adversarial framework with the minimax training objective	Data augmentation (e.g., MRI and CT segmentation), cross-modal synthesis, super-resolution	Generates sharp, realistic images; enhances the robustness of segmentation and classification pipelines	Training instability, mode collapse, requires careful tuning for convergence	Goodfellow et al. (2014) [27]; Bowles et al. (2018) [28]; Hoffman et al. (2018) [29]
Diffusion models	Forward noise addition and learned reverse denoising process	High-resolution image synthesis; generating anatomically faithful and diverse images (e.g., glioma MRI synthesis)	Superior output fidelity and diversity; avoids mode collapse; produces anatomically precise outputs	Computationally intensive; requires hundreds of sampling steps for inference	Ho et al. (2020) [32]; Pinaya et al. (2022) [33]; Song et al. (2020) [34]; Nichol & Dhariwal (2021) [35]

representations across modalities, and impute missing information. This section explores four major application areas in multimodal neurodegenerative research and diagnostics.

4.4.1 Data Augmentation

Medical imaging datasets, especially those focused on neurodegenerative diseases such as AD and PD, are inherently bounded by many factors such as lengthy imaging protocols, huge acquisition costs, patient discomfort, and rigorous privacy regulations [36]. AI models with small sample sizes have lower statistical power, which raises the possibility of overfitting and decreases generalizability for large datasets. Generative models, particularly GANs, have been widely used to create new, realistic, and diverse data samples, which help AI to learn better.

A study [37] utilized GAN-based data augmentation to synthesize abnormal brain MRI images with tumors, demonstrating improved tumor segmentation performance. Their study showed that using synthetic images improved Dice scores from 0.64 to 0.80. GAN-generated medical images can significantly improve.

4.4.2 Cross-modal Synthesis

Cross-modal synthesis helps generate one imaging modality from another to complete a multimodal dataset from other available datasets, addressing the pervasive problem of missing modalities. This approach reduces institutional costs, avoids redundant scanning, and spares patients from invasive or radiologically burdensome procedures.

Chartists et al. [38] presented a multi-input, multi-output convolutional neural network framework for MRI modality synthesis using modality-invariant latent representation (MILR). Multiple input modalities (such as T1, T2, and FLAIR) were encoded into a common latent space by the model, which then decoded them into target modalities. This method beat earlier single-input synthesis techniques on the BRATS and ISLES datasets, showing significant gains in synthesis accuracy and the ability to produce missing contrasts without retraining individual models.

Zhan et al. [39] introduced MGM-GAN, a multi-scale gate merging-based GAN architecture, to synthesize one MRI modality from others. GANs simply add or join (concatenate) the input modalities without making any distinctions. Each modality is given adaptive spatial weights via the multi-scale gate merging technique used by MGM-GAN. The model learns which parts of each MRI input are important and emphasizes them, while ignoring or reducing less useful information. Evaluated on the BRATS2015 dataset for tasks such as FLAIR synthesis from T1 and T2, their model achieved superior performance with structural similarity index measure (SSIM) values exceeding 0.90, indicating high anatomical fidelity suitable for clinical and research applications. MGM-GAN reduces noise from irrelevant signals and intelligently focuses on diagnostically relevant features to produce more accurate and valuable synthetic MRI pictures.

4.4.3 Missing-Data Imputation

Longitudinal neuroimaging and genomic studies frequently suffer from missing data due to patient dropout, contraindications to certain imaging modalities, or equipment malfunctions [40]. To handle nonlinear and complex relationships among various types of data and modalities by earlier traditional statistical imputation methods was always a challenge. By using generative models, particularly VAEs and their multimodal variants, a probabilistic framework to infer missing data based on learned joint distributions across modalities can be predicted.

Suk et al. [19] demonstrated the utility of multimodal deep generative models for finding missing FDG-PET scans based on MRI data in AD patients. Their approach achieved high SSIM values, indicating matched structural and functional consistency with actual PET scans. Such imputation improves statistical power and lessens biases caused by listwise deletion of incomplete cases by allowing the inclusion of otherwise incomplete patient data into analysis pipelines. Crucially, tasks that depend on thorough multimodal inputs, such as disease staging, progression modeling, and cognitive decline prediction, are improved by precise imputation of missing modalities.

4.4.4 Multimodal Data Fusion

Effective integration of heterogeneous data sources such as structural MRI, functional imaging, genomic profiles, and cognitive assessments is critical for understanding complex disease mechanisms, identifying subtypes, and developing personalized interventions. As introduced in Section 2, these data types provide complementary information, and some of the computational strategies for fusing them are discussed below.

Generative models learn shared latent representations that capture intricate cross-modal relationships beyond simple feature concatenation. Huang et al. [41] introduced a multimodality 3D convolutional neural network (CNN) for the diagnosis of AD by using the integration of imaging data of structural MRI and FDG-PET. To enable the capturing of complementary metabolic and structural information, their approach processed each modality separately along distinct 3D CNN branches before fusing features at subsequent layers. By having greater classification accuracy and outperforming single-modality models, the fused multimodal model demonstrated that the fusion of several neuroimaging modalities significantly improves AD diagnostic performance.

In a similar fashion, Venugopalan et al. [42] created a multimodal model using deep learning by combining cognitive and genetic evaluation data with MRI imaging characteristics to predict AD stages. This method employed multimodal fusion layers after using 3D CNNs for MRI and stacked denoising autoencoders for non-imaging modalities. Along with improving classification metrics such as accuracy compared to unimodal models, this fusion enabled identification of important biomarkers such as hippocampal volume and cognitive test performance. These examples illustrate how multimodal fusion techniques introduced in Section 2 focus on model implementation.

These multimodal frameworks show the importance of combining data from multiple sources to enhance early detection, stage classification, and personalized treatment planning for neurodegenerative diseases.

4.5 CHALLENGES IN CLINICAL TRANSLATION

Instead of revolutionary promise, there are various barriers that affect the clinical application of generative AI for multimodal neurodegeneration diagnoses. Some of the clinical translation challenges for generative AI in neurodiagnostics are shown in Table 4.2.

4.5.1 Interpretability and Trust

Generative models, such as GANs and other diffusion architectures, are often categorized as "black boxes," meaning that physicians cannot understand the mechanisms by which outputs are generated. In clinical contexts, lack of transparency not only reduces user trust, but also makes it harder to adopt these models in practice [43]. This trust gap can be resolved by developing self-explanatory architectures that incorporate explainability directly into the model, for example, by using concept bottlenecks, attention mechanisms, and integrated uncertainty estimations [44].

4.5.2 Data Privacy Concerns

Synthetic data can dilate datasets without using real patient data, but if the algorithms unintentionally reproduce identifiable patterns, there is a risk to privacy [45]. Potential threats such as membership inference attacks were emphasized [46, 47] as possible dangers, requiring privacy-preserving training frameworks such as federated learning or differential privacy to be incurred in model training.

4.5.3 Computational Demands

Extensive GPU systems are used for high-capacity generative models, especially those employed in multimodal neuroimaging. Powerful and high-end computational infrastructure and resources

TABLE 4.2
Clinical translation challenges

References	Challenge	Description	Framework
[43, 44]	**Interpretability**	Lack of transparency in model outputs	S-XAI, attribution maps, uncertainty modeling
[45–47]	**Privacy risks**	Memory-based extraction of private data	Membership inference, DP-GANs, EHR-Safe
[48]	**Compute resources**	High GPU requirements limit access	Lightweight model design, compression strategies
[49]	**Evaluation metrics**	No standard clinical benchmarks	Metrics across fidelity, utility, and plausibility
[50]	**Ethical frameworks**	Consent, ownership, and misuse risks	Synthetic data ethics governance

are required to facilitate medical facilities smoothly and efficiently. Practical deployment in such settings requires efficient model design, utilizing methods such as model compression, robust and smart diffusion architectures, neural architecture search (NAS), and quantization to lessen the hardware demands [48].

Additionally, it is hard to detect incomplete data, and various types of diagnostic variability also complicate early detection (discussed in Section 1.2). From a clinical perspective, without standard rules and measurements, validating synthetic medical images becomes complex and challenging. Well-defined standards for defined evaluation procedures and regulatory alignment are required to determine whether synthetic imaging is safe or precise enough for diagnostic decision-making. Existing metrics often focus only on statistical similarity or performance in downstream tasks and frequently overlook important aspects such as anatomical plausibility and clinical realism [49].

4.5.4 Ethical and Legal Challenges

Synthetic patient data generation raises concerns of informed consent, data ownership, and potential misuse. The ownership of the data, whether users must give their approval for synthetic data created from their records, and its potential uses are the main issues. Strict governance systems, interdisciplinary policy cooperation, and transparent stakeholder communication procedures are required to address concerns related to synthetic patient data. Beyond the diagnostic limitations discussed in Section 1.2, ethical and legal frameworks must also define ownership, consent, and the permissible use of synthetic data to ensure safe clinical adoption. Comprehensive and robust governance frameworks are essential to manage these issues [50].

Besides diagnostic issues addressed in Section 1.2, there are mainly translational challenges that require not only technical development but also cross-disciplinary collaboration, regulation-grade testing, and incorporation into healthcare policy infrastructures. Transition of generative AI from promising research to standard clinical use in neurodegenerative diagnosis requires interpretability, privacy, computing efficiency, evaluation standardization, and ethical regulation. Generative AI in healthcare processes can be facilitated by solving these concerns through proper research and collaboration.

4.6 FUTURE DIRECTIONS

As generative AI is an emerging area nowadays and it also promises to demonstrate transformative potential in diagnostic processes, future research work should focus on having a clear vision of the system and improving interpretability, integration of multimodal inputs, model generalizability, validation metrics, data privacy, and moral deployment. The main aim is to develop reliable, secure, transparent, trustworthy, and actionable models, supported by technology advancements such as generative architectures, federated learning frameworks, and foundation models trained on large multimodal datasets. This also entails the construction of robust regulatory frameworks and standardized evaluation methodologies for how generative AI works.

4.6.1 Interpretable Generative Models With Integrated Explainability Modules

One major issue in neurodegenerative diseases is interpretability, a major obstacle to clinical adoption of generative models in the diagnostic process. Doctors need to analyze completely why a certain result occurred before they can trust and validate it. The main goal of future research is to design models that are naturally interpretable generative architectures or the enhancement of current models with integrated explainability modules. In the healthcare sector, it is very important that the professionals are able to trust and validate model behavior. Generative models such as GANs and diffusion models can be enhanced by incorporating techniques such as attention-based visualization, feature attribution maps, and counterfactual generation to offer real-time insights into the decision-making process.

For example, techniques such as generative counterfactual explanations (GCEs) allow users to visualize how minimal changes to inputs such as brain volume reduction in MRI scans influence diagnostic outputs, thereby revealing underlying disease markers [51]. Similarly, a study suggested temporal decomposition network (TDN), which merges multimodal pictures by combining a GAN-based temporal feature matcher and blending salient features spanning time or modalities with a saliency feature model. The approach makes sure that crucial features such as lesions and anatomical borders are identified during the fusion process by specifically recognizing pixel-level saliency regions during diagnosis [52].

4.6.2 Integration of Real-Time Biosensor Data With Imaging/Genomics

Generative AI with medical imaging not only helps in early detection of neurodegenerative onset but also helps personalized risk evaluation by tracking brain health. A study [53] emphasized the value of artificial intelligence and machine learning in the examination of large amounts of genomic data by highlighting advanced techniques for deciphering genetic images. In addition to addressing technical challenges and ethical and privacy concerns in data processing, this investigation also explores the challenges of genetic image analysis in the medical field.

In order to support approval, there is a requirement for establishing standardized evaluation frameworks with rigorous metrics for synthetic data validation, such as Fréchet inception distance (FID) [54], kernel inception distance (KID) [55], and clinical utility metrics [56]. Furthermore, to handle the ethical, legal, and societal implications for responsible deployment, interdisciplinary partnerships between AI researchers, neurologists, radiologists, ethicists, and legislators are essential [57].

Generative artificial intelligence has revolutionized multimodal neurodegenerative disease diagnostics by resolving significant drawbacks of conventional unimodal methods. Diagnostic accuracy, robustness, and generalizability are improved through data augmentation, cross-modal synthesis, missing-data imputation, and efficient multimodal data fusion made possible by VAEs, GANs, and diffusion models (Table 4.3). However, many challenges remain unaddressed in the areas of interpretability, privacy, computing needs, and ethical considerations. To develop generalizable, scalable, and privacy-preserving diagnostic systems, future research should mainly focus on building foundation models, federated learning frameworks, and real-time data integration. In line with precision neurology's ultimate objective, generative AI has the potential to transform early detection, disease subtyping, and tailored treatment for neurodegenerative diseases.

4.7 CONCLUSION

Neurodegenerative issues such as PD, AD, and HD are rapidly growing challenges to public health, particularly seen in the elderly population worldwide. Due to the complexity of neurodegenerative diseases and their diverse clinical symptoms, there is a need to improve diagnostic frameworks for early and efficient detection. This is required to facilitate timely intervention and to prevent any

TABLE 4.3
Potential clinical integration methods for generative models

Clinical Task	Applicable Generative Model	Integration Benefit
Early diagnosis with missing modalities	VAE-based imputation frameworks	Enables diagnosis despite incomplete scans
Dataset expansion for AI training	GAN-based data augmentation	Reduces overfitting; improves model generalizability
Synthesis of unavailable modalities (e.g., PET)	Cross-modal GANs or diffusion models	Avoids invasive or costly scans

serious consequences. Traditional unimodal diagnostic strategies, however, are not well aligned because they only use one imaging modality. More integrated and accurate diagnostic strategies are required because of limitations in sensitivity and specificity.

Multimodal diagnostic frameworks are rising as an effective technique in healthcare through the mixing of numerous data types, consisting of neuroimaging, genomic information, electrophysiological signals, and clinical analysis. By combining various modalities, researchers and clinicians can easily distinguish among sickness subtypes, and gain a deeper understanding of medical techniques. Due to variations in data types, high dimensionality, and often limited sample sizes, there are the main hindrances in integrating multimodal information, which complicate analysis and deployment in the clinical environment.

The discussed barriers can be overcome with generative AI, which incorporates diffusion models, GANs, and VAEs, and has shown revolutionary scope. GANs allow information augmentation, cross-modal synthesis, and sensible photograph technology, whereas VAEs are useful for missing data. Diffusion models are the most recent development that generates anatomically accurate synthetic information. Using generative models with multimodal frameworks makes diagnostic procedures accurate, enables scalability, and improves predictive performance for early-stage detection. Models use real-time sensor data for better monitoring, apply federated learning to protect privacy, and build foundation models trained on large multimodal datasets for reliable diagnosis. Future directions must also prioritize interdisciplinary collaborations by bringing experts from the AI field, neurologists, radiologists, ethicists, and policymakers together to address the ethical, legal, and societal implications of deploying generative AI responsibly in the healthcare sector.

Besides numerous benefits of AI, some challenges have restricted the widespread adoption and use of generative AI in healthcare, such as concerns over interpretability, privacy, security, and ethical concerns. Combining innovation with clinical expertise under a well-structured regulatory framework, these AI-based multimodal diagnostic systems can progress into reliable, accurate, and impactful tools. Through validation and responsible implementation, generative AI can transform neurodegenerative diagnostics, allowing early detection and control, improving patient treatment, and advancing neurology.

REFERENCES

1. Sun, K., Zhang, Y., Liu, J., Yu, L., Zhou, Y., Xie, F., . . . & Shen, D. (2024). Achieving multi-modal brain disease diagnosis performance using only single-modal images through generative AI. *Communications Engineering*, 3(1), 96.
2. Dolci, G., Cruciani, F., Rahaman, M. A., Abrol, A., Chen, J., Fu, Z., . . . & Alzheimer's Disease Neuroimaging Initiative. (2025). An interpretable generative multimodal neuroimaging-genomics framework for decoding Alzheimer's disease. *ArXiv, arXiv-2406.*
3. Roos, R. A. (2010). Huntington's disease: A clinical review. *Orphanet Journal of Rare Diseases*, 5, 1–8.
4. Pathak, N., Vimal, S. K., Tandon, I., Agrawal, L., Hongyi, C., & Bhattacharyya, S. (2021). Neurodegenerative disorders of Alzheimer, Parkinsonism, amyotrophic lateral sclerosis and multiple sclerosis: An early diagnostic approach for precision treatment. *Metabolic Brain Disease*, 1–38.
5. Pan, Y., Liu, M., Lian, C., Xia, Y., & Shen, D. (2019). Disease-image specific generative adversarial network for brain disease diagnosis with incomplete multi-modal neuroimages. In *Medical Image Computing and Computer Assisted Intervention–MICCAI 2019: 22nd International Conference, Shenzhen, China, October 13–17, 2019, Proceedings, Part III 22* (pp. 137–145). Springer International Publishing.
6. Khan, M., Mahajan, R. A., Sivakumar, N. R., Gulhane, M., Rakesh, N., Dey, R., Uddin, M. S., & Basheer, S. (2025). A unified hybrid model for cardiovascular risk prediction: Merging statistical, kernel-based and neural approaches. *Journal of Cellular and Molecular Medicine*. https://doi.org/10.1111/jcmm.70797
7. Huang, W., & Shu, N. (2025). AI-powered integration of multimodal imaging in precision medicine for neuropsychiatric disorders. *Cell Reports Medicine*, 6(5).
8. Akdemir, Ü. Ö., Bora, H. A. T., & Atay, L. Ö. (2021). Dopamine transporter spect imaging in Parkinson's disease and Parkinsonian disorders. *Turkish Journal of Medical Sciences*, 51(2), 400–410.
9. Major Depressive Disorder Working Group of the Psychiatric GWAS Consortium. (2012). A mega-analysis of genome-wide association studies for major depressive disorder. *Molecular Psychiatry*, 18(4), 10–103.

10. Romo-Gutiérrez, D., Yescas, P., López-López, M., & Boll, M. C. (2015). Genetic factors associated with dementia in Parkinson's disease (PD). *Gaceta Médica de México*, 151(1), 110–118.
11. Khan, M., Mahajan, R. A., Katukam, R., Dey, R., Rana, A., & William, P. (2025). Smart insights: Multimodal deep learning techniques for accurate disease identification. In *2025 International Conference on Quantum Photonics, Artificial Intelligence, and Networking (QPAIN)* (pp. 1–5). Rangpur, Bangladesh. https://doi.org/10.1109/QPAIN66474.2025.11171928
12. Li, L., Chen, R., Zhang, H., Li, J., Huang, H., Weng, J., . . . & Xie, J. (2024). The epigenetic modification of DNA methylation in neurological diseases. *Frontiers in Immunology*, 15, 1401962.
13. Nakamura, A., Cuesta, P., Fernández, A., Arahata, Y., Iwata, K., Kuratsubo, I., . . . & Kato, T. (2018). Electromagnetic signatures of the preclinical and prodromal stages of Alzheimer's disease. *Brain*, 141(5), 1470–1485.
14. Lizio, R., Vecchio, F., Frisoni, G. B., Ferri, R., Rodriguez, G., & Babiloni, C. (2011). Electroencephalographic rhythms in Alzheimer's disease. *International Journal of Alzheimer's Disease*, 2011(1), 927573.
15. Pal, M., Dey, R., Mahajan, R. A., Khan, M., Syed, A. A., & Karimullah, S. (2025). Edge intelligence: Unique machine learning strategies for enhancing real-time IoT data processing. In *2025 International Conference on Quantum Photonics, Artificial Intelligence, and Networking (QPAIN)* (pp. 1–5). Rangpur, Bangladesh. https://doi.org/10.1109/QPAIN66474.2025.11171994.
16. Mahendran, R., Chua, J., Feng, L., Kua, E. H., & Preedy, V. R. (2015). The mini-mental state examination and other neuropsychological assessment tools for detecting cognitive decline. In *Diet and Nutrition in Dementia and Cognitive Decline* (pp. 1159–1174). Academic Press.
17. Mahajan, R. A., Dey, R., Khan, M., Su'ud, M. M., Alam, M. M., & Jadhav, P. (2025). Enhancing personalization in IoT-based health monitoring via generative AI and transfer learning. *Egyptian Informatics Journal*, 32, 100788. ISSN 1110-8665. https://doi.org/10.1016/j.eij.2025.100788. https://www.sciencedirect.com/science/article/pii/S1110866525001811
18. Wu, L. T., Gersing, K. R., Swartz, M. S., Burchett, B., Li, T. K., & Blazer, D. G. (2013). Using electronic health records data to assess comorbidities of substance use and psychiatric diagnoses and treatment settings among adults. *Journal of Psychiatric Research*, 47(4), 555–563.
19. Suk, H. I., Lee, S. W., Shen, D., & Alzheimer's Disease Neuroimaging Initiative. (2014). Hierarchical feature representation and multimodal fusion with deep learning for AD/MCI diagnosis. *NeuroImage*, 101, 569-582. https://doi.org/10.1016/j.neuroimage.2014.06.077
20. Mosconi, L., Perani, D., Sorbi, S., Herholz, K., Nacmias, B., Holthoff, V., . . . & Pupi, A. (2004). MCI conversion to dementia and the APOE genotype: A prediction study with FDG-PET. *Neurology*, 63(12), 2332–2340.
21. Kingma, D. P., & Welling, M. (2014). Auto-encoding variational Bayes. *arXiv Preprint arXiv:1312.6114*. https://doi.org/10.48550/arXiv.1312.6114
22. Chen, K., Liu, M., & Zhang, D. (2020). Multimodal variational autoencoder for semi-supervised learning in Alzheimer's disease diagnosis. *IEEE Journal of Biomedical and Health Informatics*, 24(9), 2617–2626. https://doi.org/10.1109/JBHI.2020.2988042
23. Das, P., Paul, S., Ghosh, J., PalBhowmik, S., Neogi, B., & Ganguly, A. (2017). An approach towards the representation of sign language by electromyography signals with fuzzy implementation. *International Journal of Sensors, Wireless Communications and Control*, 7(1), 26–32. https://doi.org/10.2174/22103279 07666170222093839
24. Sohn, K., Lee, H., & Yan, X. (2015). Learning structured output representation using deep conditional generative models. In *Advances in Neural Information Processing Systems* (Vol. 28). https://proceedings.neurips.cc/paper/2015/file/b5b5c3b6d8523b7f19a10e2eeb62f9b8-Paper.pdf
25. Wang, X., Zhao, K., Zhou, R., Leow, A., Osorio, R., Zhang, Y., & He, L. (2022). Normative modeling via conditional variational autoencoder and adversarial learning to identify brain dysfunction in Alzheimer's disease. *arXiv Preprint arXiv:2211.08982*. https://arxiv.org/abs/2211.08982
26. Paul, S., Ojha, S. K., Barui, S., Ghosh, S., Ghosh, M., Neogi, B., & Ganguly, A. (2018). Technical advancement on various bio-signal controlled arm: A review. *Journal of Mechanics of Continua and Mathematical Sciences*, 13(2), 16–30. https://doi.org/10.26782/jmcms.2018.06.00007
27. Goodfellow, I., Pouget-Abadie, J., Mirza, M., Xu, B., Warde-Farley, D., Ozair, S., Courville, A., & Bengio, Y. (2014). Generative adversarial nets. In *Advances in Neural Information Processing Systems* (Vol. 27). https://proceedings.neurips.cc/paper/2014/file/5ca3e9b122f61f8f06494c97b1afccf3-Paper.pdf
28. Bowles, C., Chen, L., Guerrero, R., Bentley, P., Gunn, R., Hammers, A., Dickie, D. A., Hernández, M. V., Wardlaw, J., & Rueckert, D. (2018). GAN augmentation: Augmenting training data using generative adversarial networks. *arXiv Preprint arXiv:1810.10863*. https://arxiv.org/abs/1810.10863

29. Hoffman, J., Tzeng, E., Park, T., Zhu, J. Y., Isola, P., Saenko, K., Efros, A. A., & Darrell, T. (2018). CyCADA: Cycle-consistent adversarial domain adaptation. In *Proceedings of the 35th International Conference on Machine Learning* (pp. 1989–1998). https://doi.org/10.48550/arXiv.1711.03213
30. Arjovsky, M., Chintala, S., & Bottou, L. (2017). Wasserstein GAN. *arXiv Preprint arXiv:1701.07875*. https://arxiv.org/abs/1701.07875
31. Karras, T., Aila, T., Laine, S., & Lehtinen, J. (2018). Progressive growing of GANs for improved quality, stability, and variation. In *International Conference on Learning Representations*. https://openreview.net/forum?id=Hk99zCeAb
32. Ho, J., Jain, A., & Abbeel, P. (2020). Denoising diffusion probabilistic models. In *Advances in Neural Information Processing Systems* (Vol. 33, pp. 6840–6851). https://proceedings.neurips.cc/paper/2020/file/4c5bcfec8584af0d967f1ab10179ca4b-Paper.pdf
33. Pinaya, W. H. L., Tudosiu, P. D., Dafflon, J., Da Costa, P. F., Fernandez, V., Nachev, P., & Cardoso, M. J. (2022). Brain imaging generation with latent diffusion models. In *MICCAI Workshop on Deep Generative Models* (pp. 117–126). https://doi.org/10.1007/978-3-031-22360-3_12
34. Song, J., Meng, C., & Ermon, S. (2020). Denoising diffusion implicit models. *arXiv Preprint arXiv:2010.02502*. https://arxiv.org/abs/2010.02502
35. Nichol, A., & Dhariwal, P. (2021). Improved denoising diffusion probabilistic models. In *Proceedings of the 38th International Conference on Machine Learning* (Vol. 139, pp. 8162–8171). https://proceedings.mlr.press/v139/nichol21a.html
36. Bron, E. E., Smits, M., Niessen, W. J., & Klein, S. (2015). Feature selection based on the SVM weight vector for classification of dementia. *Medical Image Analysis*, 18(2), 249–258. https://doi.org/10.1016/j.media.2013.12.003
37. Shin, H. C., Tenenholtz, N. A., Rogers, J. K., Schwarz, C. G., Senjem, M. L., Gunter, J. L., Andriole, K. P., & Michalski, M. (2018). Medical image synthesis for data augmentation and anonymization using generative adversarial networks. *Lecture Notes in Computer Science*, 11037, 1–11. https://doi.org/10.1007/978-3-030-00934-2_1
38. Chartsias, A., Joyce, T., Giuffrida, M. V., & Tsaftaris, S. A. (2017). Multimodal MR synthesis via modality-invariant latent representation. *IEEE Transactions on Medical Imaging*. https://doi.org/10.1109/TMI.2017.2764326
39. Zhan, B., Li, D., Wu, X., Zhou, J., & Wang, Y. (2021). Multi-modal MRI image synthesis via GAN with multi-scale gate mergence. *IEEE Journal of Biomedical and Health Informatics*. https://doi.org/10.1109/JBHI.2021.3088866
40. Dwyer, D. B., Falkai, P., & Koutsouleris, N. (2018). Machine learning approaches for clinical psychology and psychiatry. *Annual Review of Clinical Psychology*, 14, 91–118. https://doi.org/10.1146/annurev-clinpsy-032816-045037
41. Huang, Y., Xu, J., Zhou, Y., Tong, T., Song, T., & Zhang, J. (2020). Diagnosis of Alzheimer's disease via multi-modality 3D convolutional neural network. *Frontiers in Neuroscience*, 14, 509. https://doi.org/10.3389/fnins.2020.00509
42. Venugopalan, J., Tong, L., Hassanzadeh, H. R., & Wang, M. D. (2021). Multimodal deep learning models for early detection of Alzheimer's disease stage. *Scientific Reports*, 11(1), 3254. https://doi.org/10.1038/s41598-020-74399-
43. Muhammad, D., & Bendechache, M. (2024). Unveiling the black box: A systematic review of Explainable Artificial Intelligence in medical image analysis. *Computational and Structural Biotechnology Journal*, 24, 542–560.
44. Hou, J., Liu, S., Bie, Y., Wang, H., Tan, A., Luo, L., & Chen, H. (2024). Self-explainable ai for medical image analysis: A survey and new outlooks. *arXiv preprint arXiv:2410.02331*.
45. Bawal, M. K., Lin, C. C., Liu, C. L., & Chen, K. T. (2019). Synthesizing electronic health records using improved generative adversarial networks. *Journal of the American Medical Informatics Association*, 26(3), 228–241.
46. Wang, Y., Wang, Q., Zhao, L., & Wang, C. (2023). Differential privacy in deep learning: Privacy and beyond. *Future Generation Computer Systems*, 148, 408–424.
47. Zhang, Z., Yan, C., & Malin, B. A. (2022). Membership inference attacks against synthetic health data. *Journal of Biomedical Informatics*, 125, 103977.
48. Qian, Z., Callender, T., Cebere, B., Janes, S. M., Navani, N., & van der Schaar, M. (2024). Synthetic data for privacy-preserving clinical risk prediction. *Scientific Reports*, 14(1), 25676.
49. Adams, T., Birkenbihl, C., Otte, K., Ng, H. G., Rieling, J. A., Näher, A. F., . . . & Fröhlich, H. (2025). On the fidelity versus privacy and utility trade-off of synthetic patient data. *iScience*, 28(5).

50. Kumar, A. (2024). The role of synthetic data in advancing AI models: Opportunities, challenges, and ethical considerations. *Journal of Artificial Intelligence General Science (JAIGS)*, 5(1), 443–459. ISSN: 3006–4023
51. Hellemans, S., Algaba, A., Verboven, S., & Ginis, V. (2025). Flexible counterfactual explanations with generative models. *arXiv preprint arXiv:2502.17613*.
52. Albekairi, M., Mohamed, M. V. O., Kaaniche, K., Abbas, G., Alanazi, M. D., Alanazi, T. M., & Emara, A. (2025). Multimodal medical image fusion combining saliency perception and generative adversarial network. *Scientific Reports*, 15(1), 10609.
53. Gautam, M., Choudhary, A., & Agrawal, D. (2025). Machine learning–based calibration of commercial continuous glucose monitoring sensor in nonserum solutions: An in vitro validation study. *Indian Journal of Neurotrauma*, 22(4). https://doi.org/10.1055/s-0045-1806943
54. Borji, A. (2022). Pros and cons of GAN evaluation measures. *Computer Vision and Image Understanding*, 215, 103329.
55. Bińkowski, M., Sutherland, D. J., Arbel, M., & Gretton, A. (2018). Demystifying MMD GANs. In *International Conference on Learning Representations (ICLR).* https://openreview.net/forum?id=r1lUOzWCW
56. Mongan, J., Moy, L., & Kahn, C. E. Jr. (2020). Checklist for artificial intelligence in medical imaging (CLAIM): A guide for authors and reviewers. *Radiology: Artificial Intelligence*, 2(2), e200029.
57. Topol, E. J. (2019). High-performance medicine: The convergence of human and artificial intelligence. *Nature Medicine*, 25(1), 44–56.

5 Introduction to Neurodegenerative Diseases

Abraham Olufemi Asuku

5.1 INTRODUCTION

Neurodegenerative disorders (NDDs) are in the list of the commonest causes of mortality in the world because of their significant influence on the aging population. This mainly resulted from an overall decline in neuronal functions, and this causes brain damage. Some of the most common NDDs, which are now known, are discussed in this chapter: Alzheimer disease (AD), amyotrophic lateral sclerosis (ALS), multiple sclerosis (MS), Parkinson disease (PD), and Huntington disease (HD) [1]. Khan et al. (2025) introduced a hybrid statistical-kernel-neural model for cardiovascular risk, paralleling the multifaceted predictive challenges posed by progressive neurodegenerative pathologies [2]. Different NDDs can influence similar cellular and molecular processes; however, each has an etiological difference and occurs in different areas of the brain. NDDs are characterized by the gradual death of neurons in the central nervous system (CNS) or peripheral nervous system (PNS), and NDDs adversely affect millions of people in the world. The death of the neurons that are terminally differentiated and unable to effectively rejuvenate themselves and the degradation of the structure and functionality of neural networks lead to the interference with the basic circuitry of communication, which in turn influences memory, cognition, behavior, and/or the senses and/or motor activity.

As the population grows old, NDDs are becoming more prevalent in the world and are becoming an important issue in healthcare among the population. AD is the commonest form of dementia, and it affects around 50 million people worldwide. While HD and ALS affect lesser, but still important, percentages of the population, PD affects about 10 million individuals [3]. Khan et al. (2025) developed multimodal deep learning for disease identification, offering foundational insights into integrating diverse biomarkers relevant to early neurodegenerative detection [4]. The disorders have posed a massive financial dilemma in the society in regard to their emotional and social cost on patients, relatives, and carers in addition to the medical expenses that are needed to treat such disorders. As NDDs aggravate, a person is likely to become incapable of carrying out their usual jobs and become even more dependent on others [5]. The pharmacology of NDDs is not successful even with the intensive research and is focused on the symptom management, without the delay of the disorder process. The currently used therapies of ALS, HD, PD, and AD are not always sufficient and only slightly improve symptom management [6]. The absence of efficient disease-modifying therapy is still one of the biggest problems in the field of neurodegenerative medicine. The necessity to produce efficient drugs with therapeutic significance is immense despite the growing attempts to determine proper therapeutics to NDDs. Nevertheless, there is still a considerable number of problems to be solved. The mechanisms through which the cellular and molecular systems end up being tuned to the progression of various diseases remain unclear to date. Moreover, there are challenges with early and accurate diagnosis, as well as personalized disease monitoring. Asaku et al. [7] explain how Multimodal artificial intelligence (AI) possesses the ability to surmount the challenges. This is a chapter in the book *Multimodal Generative AI for Neurodegenerative Disease Management* with a focus on diverse types of neurodegenerative diseases, their pathogenesis, common risk factors, biomarkers, and interventions. Mahajan et al. (2025) harnessed generative AI and

DOI: 10.1201/9781003667360-5

transfer learning for personalized IoT health monitoring, underscoring adaptive AI's role in managing chronic neurodegenerative conditions [8].

5.2 COMMON MECHANISMS ACROSS NDDS

The clinical manifestation of NDDs depends on the increase in the malfunction of specific groups of neurons. Accumulation of the misfolded protein either in the cell or outside the cell is linked to neuronal death and is a feature of different NDDs. They involve key fundamental mechanisms, including the free radical generation and oxidative stress (OS), bioenergetic dysfunction, mitochondrial dysfunction, neuroinflammation, and cellular protein dynamics caused by the loss of the ubiquitin-proteasome-autophagy system, and the loss of axonal and Golgi apparatus transport in neurons (Figure 5.1). The processes associated with them lead to apoptosis in the long run. Although the classification of NDDs is based on the components of primary protein deposits or commonly known genetic pathways, the available research observed an intra-individual variation and also a crossover and overlap of different symptoms.

5.3 MAJOR TYPES OF NDDS

5.3.1 Alzheimer's Disease

AD is the commonest type of dementia and NDD [9]. The first symptoms are not always obvious until 20 years after the appearance of this degenerative disease. Among its symptoms, there are loss of memory, aphasia, and the inability to learn new things, abnormal sleeping patterns, and severe memory difficulties. The first characteristic of AD is the decline in cognitive abilities, which is the most common feature of the disorder. Brain atrophy is brought on by the loss of neurons and disintegration of the synapses in the brain area that is responsible for the processing of learning, emotions, spatial orientation, and formation of memory, which happens to be the hippocampus.

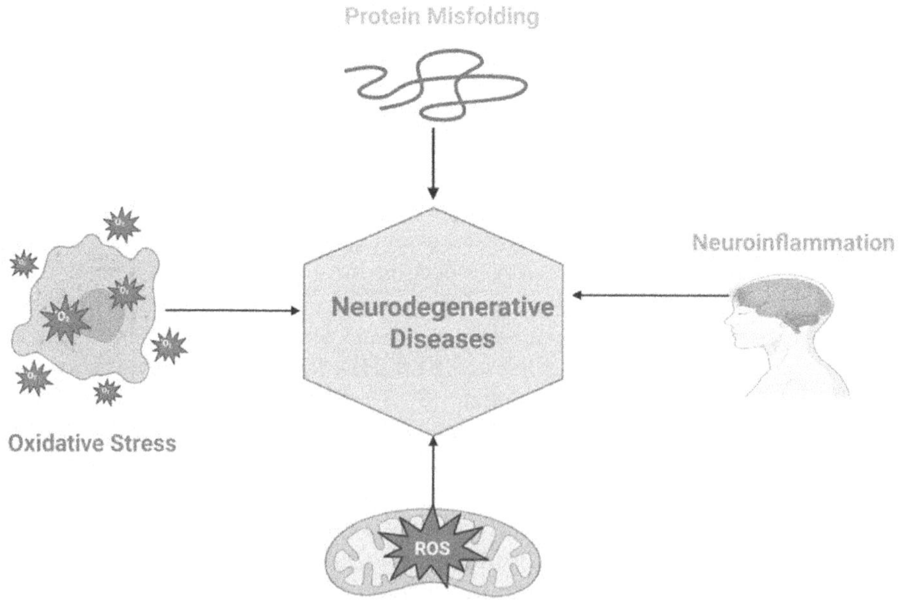

FIGURE 5.1 Common mechanisms across NDs (oxidative stress, protein misfolding, neuroinflammation, mitochondrial dysfunction)

The characteristics of AD pathogenesis are intracellular accumulation and aberrant deposition of neurofibrillary tangles (NFTs) of tau due to aggregated amyloid-beta (Aβ). These processes can be attributed to the key factor, which is OS. It may be brought on by an increase in the free radicals or a decrease in antioxidant defense molecules [10]. The AD brain can also undergo lipid peroxidation, which can destroy the synaptic functions that control memory and learning, including long-term potentiation [11]. It has been noted that the presence of the accumulation of Aβ that aggravates the dysfunction of the mitochondria can help to improve OS even in the individuals who are at the very lower levels of the disorder. Dey et al. (2025) engineered ML frameworks fusing technical indicators for financial forecasting, demonstrating how multi-signal analysis principles apply to tracking neurodegenerative progression trajectories [12].

According to research findings, the Aβ-induced OS imbalance results in a great number of by-products (such as protein and oxidation of DNA/RNA), in contrast to the low quantities of antioxidants seen in persons with AD. Furthermore, it has been noted that issues with antioxidant defense mechanisms result in elevated OS, which in turn promotes Aβ formation and deposition [13]. Paul et al. (2018) reviewed bio-signal advancements in prosthetic control, highlighting physiological signal integration strategies applicable to neurodegenerative disease monitoring [14].

5.3.2 Parkinson's Disease

PD comes second in terms of the prevalence of NDDs in the global community, as reported by [13]. This is a degenerative motor disorder that damages the nigrostriatal dopaminergic system. The neurons that take part in motor and nonmotor activities are, however, involved in PD. Resting tremor, bradykinesia, unstable posture, limb stiffness, imbalance, and lack of coordination are in the list of motor symptoms. The examples of such nonmotor symptoms include sleep problems, hyposmia, and constipation and might even be a precondition of the identified movement problems. PD has two histological features: an accumulation of misfolded and insoluble α-synuclein capable of forming Lewy bodies and the formation of aberrant neurites, which encourage neurodegeneration [15].

PD is among the first two disorders in persons who are more than 60 years old when compared to other NDDs. According to statistics, PD is uncommon in people under 50; in people over 65, it affects about 2% of the population, while in those over 80, it affects more than twice as many (i.e., 5%) of the population [16]. Diagnosis of PD is evidenced by the loss of dopaminergic neurons in the substantia nigra. The overproduction of reactive oxygen species (ROS) has been associated with this dopaminergic neuron degeneration.

Both inflammatory processes and mitochondrial dysfunction may be contributing factors to the large production of ROS. Neuroglia, which are non-neuronal cells but nonetheless provide protection, and the mitochondria in neurons are the brain's major sites where ROS is produced. Aging, high amounts of iron and calcium, neuroinflammation, mitochondrial dysfunction, and dopamine degradation are the key causes that lead to the intensification of the ROS production in this neurodegenerative disease. Moreover, the excessive exposure to neurotoxins and pesticides in the air could also aggravate the synthesis of ROS.

5.3.3 Huntington's Disease

Huntington's disease is among the genetic NDDs, and it causes muscle and other aligned psychological symptoms and mental degradation. The disease can start in people as young as 35 years of age. Most of the proteins assume certain three-dimensional structures so as to execute their functions. Protein chains can, however, assume varying states of conformation. In addition, the original structure of the protein chain tends to be stable, at best, only partially under physiological conditions. It implies that there can be some folding errors that cause incorrect folds. Probably, these unstable proteins may create aggregates, and this is an indicator of cellular toxicity. Additionally, the report had it that in HD, PD, and AD, it is thought that these protein pileups may be caused by mutations that were inherited [17]. Huntington's disease is classified as a disorder of abnormal folding of protein in which the HTT protein, a huntingtin-producing protein generated by the HTT gene, interacts with other proteins to disrupt regular biological processes. One of the primary issues is that ROS-induced protein misfolding results in the development of bodies that cluster alongside neuronal axons and dendrites, obstructing neurotransmitter transmission. The cognitive and motor problems that people with HD experience may be attributed to the disturbances that are caused by the accumulation that is produced by mutant HTT (mHTT). Das et al. (2017) proposed fuzzy-based EMG signal decoding for sign language, exemplifying bio-signal pattern recognition techniques extendable to neural degradation analysis [18].

To be more precise, the abnormally curved mHTT monomer is subjected to proteolysis that results in the formation of fragments with a given 17-amino-acid sequence (N17), which triggers the aggregation process. Although the cytoplasm also contains the aggregates, N17 is a nuclear import signal that induces their assembly in the nucleus. The alternative way through which nuclear aggregates result in unsuitable transcriptional dysregulation is via the sequestration of significant elements that govern antioxidant genes. Besides, N17 codes for a specific area that controls phosphorylation and positioning of HTT due to the action of a ROS sensor [8]. Neuronal degeneration is, however, primarily observed in the brain, particularly the cortex and the striatum, though aberrant HTT appears in all body parts [19].

5.3.4 Amyotrophic Lateral Sclerosis

Amyotrophic lateral sclerosis (ALS) is a progressive NDD in the CNS that develops in children and adults. Another neurodegenerative disease that is associated with motor neurons is ALS, and its prognosis is disastrous. Most ALS patients have a 2–5-year survival rate after symptoms start, with the disease progressing more quickly in older adults. But only 5% of patients live for 20 years or more [20]. ALS is a wretched disorder causing muscle rigidity, spasticity, and twitching due to the progressive loss of lower and upper neurons. At the complete degeneration stage, the last phase of neuromuscular dysconnectivity during the disease is atrophy of the muscles. Moreover, cognitive impairment is seen in half of the patients [21]. The piling up of the abnormally folded proteins, which are altered in a number of pathological conditions, including mislocalization and phosphorylation, is another characteristic of ALS that is shared by other NDDs. This accumulation also takes place in the neurons responsible for motor activity. Furthermore, neuroinflammation, which manifests as microgliosis and astrogliosis, coexists with neurodegeneration [22].

5.3.5 Multiple Sclerosis

An autoimmune response may cause MS; it is a nondestructive, demyelinating, chronic, and inflammatory disease. Most of the adults who are affected are between the ages of 20 and 40 years, with women being the apparent ones. Despite the pathophysiology of MS not being well known, it has been proposed that activated lymphocytes B and T bypass the blood-brain barrier (BBB) and enter the CNS, leading to neuroinflammatory processes and CNS damage, particularly the myelin sheath [23].

Close relationship exists between the development of diseases and environmental factors. The most common are the deficiency of vitamin D and the infection of the Epstein-Barr virus (EBV) [24]. Individuals who contracted EBV in childhood are 15 times and those in adolescence are 30 times predisposed to MS. Though the course of MS varies in each one of them, there are some general characteristics of the disease one may observe. MS attacks are only mild and asymptomatic at the onset and are later on regarded as MS events. The disease can progress further in two ways, namely relapses and periods of remission or slow progression of the symptoms. In addition to chronic pain and speech problems, the majority of patients have standard manifestations of muscle weakness, extremity numbness, and blurred vision [25].

5.4 NDDS DEVELOPMENTAL STAGES

The development of NDDs is shown in stages, as demonstrated in Figure 5.2.

5.4.1 Retrogenesis

The causes of NDDs are the impairment of the cholinergic system of the basal forebrain and the continuation of the impairment to the hippocampus and entorhinal cortex (EC). The main observable sign of NDDs is neglect or a few problems with present-moment memory. This is the natural progression of such changes in the brain that usually starts one or two decades before. The impaired memory and loss of knowing family members and other side effects are possible. The development of the disorder causes it to start negatively influencing the cerebral cortex and, therefore, further worsens the balance and thinking. The pathological symptoms of the NDDs in the sick individuals are related to the stage of retrogenesis that presupposes the shift of the mood and character, exaggerated feeling of being in discomfort, and lack of recognizable locations, choice, and other important objects. The next decline of the selected section of the brain results in the nature of conflict problems of thoughts, language, and physical neurons [26].

5.4.2 Intellectual Dysfunction

This occurs because the neurodegeneration has been caused by death-causing proteins. It is linked to the increase in the number of tangles and neurofibrillary plaques in the substantia nigra, EC, and caudate. As the NDDs advance, these proteins adopt pathogenic roles that lead to the degeneration of neurons and intellectual retardation. The affected area in regard to AD is the EC. The communication between the hippocampus and the EC has been documented to play a very remarkable function in the maintenance of memories and in a situation where either of the two regions fails to perform its function, there is disruption of the communication between the two, which would lead to confusion and loss of memory. It is argued that NDDs spread across the neuronal system and that the EC is the basic center that is becoming less and less effective in combating them [27].

5.4.3 Stride Abnormality

An unsettling effect in intellectual capacities is demonstrated by the ability to predict an unsettling influence in step action. This incredible plasticity of neural circuits that develop later in the

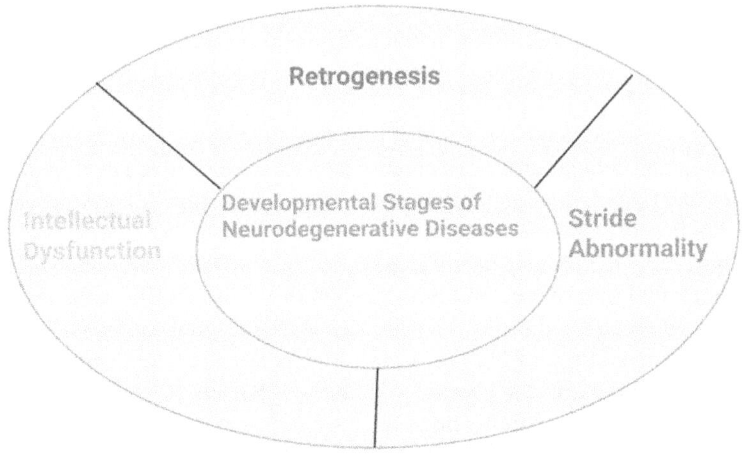

FIGURE 5.2 The developmental stages of NDDs

formative life cycle to increasingly become pathetic in the clutches of neurodegeneration is termed the "Last-in-first-out" connection. The notion is applicable in the early detection of any form of NDD and offers that adequate movement style demands a role of the neurological undertaking associated with both tangible and motor neurons and a role of the cortical tasks such as functions of judgment, planning, and spatial mindfulness [28].

5.5 RISK FACTORS AND CAUSES

5.5.1 Aging

An unsettling effect in intellectual capacities is demonstrated by the ability to predict an unsettling influence in step action. Numerous age-related health conditions develop in people as they get older, negatively affecting their quality of life and lifespan, as well as their capacity to carry out everyday tasks [11]. According to a molecular research, aberrant deposits of aggregated proteins such as α-synuclein, Aβ, and hyperphosphorylated tau (p-tau) have been found in the brain tissue of elderly people. It is still unknown, nevertheless, if the cognitive decline rate is commensurate with the levels of these deposits [30].

It is common knowledge that oxidative damage of the DNA, deletions in the mitochondria, and point mutations in the mitochondria lead to a cascade of NDDs that compound with age. The risk factor of AD is mostly aging, and nearly half of the population over 85 years old is developing the disease. Besides, women are more susceptible to being impacted by AD compared to men because the levels of estrogens decline during menopause, and life expectancy is longer [31].

5.5.2 Gene and Environmental as a Risk Factor

The recent association studies conducted on genome-wide have illuminated the contribution of immunological molecules to a number of NDDs. A number of genes that raise the vulnerability to NDDs, such as C9ORF72 in ALS, TREM2 and CD33 in AD, and SCNA, PRKN, HLA, and LRRK2 in PD, have been reported to be involved in the functions of the immune system, which include microglial activation, phagocytosis, expression of major histocompatibility complex (MHC) class II, complement activation, and formation of blood cells [32]. Since not all carriers of the said genetic risk factors result in disease, it is assumed that it is the variables of the environment that cause inflammatory processes that could lead to the pathogenesis of the NDDs. Bacterial infections have been the focus of more attention as a potential cause of neurodegenerative pathology due to their capacity to penetrate into the CNS, activate astrocytes and microglia, and facilitate the T-cells and peripheral macrophage infiltration. Such immune responses are likely to have devastating effects on the brain in a bid to kill the invading disease, yet they are there to save it. Infectious pathogens can contribute to the pathophysiology of NDDs due to the occurrence of an inflammatory response.

Even though it is epidemiologically proven that infectious agents are involved in non-communicable diseases, the molecular and cellular processes under which they are involved are typically poorly understood. On the other hand, the individuals having NDDs are more susceptible to infection by a neurotropic agent, possibly because of a malfunctioning immune system and/or a breakup of the BBB [33].

It is assumed that heavy metals are more dangerous to human well-being than all other pollutants due to their environmental persistence and bio-accessibility. With the increase in industrialization, heavy metal levels have been on the rise. NDDs are associated with long-term exposure to transition metals. The pathophysiology of NDDs is largely dependent on conformational alterations in proteins linked to the disorders, including tau, Aβ, and α-synuclein.

The mechanism of Aβ-induced neurodegeneration depends critically on the conformational alterations and oligomerization of Aβ. Amyloid fibrils are insoluble aggregates made up of Aβ oligomers. The rate of oligomerization can be modified to enhance its influence on the AD pathophysiology. Minimal amounts of Zn^{2+}, Al^{2+}, Mn^{2+}, Cu^{2+}, and Fe^{2+} induce protein conformational change; for example, they can induce Aβ oligomerization. Many studies prove that lead, copper, cadmium, arsenic, and mercury are other neurotoxins that have the potential to damage the functioning of the brain, result in cognitive impairment, and predispose to PD and AD [34].

The purpose of pesticides is to eliminate, stop, or manage harmful pests. The use of pesticides in the world is estimated at about 3,000,000 tons annually. Pesticide-induced inflammasomes have been associated with the inflammatory predisposition of cancer, reproductive dysfunction, and CNS, and PNS abnormalities also add that rotenone crosses the BBB to induce the NLRP3 inflammasome easily. Exposure to chlorpyrifos could also cause the PD risk through changes in the expression of the proteins, which have a crucial role in preserving the integrity of the BBB such as TRPC4, ZO1, and claudin5 [35].

5.6 DIAGNOSIS AND BIOMARKERS

For several years, there has been a steady improvement in the identification of cerebrospinal fluid (CSF) neurodegenerative biomarkers. Some biomarkers are already established and used in clinical practice, such as part of diagnostic criteria; others are still being worked on to standardize analytical techniques; and yet others are anticipated to have their significance validated in subsequent research. The accumulation and aggregation of altered proteins, which are unique to particular types of diseases, are linked to neurodegenerative processes. Phosphorylated tau protein (p-tau), Aβ, α-synuclein, and prion protein (PrPSc) are specific biomarkers that represent a type of aggregating pathogenic protein [19].

The most studied non-specific CSF biomarkers include the biomarkers that indicate axonal damage and degeneration, for example, neurofilament light chains (NFL) and t-tau protein. They are pointers to glial stimulation; they participate in the intracellular protein synthesis or degradation and elimination of the abnormally misfolded proteins, and they are the indicators of the synaptic, lysosomal, and mitochondrial dysfunction among other non-specific indicators.

There are also other scientific fields that examine the functional molecules (neurotransmitter and protein metabolites) that can be involved in the process of neurodegeneration, including proteomics and metabolomics [8]. The final goal is to develop a profile, which is a collection of biological measures that is distinctive to a specific clinical unit or a cluster of disorders possessing comparable properties. The cerebrospinal fluid is believed to be the perfect biomarker because it is directly connected to the extracellular space of brain tissue. CSF is supposed to demonstrate all the metabolic changes that occur in the brain [34].

The neuroimaging method offers an in-depth knowledge of the anatomical and functional alterations of the brain, which are attributed to the NDDs of different types. These forms of imaging, beginning with the detection of white matter hyperintensities (WMH) to the exactness of the amyloid and alpha-synuclein imaging, provide an important perspective in the comprehension of the complex neurobiology of NDDs.

Radiology and neuroimaging methods such as magnetic resonance imaging (MRI) and computed tomography (CT) scans are another of the earlier fields of medical computerization that are frequently employed in the diagnosis of NDDs. Since machine learning is completely evidence-based and can objectively analyze the problem, it is also useful in the objective recognition of medical images. It is also usually quicker, more precise, and more accurate than the trained people. More so, the computer-based diagnosis systems might be improved and run under monitored learning technologies to enhance the analysis of the data from neuroimaging and assist in detecting issues in the images that are not visible to the radiologists. Other studies have applied convolutional neural networks as a means to be more specific and predictive, be it the diagnosis of AD or the analysis of cognitive aging using MRI and positron emission tomography (PET) images, with or without other clinical outputs [26].

Choi et al. 2018 [36] show how different techniques and support vector machines (SVMs) have been used to analyze MRI data and to enhance the diagnosis of the disease, and Czigler et al. 2018 [27] show how biomarkers are applied and they are commonly used with functional and structural MRI and cognitive evaluation data. SVM has also been used in assessing MRI data in the context of Parkinsonism stroke and studies of cognitive dysfunction. The machine learning processes can be able to increase the diagnostic capability of the CT even though MRI is more resolved to image [34].

One way to study brain activity is through neuroimaging, and machine learning-driven data analyses can also be helpful for other brain activity monitoring techniques, such as electroencephalography (EEG), which has been employed to differentiate AD patients from healthy persons or persons suffering from other dementia types or to identify functional alterations in dopaminergic neurons to diagnose PD.

5.7 TREATMENT AND MANAGEMENT OF NDDS

5.7.1 Current Pharmacological Approaches

Since there are no known treatments for NDDs, the main goals of pharmaceutical management are symptom relief, disease progression slowing, and quality of life enhancement.

5.7.1.1 Approved Therapies for AD

The cornerstone of symptomatic treatment for AD is acetylcholinesterase inhibitors. These medications function by preventing the breakdown of acetylcholine, which is necessary for cognitive and memory function, by the enzyme acetylcholinesterase. These inhibitors lessen the cognitive decline by raising the concentrations of acetylcholine in the brain. The most administered acetylcholinesterase inhibitor is donepezil, which has been found to be temporary but with some modest benefits toward improving the cognitive functioning and slowing down the disease process. Moreover, it has similar advantages to rivastigmine and galantamine. Memantine is an inhibitor of the N-methyl-D-aspartate (NMDA) receptor that aids in the regulation of the activity of glutamate. It is believed that the process of cell death and neuron injury is associated with the overproduction of glutamate signaling, especially in the case of AD. The overstimulation of the neurons caused by the NMDA receptors that are a part of excitotoxicity is blocked by memantine. Memantine has demonstrated to be of low positive effects in AD on cognitive and functional symptoms. It can be combined with acetylcholine-ste-inhibitors or used as a single therapy [31].

5.7.1.2 Approved Therapy for PD

The basis of PD treatment is the dopaminergic drugs. The most efficient and popular one is levodopa. Due to the loss of the dopaminergic neurons, the problem is compensated for by converting L-DOPA into dopamine in the brain. This reduces motor symptoms that include bradykinesia, tremors, and stiffness, among others. However, the use of long-term levodopa is accompanied by dyskinesias and motor variations. Carbidopa is usually used together with levodopa in order to increase its effectiveness, and such side effects as nausea are minimized. In the early phases of PD, dopamine agonists such as pramipexole and ropinirole can be independently utilized, but in the late phases, the application of levodopa together with these medications can be used. These medications are imitators of the effects of dopamine since they directly stimulate the dopamine receptors. In comparison with levodopa, dopamine agonists can be less motor disturbing, though they can develop such side effects as obsessive behaviors and drowsiness. Selegiline and rasagiline are examples of monoamine oxidase-B inhibitors, which inhibit the breakdown of dopamine (Table 5.1). This increases the amount of dopamine in the brain. The PD motor symptoms are managed using MAO-B inhibitors, particularly at early disease stages, and they have also been shown to have neuroprotective attributes. The MAO-B inhibitors are typically used in combination with levodopa to improve their effectiveness and possibly lengthen the period of taking increased doses of this drug.

5.7.1.3 Approved Therapy for HD

Tetrabenazine is an inhibitor of vesicular monoamine transporter 2 (Table 5.1) that is applied to HD-related chorea or involuntary jerk motions. Tetrabenazine inhibits the dopaminergic activity of the brain by reducing the release of dopamine by the presynaptic cells, which reduces the motor symptoms. Patients with a history of mood issues or depression need to be careful with the use of these medications, as they not only result in drowsiness, Parkinsonism, and depression but also have other undesirable side effects.

Although antisense oligonucleotides (ASOs) are still not approved to be used commercially, experimental research has shown that they have potential therapeutic value in modifying HD. Because the mutant huntingtin gene causes harmful proteins to aggregate in HD and suppresses the mutant protein expression, ASOs are made to attach to it. ASOs have the potential to be an effective approach because they prevent the pathogenic action of the mutant protein rather than partially alleviate its symptoms.

5.7.1.4 Approved Therapy for ALS

The first medication licensed for ALS, kilomole, had a slight impact on survival. It is believed to reduce excitotoxicity and neuronal injury by blocking postsynaptic glutamate receptors and limiting glutamate release. However, riluzole does not considerably enhance motor function and only marginally slows the disease progression. Darvon is a potent antioxidant that scavenges ROS, and it contributes to the modulation of ALS pathogenesis. The use of dracone also has the potential of preventing the destruction of motor neurons, as well as minimizing the progress of the disease through the reduction of OS. It neither fully prevents the disease nor has it shown some slight improvements in the functional assessments, including the ALS functional rating scale.

5.7.2 Emerging Pharmacological Approaches for NDDs

The existing pharmacological interventions of the NDDs only alleviate the symptoms; they do not deal with the causative factors or mitigate the course of the disorder. Therapies involving the use of stem cells, genetic materials, and deep brain stimulation are among the emerging techniques that are promising for potency and modification of disease (Table 5.1).

5.7.3 Non-pharmacological Interventions for NDDs

NDDs respond to non-pharmacological interventions positively, especially in individuals with pharmacological issues. The preventive therapies involve regular exercise, which helps in grip strength and pain relief; manual therapy and thermal modality, which lessen the symptoms and improve the functions of the joint; and cognitive behavioral therapy, which helps patients deal with fatigue and prolonged pain. Besides the physical analgesic and relaxing effect, yoga (as well as magnetotherapy) may be used in the treatment of nonmotor issues, including melancholy, anxiety, cognitive dysfunction, and constipation. Other methods featured in the research are low-level laser therapy and treating the patient in mineral baths, known as balneotherapy [27, 29]. Cognitive therapies, which are noninvasive, are effective and can be offered to patients with NDDs. These treatments comprise cognitive stimulation, which enhances social contact to advance the thinking and memory abilities and cognitive training, which involves performing activities to enhance cognitive operations such as attention, memory, and problem-solving capacities. Physical activity and exercise are also suggested as non-pharmacological therapies that are successful in AD management and contribute to cognitive improvement. Age-related diseases develop as a result of little exercise and physical activity. The role of non-pharmacological treatment of cognitive issues in PD and AD is on the increase, and physical therapy and cognitive training are in the limelight. These techniques are beneficial to the brain through mechanisms such as improved glucoregulation and cardiovascular well-being, neurotransmitter production, and nerve growth factor up-regulation.

A novel approach to dementia therapy, brain-activating rehabilitation implements preventive measures in a welcoming and enjoyable setting. In order to increase motivation, close communication gaps, delegate social assignments, and sustain error-free engagements, measures are administered to the patients to increase autonomy and offer encouragement. By identifying patients' residual talents and preventing brain function from being misused, these treatments seek to improve cognitive function, motivation, and self-worth. Patients with NDDs also experience changes in their sleep patterns as a result of exercise, including a decrease in rapid eye movement (REM) sleep, a delay in REM periods, an improvement in overall sleep duration, and an increase in slow-wave sleep. Long-term exercise increases slow-wave sleep, sleep duration, and sleep efficiency. NDDs, including AD and PD, frequently cause sleep disturbances, which manifest as symptoms including trouble starting or sustaining sleep, a late initiation of REM sleep, and decreased proportions of REM sleep and slow-wave sleep.

5.8 CONCLUSION AND FUTURE DIRECTIONS

We often consider NDDs to be independent clinical entities with unique pathophysiology and symptoms that target diverse brain regions. Certain players and patterns, however, recur frequently when examined at the genetic, cellular, and molecular levels. These include, but are not limited to, early dysfunction of vessels, the accumulation and dissemination of abnormally folded proteins, the selective susceptibility of specific neurons, and the immune response activation. The primary goal of current pharmaceutical treatments is to control a disease's symptoms instead of stopping its progression, underscoring the critical necessity for more potent medicines. Although there are still many obstacles to overcome in terms of safety, long-term efficacy, and medication delivery, developments in gene therapy, monoclonal antibodies, and neuroprotective drugs present promising avenues for disease modification. Multi-target combination techniques that address many disease pathways, such as protein-specific treatments and enhanced drug delivery systems, are anticipated to be essential to the success of therapeutic approaches in the future. Optimizing clinical methods and speeding up drug discovery will be greatly aided by the integration of AI and developing technologies. Even though present treatments are limited, there is optimism for future discoveries that could delay or even reverse the progression of NDDs, thanks to continuous research and innovation.

TABLE 5.1
Treatment and management of NDDs

Pharmacotherapy Approaches	Non-pharmacotherapy Approaches	Emerging Techniques
AD	Physical exercise	Stem cell therapy
Acetylcholinesterase inhibitors: Donepezil, galantamine, and rivastigmine.	Cognitive stimulation therapy	Gene therapy
NMDA antagonists: Memantine	Bright light therapy	Deep brain stimulation
PD	Sleep management	
Levodopa, carbidopa, ropinirole, pramipexole.		
MAO-B inhibitors: Rasagiline, selegiline		
HD		
Tetrabenazine, ASO		
ALS		
Riluzole, edaravone		

Key: NMDA: N-methyl-D-aspartate, AD: Alzheimer's disease, HD: Huntington's disease, PD: Parkinson's disease, MAO-B: Monoamine oxidase-B, ALS: Amyotrophic lateral sclerosis.

REFERENCES

1. Ajagun E.J., Asuku, A.O., Ayinla M.T., Abdulsalam, T.A., Ajibare, A.J., Olajide, T.S., Hamza, Y.O., & Ganiyu, K.O. (2024). Pharmacotherapy of Parkinson's Disease and Their Limitations. In: *Zebrafish as a Model for Parkinson's Disease*. Taylor and Francis, CRC. https://doi.org/10.1201/9781003402893-17
2. Khan, M., Mahajan, R.A., Sivakumar, N.R., Gulhane, M., Rakesh, N., Dey, R., Uddin, M.S., & Basheer, S. (2025). A Unified Hybrid Model for Cardiovascular Risk Prediction: Merging Statistical, Kernel-Based and Neural Approaches. *Journal of Cellular and Molecular Medicine*. https://doi.org/10.1111/jcmm.70797
3. Ajibare, A.J., Akintoye, O.O., Oriowo, O.A., Asuku, A.O., Oriyomi, I.A., Adedara, J.F., Ayoola, A.M., & Adejumo, O.M. (2025). Dietary Virgin Coconut Exerted a Neuroprotective Effect via Upregulation of Nuclear Erythroid Factor and Downregulation of Nuclear Factor KB Expression in Acrylamide-Induced Neurotoxicity: Role of BDNF and AchE Pathways. *Tropical Journal of Natural Product Research*, 9(3): 1263–1269
4. Khan, M., Mahajan, R.A., Katukam, R., Dey, R., Rana, A., & William, P. (2025). Smart Insights: Multimodal Deep Learning Techniques for Accurate Disease Identification. In: *2025 International Conference on Quantum Photonics, Artificial Intelligence, and Networking (QPAIN)*. Rangpur, Bangladesh, pp. 1–5. https://doi.org/10.1109/QPAIN66474.2025.11171928
5. Akintoye, O.O., Ajibare, A.J., Fabunmi, O.A., Asuku, A.O., & Tajudeen R.A. (2021). Effect of Honey on Oxidative Stress in Brain Tissue of Sleep Deprived Rats. *Nigerian Journal of Basic and Applied Science*, 29(1): 83–89. http://doi.org/10.4314/njbas.v29i1.10
6. Alzheimer's Association. (2020). *Alzheimer's Facts and Figures Report*. Alzheimer's Association, Singapore, p. 1.
7. Asuku, A.O., Adeyemo, M.B., Adeyemo, R.O., Agoro, S.A., Odugbesan, O.A., & Ayoola, S.A. (2022). Applications of Stem Cell Therapy in Neurodegenerative Diseases. *European Journal of Biotechnology and Bioscience*, 10(2): 17–24, 2321–9122.
8. Mahajan, R.A., Dey, R., Khan, M., Su'ud, M.M., Alam, M.M., & Jadhav, P. (2025). Enhancing Personalization in IoT-Based Health Monitoring Via Generative AI and Transfer Learning. *Egyptian Informatics Journal*, 32: 100788, ISSN 1110-8665. https://doi.org/10.1016/j.eij.2025.100788. https://www.sciencedirect.com/science/article/pii/S1110866525001811
9. Asuku, A.O., Ayinla, M.T., Olajide, T.S., Oyerinde, T.O., Yusuf, J.A., Bayo-Olugbami, A.A., & Fajemidagba, G.A. (2024a). Coffee and Parkinson's Disease. In: *Progress in Brain Research*. Neuroscience of Coffee, Elsevier, p. 289. https://doi.org/10.1016/bs.pbr.2024.06.001
10. Asuku, A.O., Ayinla M.T., Olajide, T.S., Ajagun E.J., Ganiyu, K.O., Hamza, Y.O., Ajibare, A.J., & Abdulsalam, T.A. (2024b). Diagnosis and Biomarkers of Parkinson's Disease. In: *Zebrafish as a Model for Parkinson's Disease*. Taylor and Francis, CRC. https://doi.org/10.1201/9781003402893-15
11. Asuku, A.O., Ayinla, M.T., Ajibare, A.J., Adeyemo, M.B., & Adeyemo, R.O. (2024c). Heavy Metals and Emerging Contaminants in Food and Food Products Associated with Neurotoxicity. In: *Emerging Contaminants in Food and Food Products*. CRC Press, Taylor and Francis Group, Boca Raton, FL, pp. 236–250. https://doi.org/10.1201/9781003438236-17
12. Dey, R., Kassim, S., Khan, M., Mahajan, R.A., & William, P. (2025). Smart Trading in NIFTY-50: ML with MA, RSI & Volume Analysis. In: *2025 International Conference on Quantum Photonics, Artificial Intelligence, and Networking (QPAIN)*. Rangpur, Bangladesh, pp. 1–5. https://doi.org/10.1109/QPAIN66474.2025.11171705.
13. Asuku, A.O., Ogungbangbe, G.O., & Olajide, T.S. (2025). Effect of Happiness and Positive Emotions on Dementia. In: *Neuroscience of Feelings*. Progress in Brain Research. Elsevier. https://doi.org/10.1016/bs.pbr.2025.03.001
14. Paul, S., Ojha, S.K., Barui, S., Ghosh, S., Ghosh, M., Neogi, B., & Ganguly, A. (2018). Technical Advancement on Various Bio-Signal Controlled Arm: A Review. *Journal of Mechanics of Continua and Mathematical Sciences*, 13(2), 16–30. https://doi.org/10.26782/jmcms.2018.06.00007
15. Ayinla, M.T., Yakub, Z.M., Asuku, A.O., & Muzzamil, S.S. (2024). Ameliorative Effect of Aqueous Leaf Extract of Aqueous Leaf Extract of *Cola acuminata* on Mercury Chloride-induced Neurotoxicity In Male Wistar Rat. *Bulletin of Faculty of Pharmacy, Cairo University*, 62, 11–18. https://doi.org/10.54634/2090-9101.1049.
16. Ayinla, M.T., & Asuku, A.O. (2025). The Neurotoxic Effects of Lead Acetate and the Abrogating Actions of 6-Gingerol-Rich Extract of Ginger Via Modulation of Antioxidant Defence System, Pro-Inflammatory Markers, and Apoptotic Cascade. *Naunyn- Schmiedeberg's Arch Pharmacology*. https://doi.org/10.1007/s00210-025-03873-x
17. Badu-Mensah, A., Guo, X., & Hickman, J.J. (2021). ALS Skeletal Muscle: Victim or Culprit. *Neuroscience Chronicles*, 2(2). https://doi.org/10.46439/neuroscience.2.012.

18. Das, P., Paul, S., Ghosh, J., PalBhowmik, S., Neogi, B., & Ganguly, A. (2017). An Approach Towards the Representation of Sign Language by Electromyography Signals with Fuzzy Implementation. *International Journal of Sensors, Wireless Communications and Control*, 7(1), 26–32. https://doi.org/10.2174/22103279 07666170222093839
19. Barcelon, E.A., Mukaino, T., Yokoyama, J., Uehara, T., Ogata, K., Kira, J.I., & Tobimatsu, S. (2019). Grand Total EEG Score Can Differentiate Parkinson's Disease from Parkinson-Related Disorders. *Frontiers in Neurology*, 10, 398. https://doi.org/10.3389/fneur.2019.00398
20. Brooks, B.R., Heiman-Patterson, T., & Wiedau-Pazos, M. (2022). Edaravone Efficacy in Amyotrophic Lateral Sclerosis with Reduced Forced Vital Capacity: Post-Hoc Analysis of Study 19 (MCI186 19) [clinical trial NCT01492686]. *Public Library of Science*, 17(6), e0258614–e0258614. https://doi.org/10.1371/journal.pone.0258614
21. Brown, R.H., & Al-Chalabi, A. (2017). Amyotrophic Lateral Sclerosis. *The New England Journal of Medicine*, 377, 162–172.
22. Burberry, A., Suzuki, N., Wang, J.-Y., Moccia, R., Mordes, D.A., & Stewart, M.H. (2016). Loss-of-Function Mutations in the C9ORF72 Mouse Ortholog Cause Fatal Autoimmune Disease. *Science Translational Medicine*, 8, 347ra93. https://doi.org/10.1126/scitranslmed.aaf6038
23. Buschert, V., Bokde, A.L.W., & Hampel, H. (2010). Cognitive Intervention in Alzheimer disease. *Nature Reviews Neurology*, 6(9), 508–517.
24. Butterfield, D.A., & Halliwell, B. (2019). Oxidative Stress, Dysfunctional Glucose Metabolism and Alzheimer Disease. *Nature Reviews Neurology*, 20, 148–160.
25. Butink, M.H.P., Webers, C., Verstappen, S.M.M., Falzon, L., Betteridge, N., & Wiek, (2023). Non-Pharmacological Interventions to Promote Work Participation in People with Rheumatic and Musculoskeletal Diseases: A Systematic Review and Meta-Analysis from the EULAR Taskforce on Healthy and Sustainable Work Participation. *RMD Open*, 9(1), e002903.
26. Chopade, P., Chopade, N., & Zhao, Z. (2022). Alzheimer's and Parkinson's Disease Therapies in the Clinic. *Wiley*, 8(1). https://doi.org/10.1002/btm2.10367.
27. Czigler, B., Csikós, D., Hidasi, Z., Anna Gaál, Z., Csibri, E., Kiss, E., Salacz, P., & Molnár, M. (2008). Quantitative EEG in Early Alzheimer's Disease Patients—Power Spectrum and Complexity Features. *International Journal of Psychophysiology*, 68(1), 75–80. https://doi.org/10.1016/j.ijpsycho.2007.11.002.
28. Duchesne, S., Rolland, Y., & Vérin, M. (2009). Automated Computer Differential Classification in Parkinsonian Syndromes Via Pattern Analysis on MRI. *Academic Radiology*, 16, 61–70.
29. Cova, I., & Priori, A. (2018). Diagnostic Biomarkers for Parkinson's Disease at a Glance: Where Are We? *Journal of Neural Transmission*, 125, 1417–1432.
30. Blennow, K., & Zetterberg, H. (2018). The Past and Future of Alzheimer's Disease Fluid Biomarkers. *Journal of Alzheimer's Disease*, 62, 1125–1140.
31. Garber, C., Soung, A., Vollmer, L.L., Kanmogne, M., Last, A., & Brown, J. (2019). T Cells Promote Microglia-Mediated Synaptic Elimination and Cognitive Dysfunction During Recovery from Neuropathogenic Flaviviruses. *Nature Neuroscience*, 22, 1276–1288. https://doi.org/10.1038/s41593-019-0427-y.
32. Genç, M.E., & Özdamar, E.N. (2021). *Dopamine: The Amazing Molecule*. IntechOpen, https://doi.org/10.5772/intechopen.95444.
33. Guzman, A.C.V. de, Razzak, M.A., & Cho, J.H. (2022). Curcumin-Loaded Human Serum Albumin Nanoparticles Prevent Parkinson's Disease-like Symptoms in C. Elegans. *Multidisciplinary Digital Publishing Institute*, 12(5), 758–758. https://doi.org/10.3390/nano12050758.
34. Hartl, F.U. (2017). Protein Misfolding Diseases. *Annual Review of Biochemistry*, 86, 21–26.
35. Bono-Yagüe, J., Gómez-Escribano, A.P., Millán, J.M., & Vázquez-Manrique, R.P. (2020). Reactive Species in Huntington Disease: Are They Really the Radicals You Want to Catch? *Antioxidants*, 9, 577.
36. Choi, H., Kang, H., & Lee, D.S. (2018). Predicting Aging of Brain Metabolic Topographyusing Variational Autoencoder. *Frontiers in Aging Neuroscience*, 10, 212.

6 Personalized Treatment Planning Through AI Insights

V. Balammal, M. Malathi, V. Bharathi, M. Divya Bairavi, Preetha Ramiah, and Priyatharshini Rajaram

6.1 INTRODUCTION TO PERSONALIZED TREATMENT PLANNING

Personalized treatment planning represents a recent development in healthcare whereby medical treatment is customized to the demands of each patient. Unlike the traditional way of administering treatment via the use of a cookie-cutter methodology, this way of doing a treatment plan considers a host of individualized elements, including a person's DNA, medical history, way of living, surroundings, and the characteristics of a given medical condition [1]. Pal et al. (2025) proposed edge-intelligent machine learning (ML) strategies for real-time IoT data processing, supporting timely artificial intelligence (AI) insights that can adapt treatment plans as patients' clinical states evolve [2]. Healthcare providers, with the aid of AI and other technologies employed in the analysis of massive amounts of data, are able to prepare customized treatment plans that are more precise and effective. Subsequently, this advanced medicine results in a more satisfied patient, fewer complications, and improved overall health. Areas such as oncology, chronic disease management, and treatment of rare genetic conditions are other sectors that significantly benefit from personalized medicine [3]. Personalized treatment planning represents an important advancement in providing focused, patient-centered healthcare [4]. Zhou et al. (2021) by book. *Machine Learning*. Springer Nature Singapore [5] and Selvaraju et al. (2017). *Grad-CAM: explains Visual Explanations* [5, 6]. Khan et al. (2025) showed that integrating statistical, kernel-based, and neural models enables more precise individualized cardiovascular risk estimation, illustrating how hybrid AI architectures can support personalized treatment planning [7].

Through personalized treatment plans by telemedicine shown by Krittanawong et al. (2018) [8]: AI is transforming healthcare shown by Huang et al. (2021) [9]. AImakes it possible to put together individualized treatment plans, which in turn we are able to analyze huge amounts of medical info, including genetic development, health history, lifestyle factors, and diagnostic data. AI also improves results of treatment, by which it reduces side effects, changes medication doses, and is able to tell how a patient will do with certain therapies. Also, it gives docs access to useful info, which in turn improves their decision-making. Thus, by bringing AI into healthcare, there is an improvement in quality and a drop in costs. Khan et al. (2025) designed a multimodal deep learning framework that fuses imaging, EHR, and genomic data for accurate disease identification, demonstrating how rich patient representations drive AI-guided therapeutic decisions [10].

- A key aspect of our work is the integration of AI into personalized medicine to enable predictive and individualized treatment planning. To improve on that, we have incorporated explainable AI (XAI) techniques, such as Grad-CAM, which also presents visualizations of model decision processes in image classification and segmentation. Real-time interaction is also used in clinical and telehealth settings. Deep learning-based segmentation and classification, which are supplemented with XAI, are an improvement in user-centered design for liver cancer in the area of reliability and personalized diagnostics. In the future,

DOI: 10.1201/9781003667360-6

we will be putting more into diversity of the dataset, also including multimodal data, and development of longitudinal models for tumor growth. By combining clinical knowledge with intelligent decision-making support with AI, it promotes a transition toward more effective, patient-focused, and outcome-oriented cancer care. Mahajan et al. (2025) applied generative AI and transfer learning to personalize IoT-based health monitoring, directly motivating AI-driven tailoring of interventions to patient-specific profiles [11]. Kalinin et al. (2018) demonstrated the application of deep learning in pharmacogenomics, spanning gene regulation to patient stratification [12].

- Li et al. (2023) reviewed artificial intelligence approaches for personalized sequential decision-making in pharmaceutical research [13, 14]. According to the International Pharma Review (2024), artificial intelligence is transforming personalized medicine through advances in pharmacogenomics and drug therapy [15]. Abdelhalim et al. (2022) discussed the integration of artificial intelligence, clinical genomics, and pharmacogenomics in precision medicine [16, 17]. Mishra et al. (2025) systematically reviewed the role of generative artificial intelligence in personalized medicine [18, 19].
- Mahajan et al. (2025) proposed a generative AI and transfer learning framework to enhance personalization in IoT-based health monitoring [11]. Ghebrehiwet et al. (2024) highlighted the transformative role of generative AI in personalized medicine [20, 21].
- Rezayi et al. (2022) evaluated the effectiveness of artificial intelligence for personalized medicine in neoplasms [12, 24]. Rehan (2024) explored AI-driven personalized cancer treatment supported by cloud-based data integration [25, 26].
- Das et al. (2017) presented a fuzzy logic-based electromyography signal representation for sign language recognition [27]. Krittanawong et al. (2018) discussed the application of artificial intelligence in the prevention and management of heart failure [28].
- Huang et al. (2021) reviewed machine learning applications in genomics and pharmacogenomics [29]. Paul et al. (2018) reviewed advances in bio-signal-controlled robotic arm technologies [30]. Darwich et al. (2017) examined the challenges and future roadmap for model-informed precision dosing in clinical practice [31].

6.1.1 The Following Are the Primary Domains Where AI Brings Genuine Innovation

6.1.1.1 Data Integration and Synthesis

The most impressive capability is the AI's ability to produce a detailed, personalized digital profile of a patient, having integrated and synthesized information from disparate sources.

Genomics and other molecular data are integrated with clinical information to improve disease characterization and support personalized treatment planning.

6.1.1.2 Multi-Omics Data

Profiling DNA, RNA, and proteins to understand the biological peculiarities of diseases.

6.1.1.3 Clinical Data

Consolidation of EHRs, lab tests, and images (MRI, CT, X-ray).

6.1.1.4 Lifestyle and Environmental Data

Integration of the real-world data from wearables, patient-reported outcomes (PROs), and the environment (lifestyle, contact with HBV/Aflatoxin as illustrated in the figure).

6.1.1.5 Population-Scale Treatment Response

Comparing the patient profile with millions of anonymous patients and outcomes to determine the most effective treatment options.

6.1.2 Predictive and Prognostic Capabilities

6.1.2.1 AI Predictive Innovation: Prediction of Drug Efficacy

AI does not merely diagnose but forecasts which drug (at which dose and least probable to have side effects) works best for that patient, and with a high degree of confidence.

6.1.2.2 Prognosis Prediction

AI does not just assess the patient but employs algorithms to forecast, years ahead, the individual patient's disease progression, whether they will have a relapse, or develop complications, enabling proactive and not merely reactive care.

6.1.2.3 Lifestyle Factors

Development of liver cancer is a disease that changeable lifestyle factors can cause. The disease risk is significantly increased by chronic alcohol consumption and obesity. Alcoholic liver disease can eventually lead to liver cirrhosis, a precursor to hepatocellular carcinoma (HCC).

6.2 OVERVIEW OF PERSONALIZED TREATMENT PLANNING

Personalized treatment planning, as shown in Figures 6.1–6.3, in healthcare is an approach that designs medical care particularly for each individual's unique characteristics and attributes. This domain takes into account the following common features:

- Genetics
- Medical history
- Lifestyle and habits
- Environment
- Response to past treatments

By observing the detailed personal information, doctors and healthcare systems help in selecting the most suitable treatment with reduced side effects.

6.2.1 Feature Overview

- Personalized patient approach: It focuses on the needs, risks, and goals of each patient.
- Data-driven: Uses technologies such as AI, genomics, and data analytics to guide decisions.

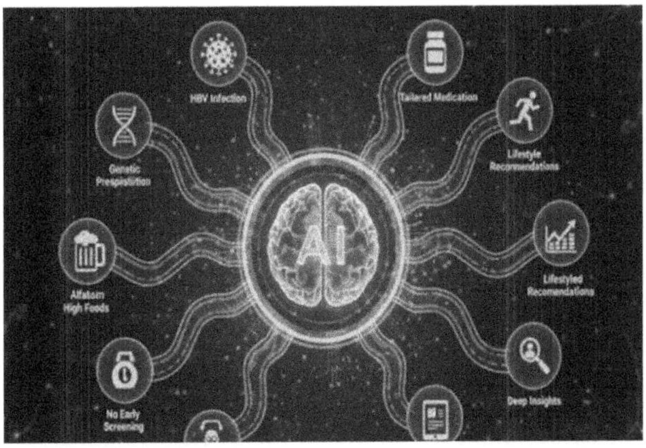

FIGURE 6.1 Personalized treatment planning through AI

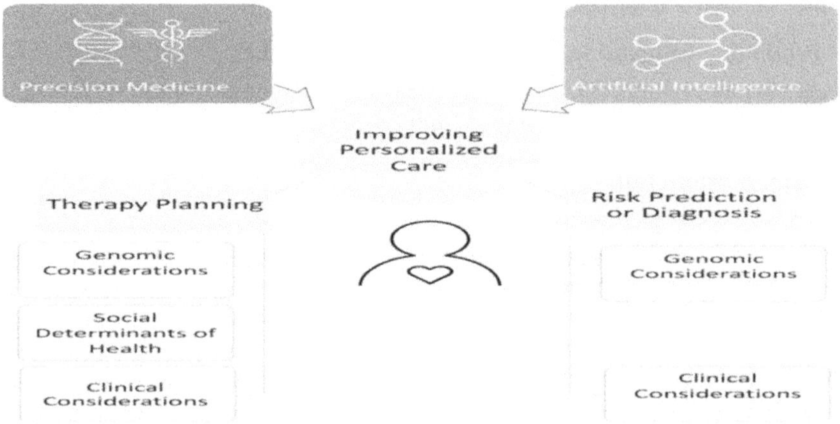

FIGURE 6.2 Improving personalized healthcare

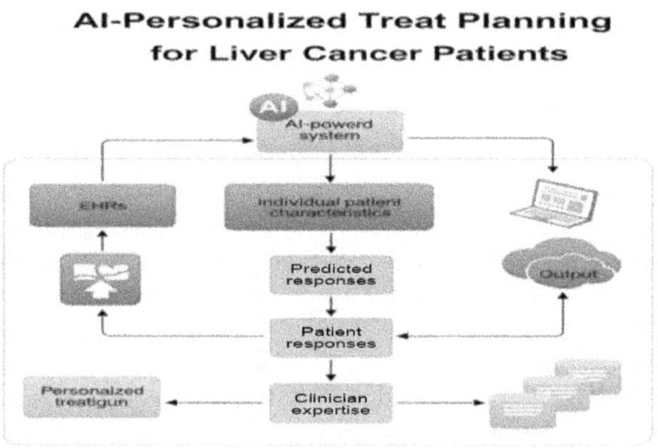

FIGURE 6.3 AI-personalized treatment planning for liver cancer patients

- Predictive: It can predict how a patient might respond to a specific therapy before it is given.
- Dynamic: Treatment plans can change over time based on ongoing monitoring and feedback.

Here are some examples:

> In cancer care, we may develop personalized plans that include genetic testing for the best chemotherapeutic agents. Diabetes management is used to create diet and exercise plans based on daily blood sugar levels.

Goal:

> Upgrade health outcomes, reduce the estimation in treatments, minimize side effects, and improve the overall quality of patient care.

6.2.2 Disease Diagnosis

In the medical field today, we see that early and accurate disease diagnosis is still an issue. It is hard at times to determine which medical conditions a patient has and what their symptoms mean. Our observations indicate that AI's data processing powers can help clinicians save time and improve accuracy. AI can play a large role in what physicians use to diagnose patients by way of its analysis of large sets of EHRs with machine learning. Also, AI may be used to help doctors in decision-making in emergency rooms (Ers) and other critical settings by looking at large numbers of similar cases and what treatments proved to be successful. Deep learning algorithms may play a role in shortening wait times and in the priority of which cases are attended. The AI-enhanced decision support systems which provide real-time electronic health records (EHRs).

The healthcare industry's digitization efforts are helped along by the industry's EHRs. Given that approximately 80% of doctors' offices utilize EHRs, many are predicting the usage of AI to analyze the information and present it in the form of new insights to doctors. The recent use of AI incorporates natural language processing (NLP). A single EHR report may report a variation of medical synonyms. For instance, one report may use the term heart attack, and another, myocardial infarction. Both are correct, but the writers may pick one term as a preference over the other. NLP works to reduce this variation to create uniformity, which is necessary for larger volumes of data to be examined. Das et al. (2017) implemented fuzzy logic–based EMG interpretation for sign language, exemplifying how AI-driven pattern recognition can be used to design highly personalized human–machine interaction and support systems [27].

Another type of NLP is that which identifies what is redundant in a doctor's notes due to repetition and which in turn reports only relevant info to improve ease of reading. In EHR improvement, that which patient is at risk for a disease is determined via AI algorithms which look at that person's past info and also their family history. For instance, we have a very general algorithm which is a rule-based system that works in a flow chart-like fashion which humans are familiar with. This system takes large amounts of data and from it develops a set of rules which in turn connect specific observations to a diagnosis. The algorithm is able to take in a new patient's data and to which it applies the rules in order to predict the chance that patient has of developing a given condition or disease. Because algorithms are capable of assessing a patient's data of record along with a set of clinical data, they can identify and highlight an issue for physician review and optimize their workflow. A study done by the research institute noted that predictive modeling of EHR data was able to attain 70–72% accuracy in forecasting individualized treatment response. Such accuracy and prediction for treatment become essential due to the prediction that the online health record data will double in volume every five years. Physicians do not have the bandwidth required to review the data, and the information can be used by AI to assist physicians in patient care.

6.2.3 Medication Conflicts

Algorithms for identification of drug interactions in medical literature were put together as a result of progress in NLP. Patients who are on multiple drugs at the same time run the risk of a drug interaction, which in turn increases with the number of drugs present. We developed machine learning algorithms to mine info on which drugs interact and what their effects are from the medical literature in order to address the issue of which known or suspected drug interactions are out there. We compared our method with existing approaches for identifying drug–drug interactions from biomedical literature. The increase of telemedicine, the treatment of patients remotely, has shown the rise of possible AI applications. AI can assist in caring for patients remotely by monitoring their information through sensors and wearable devices that may allow for constant monitoring of a patient and the ability to notice changes that may be less distinguishable by humans. The information can be compared to other data that have already been collected using AI algorithms that alert physicians if there are any issues to be aware of.

6.2.4 Healthcare Workload Optimization

Since October 2023, you have been providing your thoughts regarding AI in healthcare. AI enhances efficiency and effectiveness in healthcare delivery by streamlining workload and accelerating care coordination, since it is capable of prioritizing the needs of the patient, automating the administrative functions, and facilitating unimpeded communication in the medical workforce. Healthcare allows professionals to concentrate on patient care. Coronary artery disease (CAD) risk assessments and diagnoses have seen promising results, with AI algorithms demonstrating their use in initial patient prioritization. Some AI algorithms have been designed to predict patient mortality, clinical event outcomes, and adverse medication reactions (treatment of acute coronary syndrome). Portable technologies have also been used to remotely monitor and stream patients' cardiac data, which makes it possible to detect events outside of clinical settings and is theoretically limitless in the amount and variety of data AI models can analyze. In 2019, research found that AI was capable of predicting heart attacks with 90% accuracy. Paul et al. (2018) reviewed advances in bio-signal–controlled prosthetic arms, highlighting how decoding individual physiological patterns can inform customized assistive and rehabilitative strategies [30].

6.2.5 Overview of Skin Problems

Being able to take pictures of the skin using tools such as X-rays, along with the ability to analyze pictures using deep learning, suggests that dermatology may heavily rely on deep learning. It is certainly possible for dermatology to make significant improvements in the field and be able to use machine learning for image classification in order to enhance image-derived diagnoses. Studies have demonstrated that deep learning-based convolutional neural networks can classify skin lesion images with an accuracy of up to 94%, supporting the use of AI-assisted image analysis for skin cancer diagnosis. One issue with this work has yet to engage with the inequities of skin pigmentation and the lack of care afforded to individuals with skin color different from white.

6.2.6 Domain of Gastroenterology

In many fields of gastroenterology, AI is a great asset. Prompt detection and fast identification of abnormal tissue is a must for endoscopic practices such as colonoscopy and esophagogastroduodenoscopy (EGD). By using AI in these endoscopic practices, we see that diseases may be identified faster, determined in terms of severity, and this allows us to visualize what was unseen before. For early-stage stomach cancer, AI-based detection systems have performed in early trial work as well as very skilled endoscopists. Also, in the care of patients with chronic colitis, AI may help doctors in the detection of the micro-scale activity of the disease in patients and in the prediction of when a flare-up will present. AI uses large datasets to aid in the prediction of illness, in prevention, in diagnosis, and also in the monitoring of patients. In obstetrics, AI is utilized in magnetic resonance imaging, ultrasound, and fetal cardiotocography. AI contributes to the resolution of a variety of pregnancy-related diagnostic issues.

6.2.7 Communicable Diseases

Communicable diseases have put forth promising results in the field of infectious disease medicine, which we have seen in the lab and in clinical settings. In the case of COVID-19, we have reported that the use of AI has gone from early detection, tracking the virus's movement, to learning how it functions, yet at the time of the actual pandemic, its large-scale application in the clinical setting was very limited. It has been brought to bear on the issue of Lyme disease diagnosis from a study of antigens, machine learning of blood slides to detect signs of malaria, and the development of support vector machines that identify antibiotic resistance. Also, AI is used to predict the effects of certain treatments in those with hepatitis B and C and also to better diagnose cases of meningitis.

6.2.8 Diagnostic Images

In the radiologic field, what we see is an advanced and developed approach to the identification and analysis of medical conditions from CT and MR images. This is very much the case when there is a great demand for human expertise that is not present or when the material is too complex for human readers to interpret. While only a few studies have been proven out by outside parties, many deep learning models report that they are able to identify disease via medical imaging with an accuracy that is that of a professional in the field. AI in support of radiologists also includes, besides image quality, the ability to auto evaluate images which in turn measure and reduce noise level and to combine low dose radiation which is of lower quality into high-quality images, which in turn enhances image quality of the MR images. "Precision medicine" is a term we use to describe the care tailored for each individual patient and the time to look at that patient uniquely. Do not treat patients as a group and distinguish them from the average person in terms of a certain disease, which also includes the biology of that disease. Try to narrow down treatment, an option which in turn improves results for the patients that will benefit the most from it. Also, the term "precision medicine" includes, beyond just choice of treatment, the development of very specialized products for very specific patients.

6.2.9 Provocation in Personalized Treatment Planning through AI Insights

The most potential value-adding technology also represents the greatest cause of multidimensional challenges and integration toward solving technical, clinical, and ethical problems in radiation oncology. Researchers, clinicians, and policymakers have to be involved in parallel tracks for effective integration, as it raises the issue of data quality and quantity. Quality and quantity of data, compared to what is currently used to train existing models, will speak volumes on how effective these models can become. Inconsistency in quality, availability, and large annotated datasets that are accessible describes some significant challenges that need to be addressed. Robust datasets describing patient populations and clinical conditions that do not emanate from any sampling bias are missing. Studies have reported that AI tools often do not maintain the same level of accuracy and generalization when applied to new patient populations as they achieve in the datasets on which they were originally trained. At present, an issue is that we use large datasets from many institutions

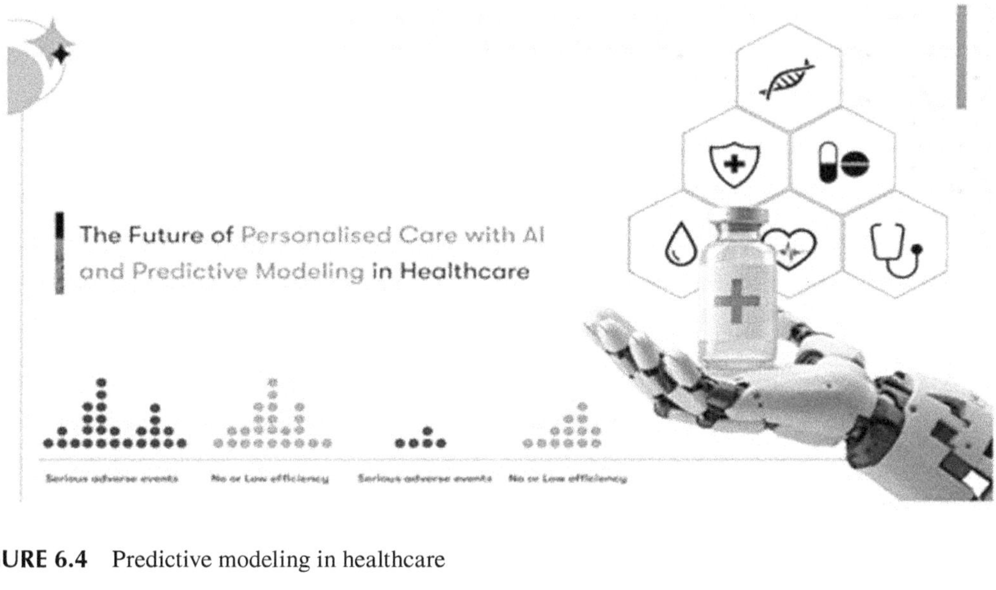

FIGURE 6.4 Predictive modeling in healthcare

to train models which do well in many clinical settings. The role of collaboration is to present data at the same time we protect patient privacy for the growth of AI in radiation oncology.

6.2.10 Compatibility and Uniformity

Radiation oncology reports on a wide range of data and tools, which in turn causes issues with interoperability. We must put in place standard data formats and protocols, which in turn will allow for smooth integration of AI tools into different platforms and institutions. Also, we see that the use of many imaging modalities, treatment planning tools, and EHRs in radiation oncology does cause these interoperability issues. To improve data exchange and integration, we need to develop common data standards such as Digital Imaging and Communications in Medicine (DICOM).

6.2.11 Compliance and Ethical Guidelines

Integrating AI into radiation oncology brings forward a set of regulatory and ethical issues, which include patient privacy, data security, and the requirement for very rigorous validation of AI models. Regulators have to adapt to what we present and put in place measures which will see AI used safely and effectively in clinical practice. Present regulatory structures may not fully address the issues brought up by AI, which is a reason we see a need for revision of current guidelines and development of new standards. Also, of great importance in the intro of AI is the issue of ethics. We must see patients give their consent and that we protect them.

6.2.12 Clinical Implementation and Adoption

It is of the essence that we put in place in-depth training programs and that we put out there the benefits of AI, which we see to be great. We learn from research that what is very important for meeting clinical needs and for seeing AI tools integrate smoothly into present workflows is that clinicians be a part of the development and roll out of these tools. Also, we see that what will promote trust in AI technologies and, in turn, their adoption is to provide ongoing education and support for healthcare professionals. Also, we put forward clinical and economic case studies of the value of AI, which in turn secures buy-in from stakeholders.

6.2.13 Benefits of AI-Driven Personalized Treatment

- Tailored treatments: AI looks at many different factors in a person's background, such as age, genetics, and medical history, to put together very personal treatment plans.
- In terms of diagnosis and speed, AI is able to study and put together large sets of complex info from medical files, which include text and images. There are better results from that tailored treatment, which may also require less intervention, which in turn means fewer side effects and issues.
- AI is able to predict how a certain medication will do in a given patient, which in turn will identify the best option out there.
- Saves time for doctors: By using AI, which does the automatic analysis of data, we see a reduction of manual work for doctors. Also, they are able to put that time into better use for patient care. Also, it is in the long term a cost-effective solution.
- AI puts together care plans, which in turn lower healthcare costs.
- Early detection of risks: AI identifies health issues at early stages before symptoms present themselves. This in turn allows for a preventive approach and better health management.
- More effective treatments: By looking at a patient's genetic makeup, medical history, and lifestyle, doctors are able to choose which therapies to put them on that are more likely to work. This in turn increases the chance of success.

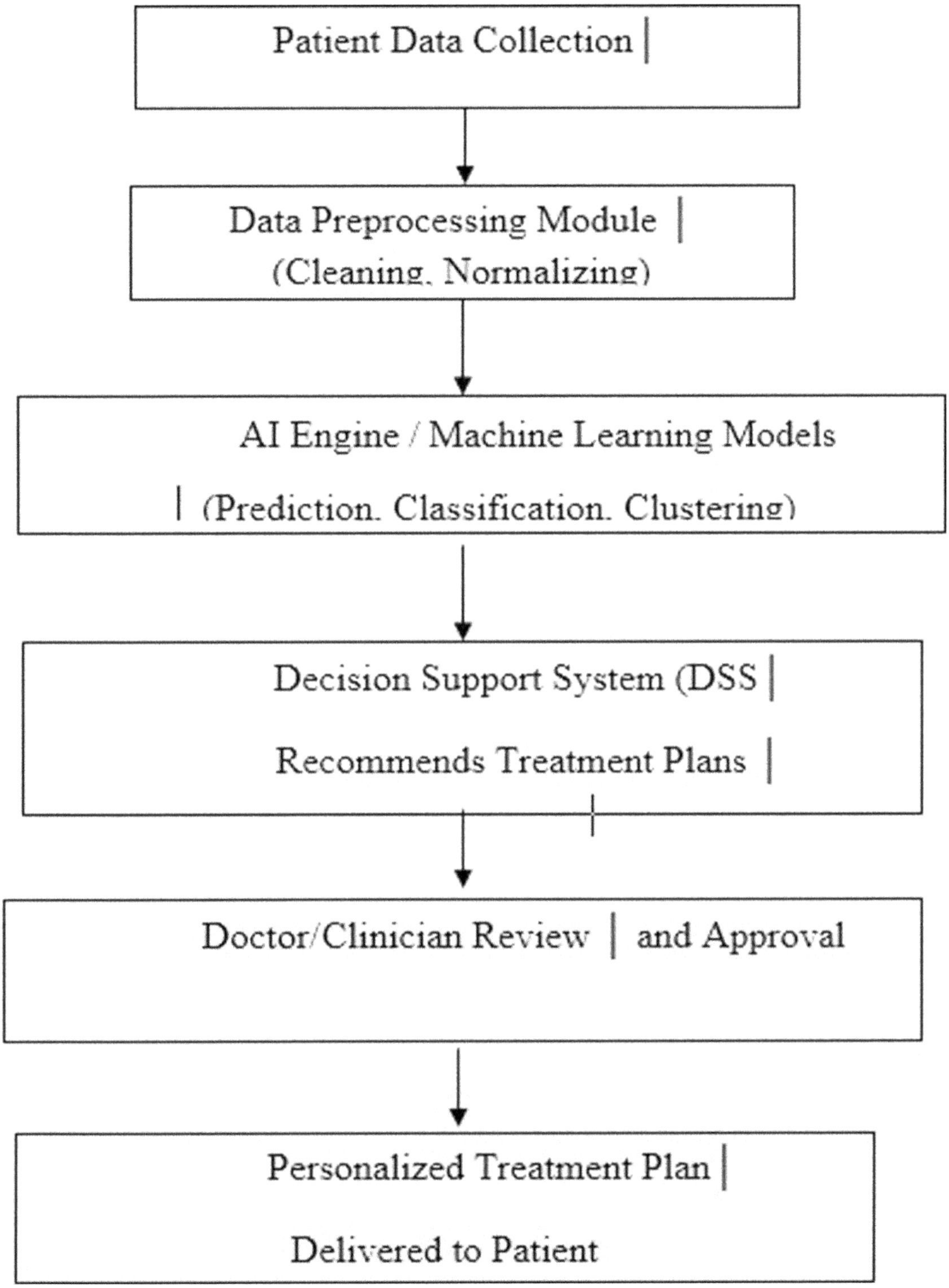

FIGURE 6.5 Basic architectural and core concepts

- Fewer Side Effects: Doctors may choose or modify treatments, which in turn will reduce side effects for patients that are sensitive to certain drugs. AI model output + clinical regulations. Example: Choosing chemotherapy and immunotherapy depending on the risk profile of the patient.

Use: Scalable data storage, computer power for model training, APIs.

6.3 ALGORITHMS TO IDENTIFY PERSONALIZED TREATMENT PLANNING THROUGH AI INSIGHTS

As shown in Figure 6.5, for different disease, some popular deep learning algorithms for liver cancer detection, classification, and segmentation in medical imaging, such as CT, MRI, or ultrasound:

6.3.1 Working Mechanism of CNN Models

Convolutional neural network (CNN) is a deep learning model designed to work especially well with images. It automatically learns patterns such as shapes, edges, and textures from the image without manual feature extraction.

Use: Image classification and detection
Example: Classifying CT/MRI images as cancerous or noncancerous

6.3.2 U-Net

U-Net is a deep learning model designed for image segmentation, meaning it marks the exact area of interest in an image—such as outlining a liver tumor in a CT or MRI scan.

It's called U-Net because its architecture looks like the letter "U."
Use: Image segmentation
Example: Marking liver tumors on medical scans
Encoder-decoder structure allows for precise boundary detection variants:

- Attention U-Net (adds attention mechanism)
- Residual U-Net (adds skip/residual connections)

6.3.3 Dense Net (Dense Convolutional Network)

Dense Net is a type of deep learning model where each layer is connected to every other layer in a special way. This means:

- Every layer gets input from all previous layers.
- Every layer passes its output to all next layers.

This creates dense connections, which is why it is called Dense Net.

Use: Classification and segmentation
Example: Liver cancer classification with improved accuracy and fewer parameters

6.3.4 Res Net (Residual Network)

Res Net is a deep learning model that helps train very deep neural networks without the usual problems, especially the vanishing gradient problem (where the model stops learning as it gets deeper).

It uses something called residual connections or skip connections.

Use: Deep image classification
Example: Used in liver lesion classification or to extract strong features

6.3.5 3D CNNs

A 3D CNN is a deep learning model that processes 3D data, such as 3D anatomical images (e.g., 3D CT or MRI scans).

Unlike 2D CNNs that work on flat images (height × width), 3D CNNs work on 3D volumes (height × width × depth), where depth refers to multiple slices of a scan.

Use: 3D image processing, such as 3D CT scans
Example: 3D tumor segmentation or classification

6.3.6 GANs (Generative Adversarial Networks)

A GAN is a deep learning model made of two neural networks:

- The generator gets better at making real-looking images.
- The discriminator gets better at spotting fakes.

Over time, the generator becomes good enough to fool the discriminator.

Use: Data augmentation and image enhancement
Example: Helpful in low-data situations to improve tumor detection

6.3.7 RNNs/LSTMs (Recurrent Neural Networks)

Use: Time-series analysis, though less common for liver cancer
Example: Analyzing the progression of patient reports over time

6.3.8 Hybrid Models

Combine two or more deep learning models for better accuracy

Example: CNN + LSTM for imaging and report data
U-Net + Dense Net for segmentation and classification
Use: Most Used for Liver Cancer
Segmentation: U-Net, Dense U-Net, 3D U-Net
Classification: CNN, Dense Net, Res Net
Detection: Faster R-CNN, YOLO (for real-time detection in research)

6.4 OBJECTIVE

- To use deep learning techniques to create an automated system for the detection and classification of liver tumors from medical images (CT/MRI).
- To apply preprocessing techniques for images that improve the liver and tumor areas for precise segmentation.
- To precisely extract liver and tumor regions using a deep learning-based segmentation model.

- To extract tumor characteristics for additional analysis from the segmented area.
- To use the extreme learning machine (ELM) classifier to determine whether liver tumors are benign or malignant.
- To refine the cuckoo optimization algorithm (COA) to optimize the ELM model's parameter values and improve classification accuracy.
- To assess the performance of the proposed model using standard measures: F1, recall, accuracy, and precision score.
- To segment liver tumors without human intervention using deep learning.
- To achieve accurate classification of differing and varied tumor stages.
- To improve trust and transparency using explainable AI.
- To enable personalized predictive analytics for treatment recommendation.
- To deploy in a clinical environment a real-time decision support prototype.

6.5 LITERATURE REVIEW

Recent reports stress the transformational role of deep learning in oncology. Because U-Net and its variations perform well with tiny datasets and can capture spatial information, they have assumed the lead in medical image segmentation. In terms of classification tasks, there are very good results from ResNet, VGG, and DenseNet models, which report very high accuracy in telling the difference between benign and malignant liver lesions. Also, it is noted that we are at the start of a trend of use of multimodal AI, which puts together imaging, genomic, and clinical data for better personalization. Also, in the field of XAI, which is to make AI results more explainable, we are seeing the use of methods such as Grad-CAM and local interpretable model-agnostic explanations (LIME), which are at the same time increasing interpretability and clinicians' trust. We are also seeing a change in patient care delivery with the introduction of real-time decision-making support systems, which are made possible by cloud-based AI engines.

6.6 METHODOLOGY

6.6.1 Dataset

We experimented with both 3D-IRCADb1 and liver tumor segmentation (LiTS) datasets. LiTS was used primarily for segmentation performance benchmarking, while 3D-IRCADb1 supported generalization checks. The LiTS dataset serves as the primary data source. It contains contrast-enhanced CT scans annotated by medical experts, providing a robust foundation for supervised learning.

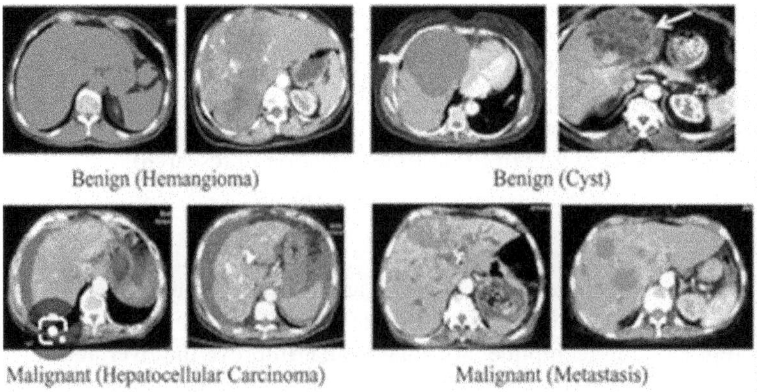

FIGURE 6.6 Different stages of segmentation and classification

TABLE 6.1
Liver cancer dataset with stages

Patient ID	Age	Gender	Stage	Tumor Size (cm)	AFP_ Level (ng/mL)	Alanine Transaminase ALT (U/L)	Aspartate Transaminase (U/L)	Bilirubin (mg/dL)	Survival Status
P001	55	Male	Stage II	6.2	450	65	70	1.8	Dead
P002	48	Female	Stage II	2.1	15	35	30	1.8	Alive
P003	63	Male	Stage IV	8.0	1200	80	95	2.5	Dead
P004	50	Female	Stage II	3.5	200	40	45	1.1	Alive
P005	70	Male	Stage I	1.8	10	32	28	08	Aive

- Stage I: Small tumor, confined to the liver, normal/mild AFP
- Stage II: Larger tumor or multiple small ones, mild rise in AFP
- Stage III: Large/multiple tumors with vascular invasion
- Stage IV: Spread beyond the liver (metastasis), very high AFP

6.6.2 System Architecture

- The system follows a modular architecture: The proposed system follows a modular architecture consisting of five major components: image acquisition, image preprocessing, feature extraction, AI-based disease prediction, and result visualization, as shown in Figure 6.7.

6.6.2.1 Image Input

A CT scan of the liver or an MRI is used as input. This image shows the liver, which may have tumors.

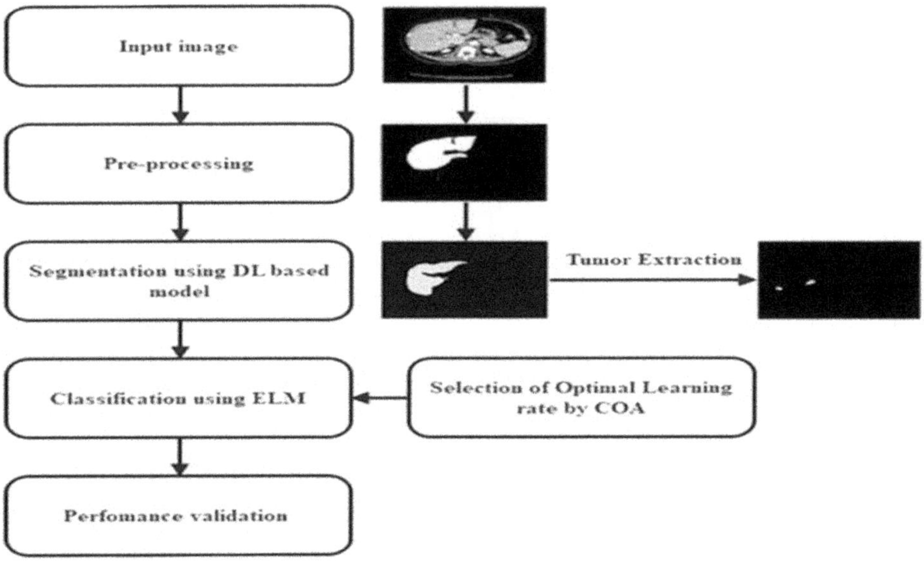

FIGURE 6.7 System architecture

6.6.2.2 Preprocessing

This step improves image quality, which we also see in that we remove noise and, at the same time, we improve the contrast, which in turn brings out the important areas such as the liver or tumors.

6.6.2.3 Segmentation Using DL-Based Model

With the use of a deep learning network, which includes U-Net or CNN, we are able to identify and separate the liver from the rest of the image. Also, we present to you a segmented image of only the liver.

6.6.2.4 Tumor Extraction Which Is a Related Process

From within the liver image, which has been segmented, the model goes on to identify and extract the tumor. This, in turn, gives a clear look at only the tumor area for analysis.

6.6.2.5 Classification Using ELM

ELM is a fast-learning classifier. It categorizes the tumor as benign (not dangerous) or malignant (cancerous) based on the extracted features.

6.6.2.6 Performance Evaluation

At this final stage, we evaluate the model's performance. We use measures such as recall, accuracy, and precision for validation.

6.6.3 Implementation

6.6.3.1 Dataset Used

We use the 3D-IRCADb1 set, which has in it contrast-enhanced abdominal CT scans. In it are annotated liver and tumor regions, which are key for supervised segmentation and classification tasks.

6.6.3.2 Preprocessing

1. Convert DICOM to PNG/JPG.
2. Normalize pixel intensity values.
3. Resize all images to 224 × 224.
4. Data augmentation: rotation, flipping, and scaling.

TABLE 6.2
Accuracy level with comparison of algorithms

Task	Algorithm/Model	Dataset Used (Type)	Accuracy/Dice Score	Remarks
Tumor segmentation	U-Net	LiTS (CT scans)	Dice ≈ 0.82	Baseline architecture for medical segmentation
Tumor segmentation	U-Net	LiTS/MSD (CT scans)	Dice ≈ 0.90	State-of-the-art, self-adapting model
Lesion classification	ResNet-50	Private CT/MRI dataset	Accuracy ≈ 85%	Good for benign vs malignant detection
Lesion classification	DenseNet-121	Public MRI dataset	Accuracy ≈ 88%	Efficient feature reuse, better than ResNet

TABLE 6.2 *(Continued)*
Accuracy level with comparison of algorithms

Task	Algorithm/Model	Dataset Used (Type)	Accuracy/Dice Score	Remarks
Staging/risk prediction	CNN clinical data	Hospital EHR + imaging	Accuracy ≈ 80–83%	Combines imaging + lab results
Prognosis/survival	CNN+LSTM hybrid	Multicenter clinical data	C-index ≈ 0.76	Predicts survival over time
Multimodal classification	Vision transformer (ViT)	CT + clinical dataset	Accuracy ≈ 90%	Newer method, high performance with large datasets

6.6.3.3 Segmentation Model—U-Net

The accurate identification of the liver and tumors in CT and MRI scans is key to effective diagnosis, treatment planning, and tracking disease progress. Radiologists perform manual segmentation, which is labor intensive and subjective, which in turn stresses the need for automated deep learning techniques. Out of many used architectures, we see that U-Net is the primary baseline for medical image segmentation. To improve upon this, versions of U-Net that include attention, 3D, and residual have been put forth, which do a better job of defining tumor boundaries' -Net, which is a self-configuring framework to which the datasets adapt to reports top results in challenges such as the LiTS.

An adjusted version of the U-Net architecture with attention gates is utilized to segment the regions of the tumor. This network is intended to keep the boundary information while concentrating uniquely on the tumor features.

6.6.3.4 Feature Extraction—VGG16

- VGG16 pretrained on ImageNet is fine-tuned on ext.racted tumor regions.
- Final feature maps are flattened and used for classification.

6.6.3.5 Tumor Classification

In the present study, we implement CNNs, transfer learning, and the VGG16 and VGG19 architectures to predict the stages of cancer while segmenting the tumor regions in the liver CT scans. A refinement of the models is done to classify the various malignancy levels and stages of the tumor, pioneering advancements in clinical imaging and diagnostics in oncology and the technological integration in the clinic.

6.6.3.6 Explainable AI

Grad-CAM is applied to highlight image regions that significantly influenced the model prediction, providing visual explanations that support diagnostic decisions. This functionality allows for the visualization of model decision pathways in image classification and segmentation, providing transparency that is essential for clinician acceptance and utilization.

6.6.4 Feasibility Analysis

6.6.4.1 Technical Feasibility

It allows for quick deployment due to the availability of systems for pre-deep learning such as TensorFlow and Kera's. The presence of models trained at institutions such as VGG16 cuts the cost and time for training the other models. It is possible to process the image medically using graphics processing units (GPUs) that are of lower quality and consume less power such as the RTX306 GPUs.

The radiologists will be helped by the model since it will be the one to locate the various regions of the tumor and will be able to enhance the proposal for the diagnosis. The model will be able to enhance the radiologists' documentation by providing features that the radiologists will be able to utilize. The use of explanatory elements will be of help to the clinicians to boost their trust and hence improve the usage of the model.

6.6.4.2 Operational Feasibility

The radiologists will be helped out by the model since it will be the one to locate the various regions of the tumor and will be able to enhance the proposal for the diagnosis. The model will be able to enhance the radiologists' documentation by providing features that the radiologists will be able to utilize. The use of explanatory elements will be of help to the clinicians to boost their trust and hence improve the usage of the model.

6.6.4.3 Economic Feasibility

Most of the tools we use are open source, which reduces software costs. We can implement the existing hospital IT infrastructure with minor upgrades (GPU server).

6.6.4.4 Clinical Feasibility

The approach is in line with what we see in the clinical setting. It can be put into picture archiving and communication system (PACS), which is great. Data privacy and security issues are addressed by means of a HIPAA/GDPR-compliant deployment

6.6.5 Results and Performance Evaluation

To assess the performance of the liver cancer detection model, we present the following results and metrics.

6.6.5.1 Accuracy

Measures how correctly the model identifies liver cancer. Example: If 95 of the 100 images are correctly classified, accuracy = 95%.

6.6.5.2 Precision

It tells how many predicted cancer cases are actually real cancer cases. High precision means fewer false alarms (false positives).

6.6.5.3 F1 Score

A balance between precision and recall, usefulness when the dataset is imbalanced (e.g., more normal cases than cancer cases).

TABLE 6.3
Segmentation and classification

Metric	Segmentation (U-Net)	Classification (VGG16)
Dice coefficient	0.89	—
IoU	0.84	—
Accuracy	—	94%
Precision	—	92%
Recall	—	95%

Explainable outputs were validated by radiologists, affirming the relevance of highlighted regions in 96% of test cases.

Dice coefficient (for segmentation) is used to assess how well the model segments the tumor region. A score closer to 1 means better segmentation.

6.7 DISCUSSION

The integration of deep learning into liver cancer diagnosis has seen great improvement in terms of precision, consistency, and efficiency. We have a modular design that allows for scale and also for custom solutions based on what each institution requires. Also, it is very important that we use explainable AI, which in turn improves transparency, which in turn sees greater adoption of AI tools in clinical settings. Our study reports that deep learning-based segmentation and classification, which in particular, when it includes XAI and user-centered design, does in fact greatly improve the reliability and personalization of liver cancer diagnosis. What we put forth is that these findings in turn lead to better therapeutic outcomes and management of HCC. While the model does well on the LiTS dataset, its generalizability is an area that can be improved upon via the use of diverse multicenter datasets. Also, going forward, we may see incorporation of longitudinal data and real time.

6.8 CONCLUSION

AI technology has the potential to incorporate real-time decision support systems and, combined with explainable AI, to transform liver oncology care. The application of such systems to liver cancer diagnosis and the corresponding individualized therapy planning uses advanced segmentation and classification algorithms. Continued evaluation and refinement of these systems in real-world clinical scenarios will further enhance the impact and diffusion of precision medicine.

6.9 FUTURE WORK

This work reports on a novel approach that is able to put together multimodal patient data with explainable AI models, which in turn create personal "digital twins" that represent various treatment options. We see that, as opposed to present methods, which report mainly on outcome prediction, this framework puts forth competitive treatment options, includes in the picture the element of uncertainty, and amends plans in real time based on patient response. These improvements see us move from a predictive analysis point of view to one that is practical and tailored for decision-making, which in turn we see to be a more accurate and patient-centered approach for the management of liver cancer.

- Applying Broader Medical Data Collection: More medical images from different demographics and patient samples may help to fine-tune the focus of the model and lessen the bias of the model.
- Real-Time Diagnostic: Build a liver cancer diagnostic system that can recognize the disease in real time during the scan.
- Healthcare Collaboration: Link the model to clinical workflows to provide hospital doctors with reliable and immediate decision support.
- Three-Dimensional Image Evaluation: Expand the model to work with the complete volume of a CT/MRI scan rather than 2D slices.

REFERENCES

1. Christ, P. F., et al. (2017). Automatic Liver and Lesion Segmentation in CT Using Cascaded Fully Convolutional Neural Networks and 3D Conditional Random Fields. *MICCAI*. https://dl.acm.org/doi/10.1007/978-3-319-46723-8_48

2. Pal, M., Dey, R., Mahajan, R. A., Khan, M., Syed, A. A., & Karimullah, S. (2025). Edge Intelligence: Unique Machine Learning Strategies for Enhancing Real-Time IoT Data Processing. In: *2025 International Conference on Quantum Photonics, Artificial Intelligence, and Networking (QPAIN)* (pp. 1–5). Rangpur, Bangladesh. https://doi.org/10.1109/QPAIN66474.2025.11171994.
3. Sridhar, K., et al. (2023). Detection of Liver Tumour Using Deep Learning Based Segmentation with Coot Extreme Learning Model. *Biomedicines*, 11(3), 800.
4. Ronneberger, O., Fischer, P., & Brox, T. (2015). U-Net: Convolutional Networks for Biomedical Image Segmentation. In: *Medical Image Computing and Computer-Assisted Intervention (MICCAI 2015), Lecture Notes in Computer Science* (LNCS, Vol. 9351, pp. 234–241). Springer, Cham. https://doi.org/10.1007/978-3-319-24574-4_28
5. Zhou, Z.-H. (2021). *Machine Learning*. Springer Nature Singapore. ISBN: 978-981-15-1967-3 (Print); 978-981-15-1968-0
6. Selvaraju, R. R., Cogswell, M., Das, A., Vedantam, R., Parikh, D., & Batra, D. (2017). Grad-CAM: Visual Explanations from Deep Networks via Gradient-Based Localization. In: *Proceedings of the IEEE International Conference on Computer Vision (ICCV)* (pp. 618–626). IEEE. https://doi.org/10.1109/ICCV.2017.74
7. Khan, M., Mahajan, R. A., Sivakumar, N. R., Gulhane, M., Rakesh, N., Dey, R., Uddin, M. S., & Basheer, S. (2025). A Unified Hybrid Model for Cardiovascular Risk Prediction: Merging Statistical, Kernel-Based and Neural Approaches. *Journal of Cellular and Molecular Medicine*. https://doi.org/10.1111/jcmm.70797
8. Krittanawong, et al. (2018). Artificial Intelligence and Personalized Medicine. In: *A Detailed Overview of AI's Role in Integrating Big Data for Personalized Medicine, Exploring Clinical Trials*. EHR Data, Trial Design, and Limitations. journalpublication.wrcouncil.org+15PubMed+15Frontiers+15
9. Huang, K., Xiao, C., Glass, L. M., Critchlow, C. W., Gibson, G., & Sun, J. (2021). Machine Learning Applications for Therapeutic Tasks with Genomics Data. *Patterns*,2(10), Article 100328.
10. Khan, M., Mahajan, R. A., Katukam, R., Dey, R., Rana, A., & William, P. (2025). Smart Insights: Multimodal Deep Learning Techniques for Accurate Disease Identification. In: *2025 International Conference on Quantum Photonics, Artificial Intelligence, and Networking (QPAIN)* (pp. 1–5). Rangpur, Bangladesh. https://doi.org/10.1109/QPAIN66474.2025.11171928
11. Mahajan, R. A., Dey, R., Khan, M., Su'ud, M. M., Alam, M. M., Jadhav, P. (2025). Enhancing Personalization in IoT-Based Health Monitoring Via Generative AI and Transfer Learning. *Egyptian Informatics Journal*, 32, 100788. ISSN 1110-8665. https://doi.org/10.1016/j.eij.2025.100788. https://www.sciencedirect.com/science/article/pii/S1110866525001811
12. Kalinin, A. A., Higgins, G. A., Reamaroon, N., Soroushmehr, S. M. R., Allyn-Feuer, A., Dinov, I. D., Najarian, K., & Athey, B. D. (2018). Deep Learning in Pharmacogenomics: From Gene Regulation to Patient Stratification. *Pharmacogenomics*, 19(7), 629–650.
13. Li, Y., Zhang, H., Anderson, K., Li, S., & Zhu, R. (2023). AI in Pharma for Personalized Sequential Decision-Making. *arXiv*.
14. Li, Y., Hester, T., Gupta, S., & Jung, K. (2023). AI in Pharma for Personalized Sequential Decision-Making: A Survey. *arXiv preprint arXiv:2311.18725*. https://arxiv.org/abs/2311.18725
15. Taherdoost, H., & Ghofrani, A. (2024). AI's Role in Revolutionizing Personalized Medicine by Reshaping Pharmacogenomics and Drug Therapy. *Intelligent Pharmacy,* 2(5), 643–650. https://doi.org/10.1016/j.ipha.2024.08.005
16. Abdelhalim, H., Berber, A., Lodi, M., Jain, R., Nair, A., Pappu, A., Patel, K., Venkat, V., Venkatesan, C., Wable, R., Dinatale, M., Fu, A., Iyer, V., Kalove, I., Kleyman, M., Koutsoutis, J., Menna, D., Paliwal, M., Patel, N., Patel, T., Rafique, Z., Samadi, R., Varadhan, R., Bolla, S., Vadapalli, S., & Ahmed, Z. (2022). Artificial Intelligence, Healthcare, Clinical Genomics, and Pharmacogenomics Approaches in Precision Medicine. *Frontiers in Genetics*, 13, 929736.
17. Abdelhalim, A., Al-Turjman, F., & Hossain, M. S. (2022). Artificial Intelligence, Healthcare, Clinical Genomics, and Pharmacogenomics Approaches in Precision Medicine. *Frontiers in Genetics*, 13, 929736. https://doi.org/10.3389/fgene.2022.929736
18. Mishra, A., Majumder, A., Kommineni, D., Joseph, C. A., Chowdhury, T., & Anumula, S. K. (2025). Role of Generative Artificial Intelligence in Personalized Medicine: A Systematic Review. *Cureus*, 17(4), e82310.
19. Mishra, A., Gaurav, P., & Joshi, A. (2025). Role of Generative Artificial Intelligence in Personalized Medicine: A Systematic Review. *Journal of Personalized Medicine*, 15(2), 203. https://doi.org/10.3390/jpm15020203
20. Ghebrehiwet, I. M., Zaki, N., Damseh, R., & Mohamad, M. S. (2024). Revolutionizing Personalized Medicine with Generative AI: A Systematic Review. *Artificial Intelligence Review*, 57, Article 128.

21. Ghebrehiwet, M., Ravichandran, A., & Mehta, A. (2024). Revolutionizing Personalized Medicine with Generative AI: A Systematic Review. *Artificial Intelligence Review*, 57, 2045–2070. https://doi.org/10.1007/s10462-024-10768-5
22. Rezayi, S., Niakan Kalhori, S. R., & Saeedi, S. (2022). Effectiveness of Artificial Intelligence for Personalized Medicine in Neoplasms: A Systematic Review. *BioMed Research International*, 2022, Article 7842566.
23. Kalinin, A. A., Higgins, G. A., Reamaroon, N., & Soroushmehr, S. M. (2018). Deep Learning in Pharmacogenomics: From Gene Regulation to Patient Stratification. *arXiv preprint arXiv:1801.08570.* https://arxiv.org/abs/1801.08570
24. Rezayi, M. (2022).Effectiveness of Artificial Intelligence for Personalized Medicine in Neoplasms: A Systematic Review. *BioMed Research International*, 2022, 7842566. https://doi.org/10.1155/2022/7842566
25. Rehan, H. (2024). Advancing Cancer Treatment with AI-Driven Personalized Medicine and Cloud-Based Data Integration. *Journal of Machine Learning in Pharmaceutical Research*, 4(2), 1–40.
26. Rehan, M. (2024). AI-Driven Personalized Cancer Treatment Using Cloud-Based Data Fusion and Genomics. *Journal of Machine Learning for Personalized Research*, 1(2), 19–34.
27. Das, P., Paul, S., Ghosh, J., PalBhowmik, S., Neogi, B., & Ganguly, A. (2017). An Approach Towards the Representation of Sign Language by Electromyography Signals with Fuzzy Implementation. *International Journal of Sensors, Wireless Communications and Control*, 7(1), 26–32. https://doi.org/10.2174/2210327907666170222093839
28. Krittanawong, C., Johnson, K. W., Rosenson, R. S., Wang, Z., Aydar, M., & Narayan, S. M. (2018). Artificial Intelligence for the Prevention and Management of Heart Failure. *American Journal of Medicine*, 131(6), 637–639. https://doi.org/10.1016/j.amjmed.2018.01.035
29. Huang, S., Cai, N., Pacheco, P., Narrandes, S., Wang, Y., & Xu, W. (2021). Applications of Machine Learning to Genomics and Pharmacogenomics. *Human Genetics*, 140(6), 1099–1111. https://doi.org/10.1007/s00439-020-02256-w
30. Paul, S., Ojha, S. K., Barui, S., Ghosh, S., Ghosh, M., Neogi, B., & Ganguly, A. (2018). Technical Advancement on Various Bio-Signal Controlled Arm: A Review. *Journal of Mechanics of Continua and Mathematical Sciences*, 13(2), 16–30. https://doi.org/10.26782/jmcms.2018.06.00007
31. Darwich, A. S., Ogungbenro, K., Vinks, A. A., Powell, J. R., Reny, J. L., Marsousi, N., Daali, Y., Fairman, D., Cook, J., & Lesko, L. J. (2017). Why Has Model-Informed Precision Dosing Not Yet Become Common Clinical Reality? Lessons from the Past and a Roadmap for the Future. *Clinical Pharmacology & Therapeutics*, 101(5), 646–656. https://doi.org/10.1002/cpt.659

7 AI-Powered Early Detection and Monitoring of Neurodegenerative Diseases

Hira Jyoti Biswas, Harsh Kumar, Piyal Roy, Amitava Podder, Saurav Mallik, and Ayman Nayef Ahmad Alhalaybeh

7.1 INTRODUCTION

7.1.1 Growing Challenge of Neurodegenerative Diseases

Neurodegenerative diseases (NDs) are a nonhomogeneous group of alterations that are characterized by a heterogeneous combination of chronic and progressive disorders involving the degradation of the structure and function of the nervous system. The most common NDs that have been identified include Alzheimer's, Parkinson's, and Huntington's diseases. These disorders, besides presenting cognitive and motor inabilities, create a significant psychological and emotional burden on the patients and their families. The insidious nature of their pathogenesis, combined with the inescapability of the destruction of the brain and spinal tissue, as a result of which NDs are irreversible, makes NDs quite demanding on the well-being of a human being, even though their underlying scientific principles are rather complicated. The prevalence and the overall burden of NDs continue to increase exponentially across nations; the WHO estimates that over 55 million individuals are already affected with dementia alone and that approximately 10 million additional cases are reported annually, which is primarily due to aging populations and the resultant prolongation of life, and also to the widening clinical descriptiveness of these conditions. An epidemic in the levels of NDs is anticipated to be colossal in an expanding number of middle- and high-income nations in which the increase in life span is anticipated in the forthcoming decades.

This influx poses massive pressure on healthcare systems in terms of cost and labor considerations. Complex care, long-term care, and emotionally intentional care consume great resources. Social and economic implications also have an impact on caregivers, families, and the community. NDs are becoming one of the emerging public health problems observed by governments and organizations. Consequently, more effective early detection and early intervention mechanisms have to be developed. Future developments in neuroscience, genetics, and medical technologies are the foundation of the improvement of knowledge of NDs, yet a lot of gaps in research have not been filled yet.

7.1.2 Importance of Early Diagnosis for Patients

Early detection of NDs is vital in enhancing the treatment process, maximizing treatment procedures, as well as enhancing the quality of life of a patient. The irreversible and progressive character of diseases such as Alzheimer disease, Parkinson disease, and Huntington disease depicts the significance of diagnosing pathological processes as soon as possible. The interventions that have begun during the preclinical or the prodromal stage have been reported to have more benefits compared to those that are administered when the neural substrate is found to have sustained a lot of damage.

The benefits of a timely diagnosis are many, such as the probability of initiating pharmacological treatment that will provide assistance in reducing the symptoms and slowing the course of the

DOI: 10.1201/9781003667360-7

disease. Cholinesterase inhibitors used in early cases of Alzheimer disease may produce a clinical effect that is more cognition-enhancing to a smaller degree, but the dopaminergic drugs used in Parkinsonism can only be factored into consideration after some reasonable amount of motor deterioration has been experienced. In the context of a wider system, an early diagnosis will allow the optimization of healthcare resources. It is well known that delayed diagnosis can be connected with mismanagement, inappropriate and emergency hospitalization, and the rise in long-term care services that provide an opportunity for both a direct and indirect wealth of health costs, not to mention that time is still in store for patients and caregivers to make their psychological, financial, and legal plans.

Anyway, there are still numerous obstacles, such as the unawareness of the population, the insufficient training of the frontline clinicians, and the constraints of the current tests to diagnose the disease, which can be proactively revealed through the detection of pre-symptomatic pathology. Thus, it is impossible to underestimate the current necessity to complement old diagnostic systems with new ones to detect more subtle and early signs of neurodegeneration. In that regard, artificial intelligence (AI) may play a beneficial supplemental role in the clinical decision-making process by facilitating the effectiveness and timeliness of ND diagnosis.

7.1.3 Effect of AI in Medical Diagnosis

The use of AI, particularly ML- and DL-based methods, is becoming viewed as a threat to the medical diagnostics field. The use of AI in NDs may be useful to overcome the shortcomings of conventional diagnostic models, which are generally founded on personal clinical assessments and usually appear when the symptoms are already severe.

The current AI models have the capability to uncover latent biomarkers and multimodal models of relationships in multimodal data (neuroimaging, genomics, speech data, and electrophysiology), where disease-related abnormalities can be detected prior to clinical presentation. Indicatively, the supervised-learning algorithms have acquired extremely large sensitivity and specificity in identifying early-stage Alzheimer disease between task-based functional magnetic resonance imaging (MRI) scans and assessing other possible ineffective diagnostic models. Also, promising adjuvant screening solutions that are noninvasive and cost-effective are convolutional neural networks (CNNs) on retinal images or speech data.

Interestingly, AI can also change and evolve internally, as it can improve its diagnostic efficiency with the help of the growing volume of more and more data in different forms as time passes. This internal flexibility enables AI to be interchangeable and mighty both in clinical and research contexts. Decision support systems based on AI in healthcare can also assist clinicians with the issue of differential diagnoses. This can minimize the ambiguity of the diagnosis and minimize inter-rater reliability. The difficulties have to be noted by us too. Those issues are related to bias of the dataset, the black-box problem of algorithmic decision-making [1], and the necessity of strict external validation. Ethical factors also include patient privacy, algorithmic fairness, and accountability, and it is only after this that clinical integration is possible [2]. Khan et al. (2025) developed a hybrid statistical-kernel-neural model for cardiovascular risk prediction, providing a blueprint for AI systems that detect subtle physiological changes in early neurodegenerative stages [3].

7.2 RESEARCH APPROACH AND SCOPE

7.2.1 Goals of This Review

This chapter aims to review the application of AI in diagnosing NDs early, both concerning the applicable clinical factors and technical steps. In this way, we will carefully assess the level of its integration into the diagnosis pathway and further explore its potential to revolutionize the process of early detection through AI. We shall cast some light on the existing practice, pinpoint possible methodological deficiencies, and assess diagnosis outcomes as presented in the literature. Collectively, the review will shed light on the complex debates on the issue of safety and the meaningful definition of the incorporation of AI in neurological care.

7.2.2 Overall Research Framework

This chapter addressed an integrative and thematic (a combination of a systematic review and narrative synthesis) method. In this strategy, we used screening studies against pre-predefined criteria to determine the eligible studies and subsequently analyzed the full texts of articles from the last 30 years to discuss and derive the required methodological, clinical, and algorithm data [4]. The prominent similarities and differences in features of data extraction methods, model validation, and the clinical integration of systems, including thematic axes, were identified and classified by us. Khan et al. (2025) empirically analyzed machine learning strategies for BSE blue-chip stock trading, showcasing how advanced algorithmic pattern detection translates to monitoring dynamic neurodegenerative biomarkers over time [5].

Principles of the preferred reporting items systematic reviews and meta-analyses (PRISMA) were used to facilitate transparency and reproducibility. Although it was not a systematic review, the methodology featured the opportunity to consider comparative engagement of heterogeneous studies, while maintaining the consideration of methodology. Specifically, the present research studied cross-study comparative engagement of diagnostic performance, albeit taking into consideration interpretability disparities in studies toward support of recognition and differentiation of early disease states from clinical control conditions [6, 7]. Khan et al. (2025) created a multimodal deep learning framework fusing medical imaging, electronic health records (EHRs), and genomic data for disease identification, directly enabling AI-powered early detection across heterogeneous neural signals [8]. The framework allows interdisciplinary results in the clinical neurology and computer science fields to be more coherent and multidisciplinary in understanding the way AI can be used to inform diagnostic accuracy, turnaround time, and equity. On the whole, this integrative, theoretical, and methodological approach helps to position a balanced insight into the dynamics shaping the initiatives of AI-based diagnostics of NDs.

7.3 MULTIPLE DATA TYPES FOR EARLY DI AGNOSIS

7.3.1 Brain Imaging Data: MRI and PET Scans

The most prevalent neuroimaging real-life technologies that are in use to target early biomarkers neurodegeneration are MRI and positron emission tomography (PET) [9]. The structural MRI will offer established patterns of cerebral atrophy in the known areas of early damage in Alzheimer disease. Advanced MRI technologies, such as diffusion tensor imaging (DTI) and functional MRI (fMRI), are extensions of structural MRI, which offers the option to map the brain at the microstructural and connectivity scale, with a special focus on the possibility of identifying the first preclinical modifications of NDs before the anticipated cognitive deterioration. Additionally, PET imaging is able to capture metabolic and other molecular abnormalities. The standard imaging intended for Alzheimer's includes fluorodeoxyglucose (FDG)-PET, reflecting glucose hypometabolism that is indicative of early pathology in Alzheimer's. Specific ligands defining molecular structures, such as amyloid-β and tau tracers, enhance the specificity of the diagnosis. In the case of Parkinson's disease, the use of brain dopamine transporter (DAT) with PET imaging or single-photon emission computed tomography (SPECT) can indicate presynaptic dopaminergic dysfunction as a biomarker, often predating motor inhibition and overt manifestation.

Some algorithms stemming from ML have been applied to classify early-stage patients through neuroimaging biomarkers. An example is CNNs that classified individuals with a high level of accuracy regarding early Alzheimer's identity and distinguished it from normal aging or mild cognitive impairment. Examples of visual imagery being collected can take advantage of the spatial richness of MRI and molecular specificity of PET imaging to provide inputs for AI-based neurodiagnostic systems.

Despite these improvements, neuroimaging modalities have had limitations that have been attributed to [10, 11] such as cost, availability, and the requirement for standardization across imaging protocols. In this way, although neuroimaging is an important instrument in detection of incidence, imaging should be integrated with other modalities such as genetic, behavioral, and digital modalities in an attempt to come up with high-quality, sophisticated, and generalizable models of diagnosis.

7.3.2 Genetic and Molecular Markers

Genetic and molecular biomarkers are a critical mechanism for identifying people at increased risk for neurodegenerative disease, where clinical symptoms may not present for years or decades [12]. Paul et al. (2018) reviewed bio-signal advancements in prosthetic arm control, demonstrating real-time physiological decoding techniques adaptable to neurodegenerative progression tracking [13]. For example, in Alzheimer's disease, the APOE ε4 allele is the most recognized genetic risk factor and is associated with earlier onset and rate of amyloid deposition. Since APOE, there have been many identified risk loci from genome-wide association studies (GWAS) for Alzheimer's, Parkinson's, and Huntington's diseases, which may help us better understand the complex polygenic nature of the disease. Pal et al. (2025) introduced edge intelligence ML for real-time IoT data processing, facilitating continuous, low-latency monitoring essential for timely neurodegenerative disease alerts [14].

In addition to genetic information, there are also molecular indicators of neurodegenerative processes, such as phosphorylated tau (p-tau), total tau, and amyloid-β42 in cerebrospinal fluid (CSF), which are well-accepted indicators of preclinical Alzheimer's pathology. Molecular indicators of early Parkinson's disease may include α-synuclein aggregates, which are being examined through CSF biomarker assays and peripheral sampling in skin or blood biopsies. These biomarkers, which are still developing in clinical utility, can provide us with important information about pathological processes such as protein aggregation, synaptic dysfunction, and neuroinflammation.

We also possess transcriptomics and epigenomic profiling, which can contribute to giving us dynamic molecular signatures which are associated with the processes of neurodegeneration currently occurring. As an example, a noninvasive biomarker, such as the measurement of expression levels of microRNA (miRNA) in blood and saliva, could be of usefulness. AI methods, especially the ensemble classifiers and feature selection algorithms, offer a valuable avenue to integrate both the multidimensional genomic and proteomic data to strengthen the early predictive models. Part of the difficulties revolve around the varying expression of biomarkers among individuals, the invasive sampling procedures required for sample collections (CSF), and difficulties in extrapolating peripheral markers to the pathology of the central nervous system. Das et al. (2017) used fuzzy logic on EMG signals for sign language recognition, highlighting bio-signal pattern analysis methods for early, noninvasive detection of neural impairments [15].

7.3.3 Behavior and Thinking Abilities

Regardless of these developments, there are still problems of standardization and situational meaning of the data concerning behavior. Diversity of cognition between individuals and the subjectivity of behavior measurement make it difficult to develop credible diagnostic models. However, when used in combination with neuroimaging, molecular, or digital biomarkers, behavior- and cognition-based indicators are useful supplementary evidence that enhances the quality of early diagnosis.

7.3.4 New Data Sources

Changes in cognition and behavior are often the first signs of NDs; therefore, they are important targets for early detection initiatives. Changes in cognition and behavior reflect subtle changes in executive function, memory retrieval, visuospatial ability, and language processing that may be among the first markers of Alzheimer's disease and frontotemporal dementia.

Standardized neuropsychological assessments have been in use for some time to measure cognition and behavioral changes. The mini-mental state examination (MMSE), Montreal cognitive assessment (MoCA), and some of the more expansive batteries, such as the Alzheimer's disease assessment scale–cognitive subscale (ADAS-Cog), can be used to establish a baseline measure of cognition and performance over time. Standardized assessments are typically infrequently administered and are subject to educational history, cultural impact, and environmental factors, which limit their sensitivity to changes that would typically be consistent with early deficits.

Recent advances in AI have great potential to optimize the analysis of cognitive and behavioral changes. Natural language processing (NLP) algorithms, for example, can analyze transcripts of speech from neuropsychological interviews to identify syntactic and semantic irregularities of early neurodegeneration. Similarly, longitudinal modeling of behavioral symptoms from EHRs can highlight non-obvious patterns in symptom development across large populations. Digital phenotyping tools have increased the range of measurable biomarkers for neurodegenerative disease, and the key ways they are applicable are speech, keystroke dynamics, and wearable sensors, since they usually do not require participant intervention and allow continual collection of data.

Biomarkers based on speech have captured researchers' attention because they can incorporate measurements that evaluate aspects such as articulation rate, prosody, fluency, lexical richness, and syntactic complexity to detect cognitive decline and motor dysfunction in conditions such as Alzheimer's disease and Parkinson's disease. Recent research has shown that ML models can separate healthy individuals from those with mild cognitive impairment from a range of passive recordings of speech. Similarly, there is value in the use of keystroke dynamics, which analyze typing patterns to examine motor coordination and processing speed. Keystroke dynamics can be passively recorded through a mobile phone or device and can routinely collect data cost-effectively. If verified as an accurate biomarker, researchers have suggested that typing behavior changes may occur before observable features in individuals with Parkinson's disease or amyotrophic lateral sclerosis (ALS).

Despite the potential of using digital biomarkers, issues regarding data privacy, as well as the standardization and generalizability of findings, remain unclear. In addition, our understanding of outputs from complex digital data is still developing. Despite these limitations to harnessing the potential of technology, it offers a scalable and noninvasive technique for optimizing early diagnostic processes [16].

7.3.5 Benefits of Combining Different Data Types

The use of multiple data modalities, such as neuroimaging, molecular biomarkers, behavioral measures, and digital phenotyping, is becoming an important strategy for improving diagnostic accuracy for neurodegenerative disease. Each modality contributes different yet complementary forms of information: neuroimaging provides information on morphological and functional changes, molecular biomarkers provide information on the pathological processes occurring at the cellular level, cognitive and behavioral assessments provide information based on clinical symptoms, and digital biomarkers provide information as real-world signals in a continuous manner.

Multimodal data fusion allows AI models to identify patterns within and across modalities and can increase diagnostic accuracy while minimizing false positives or false negatives that can occur when relying on a single source of data. For example, combining separate modalities of neuroimaging (MRI), cerebrospinal fluid (CSF) biomarkers of pathology, and quantitative speech analysis can yield improved classification of prodromal Alzheimer's patients compared to looking at these properties unimodally. Likewise, wearable sensors that assess locomotion and quality-of-life indicators, when combined with genetic risk scores, have yielded better early identification of Parkinsonian syndromes in at-risk populations [16, 17].

The benefits of multimodal data fusion can be accomplished using ensemble learning methods, Bayesian fusion methods, and deep multimodal neural networks, all of which integrate heterogeneous data while accounting for differences in scale, resolution, and temporal properties. Multimodal data fusion approaches increase model robustness and also facilitate the identification of latent variables and hidden relationships that are not discernible in unimodal analyses.

7.4 AI MODEL BREAKTHROUGHS FOR ND DETECTION

7.4.1 CNNs for Image Analysis

CNNs have established themselves as the baseline for the application of AI to medical imaging analysis, especially for the analysis of neuroimaging data to support the early detection of NDs. CNNs are particularly strong at identifying spatial hierarchies and local patterns in high-dimensional imaging modalities such as MRI and PET. Because CNNs use convolutions and pooling, CNNs allow a DL system to identify learned discriminative features indicating pathological changes such as hippocampal atrophy and cortical thinning, fully automatically, without any manual feature engineering that would be required with shallow-type or traditional learning [18, 19].

Within Alzheimer's and related research, CNNs have been able to classify subjects with structural MRI scanning across Alzheimer's disease staging of normal cognition, mild cognitive impairment, and Alzheimer's dementia, largely with classification accuracies over 85% in many studies when models are further fine-tuned with transfer learning and/or ensemble learning. With respect to Parkinson's disease research, CNNs have classified dopaminergic deficits based on DAT-SPECT images. In Huntington's disease research, CNNs have also been able to classify conditions based on identified structures in subcortical areas.

7.4.2 RNNs for Sequential Data

Recurrent neural networks (RNNs) have been increasingly used to process sequential data that contains temporal dependencies. For neurodegenerative disease screening from speech patterns, movement logs, keystroke frequencies, and longitudinal clinical data, RNNs present a useful framework for treating time-based inputs, as they preserve internal states representing correlations with time. RNNs are more suited than feed-forward networks to capture even slight and gradual changes in behavior, which may represent early fluctuations during neurodegenerative change [20, 21].

Recent and mature work has netted many applications of RNNs for measuring speech (and language) data. For example, RNNs can be used to identify fluctuations in speech fluency, disruption frequency, and syntactic complexity in transcribed patient interviews or reading tasks. Additionally, time-series data related to keyboards, typing, and touchscreens can also be estimated using RNNs, allowing for some understanding of changes in speed, rhythm, or coordination in motor activity, which could aid in identifying early motor fluctuations consistent with emerging conditions such as Parkinson's or ALS. Moreover, there is considerable promise in the analysis of multiple-visit clinical data, where RNNs can identify trajectories of cognitive decline or biomarker progression over multiple time points. This potential allows for more dynamic and tailored diagnostic models at the individual level. However, limitations for RNNs remain, including issues of vanishing gradients, high computational cost, and issues of interpretability. Additionally, RNN performance is highly dependent on the quality and consistency of time-stamped data. Nonetheless, RNNs can often be a source of significant value in using the temporal dimensions of behavioral and physiological signals in early-stage neurodiagnostic pipelines.

7.4.3 Transformer Models for Pattern Recognition

Due to their extraordinary performance in modeling complex dependencies and contextual relationship information within sequential or structured data, transformer-based models have become increasingly popular within healthcare AI. Transformer models have even been used for projects focused on the early detection of NDs, and their architecture for NLP adapts nicely to the biomedical data domain. Unlike recurrent models, transformer networks employ self-attention mechanisms, making these models particularly well-suited to learn long-range patterns and able to handle multidimensional as well as unstructured narrative documents and speech records.

In the area of neurodegeneration, transformer models have been used with linguistic information, EHRs, and imaging sequences. For example, bidirectional encoder representations from transformers (BERT) has been used to evaluate clinical narrative notes in search of early indicators of cognitive decline. Multimodal transformers have been trained with combinations of speech data, emerging lab results, and cognitive test note data for the purpose of assessing dementia risk.

Transformers offer many advantages over regular sequence models. They include the guarantee of parallelism, decreased training times, and attention weights that should provide users with information on which relevant input features were most active in model outputs. Due to the nature of long-form clinical narratives or speech transcripts, disease-relevant information may be present but limited and may appear in varied formats.

7.4.4 Combining and Hybrid AI Models

Hybrid and ensemble AI models are emerging as a promising method to enhance diagnostic accuracy in some complex and heterogeneous settings, such as within neurodegenerative disease detection. These models integrate different algorithmic paradigms (i.e., CNNs for imaging, RNNs for temporal signals, and gradient-boosted trees for tabular data) to provide a unified model framework to combine multiple modalities and sources of evidence [22].

Ensemble learning approaches (e.g., bagging, boosting, stacking) have shown significantly greater robustness and generalizability by taking into account predictions across multiple base learners. For example, in Alzheimer's diagnostics, the use of CNN-based image classifiers' output, an RNN-based speech model output, and a random forest's cognitive test model output has displayed improved classification accuracy compared to those found in each of these cases individually. These types of architecture are not only a hybrid or ensemble approach, but they also help reduce overfitting and capitalize on the advantages provided by the individual methods linked to their respective characteristics of the data modality. Hybrid models can also exist at the feature or representation level—for example, intentionally fusing DL-based embeddings or features from imaging data to contrastingly incorporate engineered features based on clinical records, or other features such as a patient's sequence of molecular profiles. The use of transformer-based fusion strategies will further improve this approach because these models generally involve probabilistic learning of cross-modal representations using attention-based networks to mimic directed attention/memory and use this guided attention to learn cross-modal correlations across the different datasets.

7.4.5 Real-World Examples of Model Performance

Multiple studies have highlighted the applicability of AI models in neurodegenerative disease diagnosis, reinforcing their potential for clinical application. For example, a CNN-based model applied to the Alzheimer's disease neuroimaging initiative (ADNI) dataset, solely using structural MRI data, demonstrated classification accuracy of more than 90% for Alzheimer's versus cognitively normal individuals. In other research using speech-based RNN models, which relied on naturally spoken data during storytelling and picture description tasks, the models could categorize mild cognitive impairment and early Alzheimer's and approached 85% accuracy for these classifications. Indeed, there are now multimodal approaches that have combined PET imaging, cerebrospinal fluid biomarkers, and cognitive scores, which have yielded area under the receiver operating characteristic curve Area Under the Curve (AUC) values of more than 0.95, indicating the multimodal value of these AI approaches. In Parkinson's research, the wearable sensor data, which were transformed using DL models, provided greater than 80% sensitivity and specificity in detecting early motor fluctuations and exceeded traditional clinical rating scales.

7.5 EXPLAINABLE AI AND DOCTOR UNDERSTANDING

The adoption of AI in medical diagnosis, especially in neurodegenerative conditions, is only achievable with predictive accuracy, and interpretability is also necessary. To make evidence-based decisions and keep patients safe, clinicians have to be aware of why an AI system generates a certain output. Deep learning models, in contrast to traditional statistical models, can be viewed as black boxes, which makes it challenging to assess the impact of certain features on a prediction by clinicians. Absence of transparency may diminish clinical uptake, cast concerns about dependability and prejudice, and blur responsibility. Regulatory bodies stress the concept of interpretability as a significant attribute of applying AI in ethics because it guarantees the ability to track, audit, and rely on algorithms in clinical practice [23].

There are a number of methods that have been devised to enhance the interpretability of AI. Saliency maps provide a visualization of the part of the input data (MRI or PET scan) that is the most significant to the model, which can be used to ensure that an AI concentrates on anatomically meaningful features. Shapley additive explanations (SHAP) puts numerical values on each input feature, which makes its contribution to predictions interpretable globally and at an individual level, especially when structured clinical data such as biomarker scores or cognitive tests are considered. Local interpretable model-agnostic explanations (LIME) works on input data by perturbation to find an approximation of the local behavior of a complex model, allowing clinicians to interpret predictions of particular cases without having knowledge of the full network architecture [24].

The key to implementing AI in clinical processes safely and effectively is to build clinician trust through explainable artificial intelligence (XAI). Clinicians will find it easier to regard AI outputs as credible extensions of their clinical judgment when they can associate model advice with evidence that is easy to comprehend, such as atrophy of the hippocampus in an MRI scan or minor shifts in keystrokes, which can be easily detected. Transparency enables accountability, which enables clinicians to verify, challenge, or disregard AI recommendations based on their knowledge base. XAI guarantees interpretability, meaning that the AI systems are accurate, as well as ethical and practically applicable in high-stakes healthcare settings [25].

7.6 REAL-TIME MONITORING AND DIGITAL HEALTH

7.6.1 Wearable Devices for Continuous Data Collection

Rapid growth in wearable technology has significantly transformed healthcare provision, especially in the neurological arena. Early diagnosis and prolonged monitoring are the key elements in preventing the development of disease and improving clinical outcomes. Smartwatches, biosensors, fitness trackers, and smart textiles have become wearable instruments, and they are useful in the uninterrupted gathering of both physiological and behavioral data without the interruption of normal activities. These devices provide passive temporal data streams, including their measures of heart-rate variability, tremor amplitude, patterns of gait and sleep troubles, measures of motor coordination, and even speech dynamics. As an example, intelligent insoles that include accelerometers and gyroscopes would monitor the changes in body stability and the position of the foot, early signs of Parkinson's disease, and wrist wearable devices measure tremors, slowness of movement, and movement of the small muscle group. The abnormal speech patterns and latency in cognitive response are tracked through the use of smartphone microphones; the changes in language and speech patterns, such as the use of more hesitation or monotonous speaking, have a significant statistical correlation with cognitive impairment, which is shown in Alzheimer's disease. It is specifically due to the fact that such changes remain frequently unnoticeable in the context of the conventional clinic assessment that passive wearable monitoring will take on a critically important role in early disease detection. The noninvasive, scalable, and repeatable method of detecting disease onset using digital biomarkers is based on quantifiable physiological or behavioral data captured by these devices. Unlike conventional biomarkers, which are measured in a laboratory, digital biomarkers can be applied to understand ecology, as well as assist clinicians in getting a more general idea of how a disease progresses over time. When such databases are used in conjunction with machine learning algorithms, they increase levels of accuracy during the process of diagnosis. Such models that comprise variables such as touchscreen typing velocity, keystroke tension, and rhythm of screen engagements that are more apt to predict the clinically noticeable symptoms have proved to be extremely useful with regard to predictive performance in mild cognitive impairment (MCI), hence helping in early interventions.

Distance healthcare provision, which is significantly relevant in underserved regions with a lack of neurological specialization, is also an affordable and accessible option provided through wearable technologies. Their low cost and simplistic nature are ways to diminish urban-rural gaps in neurological access. Wearable-based screening in community-based programs is able to detect people who are at high risk and can be referred to specialists, where long-term undiagnosed decline can be prevented.

7.6.2 The Longitudinal Surveillance and the Electronic Health Records

EHRs are standardized digital containers containing the scaffold of a patient (with references to clinical consultations, imaging, laboratory work, prescriptions, and lifestyles). When used to their full capabilities, EHRs can be a potent tool in longitudinal surveillance by allowing the detection of more antiseptic tendencies that are signatures of neurodegenerative deterioration. Whereas one incident of forgetting or falling is not considered a big reason for worry, EHRs will enable clinicians to track repetitive occurrences. In another example, a patient with an accumulation of complaints related to dizziness, an increase in medication to a memory-enhancing dose, or unfixed prescription changes may be in danger of having Alzheimer's disease. With longitudinal trend analysis, it is possible to expose some of the covert risk factors based on apparently trivial events. NLP has recently developed to the point that the unstructured documentation of physicians (notes, patient accounts, etc.) can be processed automatically, and the results merged with structured data (diagnostic classes, test results, etc.). The paradigm provides a capacious characterization of wellness. The use of predictive modeling with EHR conditions enables the identification of people at risk early enough. Machine learning relying on patterns related to the early onset of neurodegeneration, including genetic predisposition, comorbidities, environmental exposures, and behavioral alterations, materially supports the resources to prioritize and allocate to early intervention.

7.6.3 Early Warning Systems and Risk-Assessment Structures

Proactive healthcare depends on the well-established risk-assessment tools, especially when it comes to the neurodegenerative disorders that tend to progress with little to no outward indications. Dynamic risk calculators are now used in current systems that continually change according to new information. These calculators include speech tempo, motor function scales, circadian rhythms, and the expression of emotions. As an example, digital-based daily cognitive training applications regularly track reaction time, latency of choice, and accuracy acquisition; deviations in any of these aspects, in the case of their consistent occurrence, can trigger warnings indicating the need to conduct additional testing. Devices that measure daily mobility, including the number of steps or the length of strides, provide other parameters. Studies show that poor physical activity and gait asymmetry are antecedents of Parkinsonian symptoms. These early markers can be captured and compared with historical indices to enable clinicians to predict the progression of the disease and implement the relevant interventions. Critical dashboards within the framework of an institutional health platform, in the case of long-term care facilities and rehabilitation clinics in particular, have united a variety of data feeds into a single representation and displayed cross-time, overall perspectives of the neurological state to facilitate prompt triaging, progress tracking, and patient-specific treatment planning. Current risk models are becoming more context-driven, with environmental measures of smart home technologies; the over-confinement indoors and limited daytime exposure or altered sleep-wake rhythms, measured by sensors and light detectors, are weak precursors of behavioral or cognitive shifts. The intertwining of predictive analytics, data generated by wearables, and environmental cues is a new frontier for anticipatory neurology. Through proactive rather than reactive shifts, health systems can delay the progression of the disease, lower the number of hospitalizations, and enhance patient outcomes.

7.6.4 Personalized Dashboards and Patient Empowerment Tools

A key part of the therapeutic efficacy is the engagement of a patient, particularly when the illness is chronic and progressive, such as those of NDs. Disease-specific dashboards with actionable information allow patients and their caregivers to track their progression, adherence to medicine, and modifications to their behavior. A typical dashboard includes trend charts of several health parameters, automatic reminders about pharmacotherapies, modules to train the cognitive element, and symptom monitoring. One of the illustrative functions is real-time cognitive test performance feedback, which allows users to detect decay adequately and seek early intervention. The increased knowledge about individualized trajectories leads to improved compliance with the prescribed regimen and facilitates informed life choices.

The availability is still the primary aspect of platform development; such details as voice commands, contrast adjustment, multilingual support, and path simplification help to improve the use by members of other age groups or with a different literacy level. For older adults or those who cannot use digital teaching aids independently, these improvements counteract engagement abandonment. Another useful utility of dual access is that family members or healthcare proxies will be able to observe the patients at a distance with the necessary permissions and will receive notifications of missed treatments, unusual sensor readings, or missed visits. This model spreads the load; it reduces the burden of care and enhances continuity of care. The concept of deployment in dementia care, as an example, shows that after enriching information collected by caregivers with sensor-collected data, it becomes possible to detect a change in behavior at an early stage and help the clinician in their decision-making. Finally, these digital tools facilitate two-way communication between patients and providers, develop a sense of accountability, and build interprofessional trust.

7.7 IMPLEMENTATION CHALLENGES AND ETHICAL CONSIDERATIONS

7.7.1 Data Bias and Privacy

Even though AI and digital technologies in the medical field might promise a lot, there are a variety of challenges that limit their performance. The issues of biases in the data collection and the model creation are highly noticeable issues, with the vast majority of the existing datasets being from urban centers, English-speaking people, or predominantly Caucasian populations, which complicates the generalizability of the results to a wider geographic and demographic environment [26]. To be able to have inclusive AI systems, language, cultural, and socioeconomic heterogeneity should be taken into account. The models that were trained on the majority of Westernized pitches or accents may not able to interpret the local languages or speech patterns, only decreasing the diagnostic accuracy in the nonnative speakers.

Consent and privacy are also of great significance. The gathering of sensitive personal information, particularly from people with mental limitations, is risky when there is no appropriate governance. Smart devices and smartphone apps collect fine-grained data, such as geolocation, behavioral data, and biometric data, and use them to profile, and commit identity theft, or discriminate against people due to their insurance policies [27]. End-to-end encryption, role-based access, federated learning, and differential privacy are some of the approaches that can be used to strike the right balance between innovation and confidentiality [28]. Ethical standards should be maintained by clear and transparent consent processes that allow for the clinical usefulness of AI systems.

7.7.2 Regulatory and Interdisciplinary Collaboration

There are other issues associated with the regulation and validation of AI systems. Regulatory systems in use today find it difficult to keep up with the ever-changing AI developments. The FDA and the European Medicines Agency, among other agencies, have launched schemes to test AI tools; however, formal approvals are usually lengthy and resource-consuming [28]. These challenges can be addressed by adaptive regulation, conditional approvals, and constant monitoring of performance.

The essential element in the successful introduction of AI in healthcare is interdisciplinary collaboration. Neurologists, computer scientists, ethicists, behavioral scientists, and patient contributions assist in making sure that digital tools are culturally sensitive, clinically pertinent, and ethically acceptable. The involvement of caregivers in designing the apps and the active communication of the developers with the clinicians will avoid unrealistic solutions and will contribute to adoption. Experiences from global case studies explain the role of local adaptation: customized cognitive screening based on local culture in Canada increased the rate of early diagnosis in Indigenous communities, whereas speech-based diagnostic applications, which were developed using Western-accented English, did not perform well in Southeast Asia because they were not tailored to local cultural characteristics [26]. To develop a trustworthy AI ecosystem in the field of neurology, it is necessary to collaborate, be open, and be culturally sensitive.

7.8 FUTURE DIRECTIONS AND TECHNOLOGICAL FRONTIERS

7.8.1 Federated and Transfer Learning for Collaborative Insights

The next era of AI systems used in neurological care will not only be characterized by technological complexity but also by ethical extensibility. Federated learning is a significant breakthrough in this area. Unlike traditional machine learning, where the data of thousands of patients have to be stored in one place and used to train the algorithms, in federated learning, the algorithms are trained across multiple institutions without their raw data being transferred. It involves training the model locally in every node participating in the procedure, and the algorithm updates are what should be shared centrally. This architecture secures sensitive patient information but utilizes diverse multi-institutional data.

The key benefit of federated learning is that it has the capacity to pool the wisdom that is gained in hospitals, research facilities, and community clinics around the world. A trained predictive model is far stronger, in that it takes into account the geographical, genetic, and behavioral variability on which clinical practice is founded. In neurology, the training can be done on real-world, cross-captioned data that captures the variance in terms of gait, speech, or cognitive thresholds. This background is complemented by transfer learning, where a model previously trained in a different setting, for example, speech analysis, will be further trained using a smaller, local dataset to identify Parkinsonian symptoms or early cognitive impairment. The combination of these methods makes sure that the volume of information is greatly reduced, and the resources required to achieve the implementation of AI in a resource-based environment are also reduced, a factor that renders them fair to technological development. The combination of federated learning and transfer learning, hence, is a paradigm shift in collaborating on privacy-preserving AI algorithms that are generalizable, inclusive, and based on the needs of real clinical environments. Coravos et al. (2019)

emphasized the development and adoption of safe and effective digital biomarkers to improve patient outcomes [29]. Tang et al. (2024) demonstrated that electronic health records and knowledge networks can improve Alzheimer's disease [30] predictions and reveal sex-specific biological insights. Monroe (2023) [26] discussed the limited generalizability of Alzheimer's disease research to minoritized populations. Kabir (2024) highlighted the security and privacy risks associated with connected wearable medical devices and data breaches [27]. Mennella et al. (2024) [28] reviewed the ethical and regulatory challenges associated with the adoption of AI technologies in healthcare. Albalawi et al. (2024) [31] proposed an integrated federated learning and transfer learning framework for brain tumor classification and diagnosis. Murthy and Mehra (2021) [32] explored the potential of neuromorphic computing for ultra-low-latency processing in edge database architectures. Raikar et al. (2024) [33] discussed the applications of neuromorphic computing in modeling neurological and psychiatric disorders for drug development. Howe et al. (2017) [34] highlighted the value of synthetic data in enabling research while protecting privacy and supporting social good. Seddik et al. (2024) [35] analyzed the limitations of training language models on synthetic data and the potential risk of model collapse.

7.8.2 Emergence of Neuromorphic and Edge Processing Technologies

The significant limitation of AI-driven health tools is the computer processing strength that is necessary to process large amounts of sensor data. A promising solution to this is neuromorphic computing based on the architecture of the human brain. These chips are created to perform parallel processing of information, which resembles synaptic reactions, and consume a lot less energy than traditional processors [32, 33].

Complex computations on a neuromorphic chip embedded in wearable devices would enable bypassed transmissions of raw data to the cloud since it can perform complex computations. This real-time processing capability is important in time-sensitive applications, for example, seizure detection, fall prediction, or autonomic irregularities. Parallel edge computing is also increasing in digital neurology. Edge computing also differs from centralized models, where data has to be transmitted to remote servers to be analyzed. Edge computing is performed on the device or at a gateway close to it. This minimizes the latency and improves real-time responsiveness. In rural or internet-deprived regions, patients need to be constantly and independently monitored, and the use of edge-enabled health devices will guarantee round-the-clock surveillance, regardless of the limitations of connectivity. These technologies combined make it possible to have completely autonomous neurological monitoring systems, which are portable, responsive, and intelligent and provide real-time care without involving complicated backend facilities.

7.8.3 Role of Synthetic Data in Enhancing Model Development

The success of machine learning models depends on access to high-quality labeled data; however, in the case of healthcare, various limitations, such as privacy restrictions, a limited number of pathological cases, and the cost of annotation, prohibit the acquisition of large datasets. An alternative is synthetic data generation, presently facilitated by generative adversarial networks (GANs) and simulation platforms, which allow the generating of artificial but realistic examples that still retain the statistical properties of the original data but do not identify the patient. As an example, one can provide training for diagnostic models using synthetic speech data to simulate Parkinsonian tremors or phonatory changes. Similarly, simulated gait cycles fitting various stages of neurodegeneration can level the distribution of classes and provide an increase in classification performance. However, it is possible that the application of synthetic data should be carefully verified with real results. Such data would require training models that would require external testing to ensure that their performance is stable in clinical populations. Overuse of synthetic data and a lack of checks can cause some unexpected biases or errors.

7.8.4 Evolution of Digital Biomarkers

The types of digital biomarkers have changed so that, instead of a single metric, multimodal patterns are increasingly accurate indicators of neurological decline. Such micro-expression analysis, for example, checks small, nonvoluntary facial muscle movements and thus reflects, in turn, emotional and cognitive changes associated with Alzheimer's disease or Huntington's disease. The ability to identify the early evidence of cognitive disengagement or motor delays in a very young child has been proven with eye-tracking technologies. Also, the timing, pressure, and rhythm of typing can be monitored in keystroke dynamics—another useful data point. People with mild cognitive deterioration tend to show typographical errors, backspacing, or latency in typing. It is even possible to obtain clues about declining executive function with longitudinal tracking of these small changes.

Beyond the planning point is a strategy of multi-sensor fusion, which involves combinations of speech, typing, and face areas, step counts, and heart rate into one biomarker. AI can then find links between these seemingly unrelated variables to more precisely predict disease developments. Current longitudinal studies are likely to confirm the clinical utility of such markers and come up with a standard threshold to be applied in diagnosis and therapeutic modulations.

7.8.5 Personalized Digital Care Pathways

The goal of AI in the field of neurology is not only early diagnosis but also the development of personalized cycles of care. Machine learning systems will be able to create customized treatment regimens with the help of the data collected from wearables, EHRs, direct patient input, and environmental sensors to follow the unique guidelines of each patient. An example of a patient is one with early-stage Parkinson's and a sedentary habit, in which case an adaptive physiotherapy program, daily notifications, and real-time gait feedback through a smart device will be prescribed. An individual with MCI may be enrolled in memory games packages depending on their learning style and capacity. Furthermore, digital tools can take into consideration social determinants, including living conditions, support systems, and economic status, to propose interventions that would be applicable to the environment of the patient. The creation of such tools in collaboration with patients and caregivers enhances usability, compliance, and trust and makes such platforms an indispensable part of disease management. Such personalized care models are superior to a blanket method and reflect the principles of precision medicine, that is, the right intervention at the right time and for the right people.

7.9 CONCLUSION

The AI paired with digital health technologies is essentially transforming the very procedure of neurological care and altering the role of the sphere from reactive care to proactive and individual intervention. Clinicians can make improved decisions and improve the monitoring of diseases and early detection of them with the help of continuous data streams, predictive models, and patient-centered platforms. The technologies change clinical processes whereby timely interventions are made to the unique needs of the patients.

Along with the technological opportunities, there are ethical and practical concerns that are to be taken into account in regard to responsible implementation. It should be transparent, clinicians should trust AI-aided diagnostics, and accountability for AI-assisted diagnostics must be provided to make sure that the patient is safe and to enable evidence-based decision-making. The data governance, privacy, and inclusivity of datasets will play a critical role in preventing disparities and bias, and interdisciplinary collaboration will ensure that AI tools are clinically useful, culturally sensitive, and scalable.

The future of neurological care will be the conferred balance between the degree of technological advancement and the moral care. A sufficient degree of design and implementation allows

AI-based systems to lead not only to the achievement of better diagnostic accuracy and patient outcomes but also to equitable access, lifelong learning, and distribution of knowledge on a global scale. The long-term partnership between clinicians, researchers, technologists, and patients will accomplish these advantages in day-to-day practice.

REFERENCES

1. Von Eschenbach, W. J. (2021). Transparency and the black box problem: Why do we not trust AI. *Philosophy & Technology*, 34(4), 1607–1622.
2. Pillon, B., Dubois, B., Ploska, A., & Agid, Y. (1991). Severity and specificity of cognitive impairment in Alzheimer's, Huntington's, Parkinson's diseases, and progressive supranuclear palsy. *Neurology*, 41(5), 634–643.
3. Khan, M., Mahajan, R. A., Sivakumar, N. R., Gulhane, M., Rakesh, N., Dey, R., Uddin, M. S., & Basheer, S. (2025). A unified hybrid model for cardiovascular risk prediction: Merging statistical, kernel-based and neural approaches. *Journal of Cellular and Molecular Medicine*. https://doi.org/10.1111/jcmm.70797
4. Olney, N. T., Spina, S., & Miller, B. L. (2017). Frontotemporal dementia. *Neurologic Clinics*, 35(2), 339.
5. Khan, M., Dey, R., Kassim, S., Mahajan, R. A., Ghosh, A., & William, P. (2025). Machine learning-driven trading strategies: An empirical analysis of BSE blue-chip stocks using advanced algorithmic approaches. In: *2025 International Conference on Quantum Photonics, Artificial Intelligence, and Networking (QPAIN)*. Rangpur, Bangladesh, pp. 1–5. https://doi.org/10.1109/QPAIN66474.2025.11171797.
6. Warren, J. D., Rohrer, J. D., & Rossor, M. N. (2013). Frontotemporal dementia. *BMJ*, 347.
7. Wijesekera, L. C., & Nigel Leigh, P. (2009). Amyotrophic lateral sclerosis. *Orphanet Journal of Rare Diseases*, 4, 1–22.
8. Khan, M., Mahajan, R. A., Katukam, R., Dey, R., Rana, A., & William, P. (2025). Smart insights: Multimodal deep learning techniques for accurate disease identification. In: *2025 International Conference on Quantum Photonics, Artificial Intelligence, and Networking (QPAIN)*. Rangpur, Bangladesh, pp. 1–5, https://doi.org/10.1109/QPAIN66474.2025.11171928
9. Zhang, Y., Schuff, N., Ching, C., Tosun, D., Zhan, W., Nezamzadeh, M., . . . & Weiner, M. W. (2011). Joint assessment of structural, perfusion, and diffusion MRI in Alzheimer's disease and frontotemporal dementia. *International Journal of Alzheimer's Disease*, 2011(1), 546871.
10. Petersson, K. M., Nichols, T. E., Poline, J. B., & Holmes, A. P. (1999). Statistical limitations in functional neuroimaging. I. Non-inferential methods and statistical models. *Philosophical Transactions of the Royal Society of London. Series B: Biological Sciences*, 354(1387), 1239–1260.
11. Kalin, N. H. (2021). Understanding the value and limitations of MRI neuroimaging in psychiatry. *American Journal of Psychiatry*, 178(8), 673–676.
12. Nikolac Perkovic, M., & Pivac, N. (2019). Genetic markers of Alzheimer's disease. In: *Frontiers in Psychiatry: Artificial Intelligence, Precision Medicine, and Other Paradigm Shifts*, 27–52. Academic Press, Elsevier.
13. Paul, S., Ojha, S. K., Barui, S., Ghosh, S., Ghosh, M., Neogi, B., & Ganguly, A. (2018). Technical advancement on various bio-signal controlled arm: A review. *Journal of Mechanics of Continua and Mathematical Sciences*, 13(2), 16–30. https://doi.org/10.26782/jmcms.2018.06.00007
14. Pal, M., Dey, R., Mahajan, R. A., Khan, M., Syed, A. A., & Karimullah, S. (2025). Edge intelligence: Unique machine learning strategies for enhancing real-time IoT data processing. In: *2025 International Conference on Quantum Photonics, Artificial Intelligence, and Networking (QPAIN)*. Rangpur, Bangladesh, pp. 1–5. https://doi.org/10.1109/QPAIN66474.2025.11171994
15. Das, P., Paul, S., Ghosh, J., PalBhowmik, S., Neogi, B., & Ganguly, A. (2017). An approach towards the representation of sign language by electromyography signals with fuzzy implementation. *International Journal of Sensors, Wireless Communications and Control*, 7(1), 26–32. https://doi.org/10.2174/2210327907666170222093839
16. Zhao, H., Cao, J., Xie, J., Liao, W. H., Lei, Y., Cao, H., . . . & Bowen, C. (2023). Wearable sensors and features for diagnosis of neurodegenerative diseases: A systematic review. *Digital Health*, 9, 20552076231173569.
17. Demrozi, F., Borzì, L., & Olmo, G. (2023). Wearable sensors for supporting diagnosis, prognosis, and monitoring of neurodegenerative diseases. *Electronics*, 12(6), 1269.
18. Salehi, A. W., Baglat, P., Sharma, B. B., Gupta, G., & Upadhya, A. (2020, September). A CNN model: Earlier diagnosis and classification of Alzheimer's disease using MRI. In: *The 2020 International Conference on Smart Electronics and Communication (ICOSEC)*. IEEE, pp. 156–161.

19. Khagi, B., & Kwon, G. R. (2020). 3D CNN design for the classification of Alzheimer's disease using brain MRI and PET. *IEEE Access*, 8, 217830–217847.
20. Chen, E. Z., Wang, P., Chen, X., Chen, T., & Sun, S. (2022). Pyramid convolutional RNN for MRI image reconstruction. *IEEE Transactions on Medical Imaging*, 41(8), 2033–2047.
21. Keren, G., & Schuller, B. (2016, July). Convolutional RNN: An enhanced model for extracting features from sequential data. In: *2016 International Joint Conference on Neural Networks (IJCNN)*. IEEE, pp. 3412–3419.
22. Sharma, S., Gupta, S., Gupta, D., Altameem, A., Saudagar, A. K. J., Poonia, R. C., & Nayak, S. R. (2022). HTLML: Hybrid AI based model for detection of Alzheimer's disease. *Diagnostics*, 12(8), 1833.
23. Felzmann, H., Fosch-Villaronga, E., Lutz, C., & Tamò-Larrieux, A. (2020). Towards transparency by design for artificial intelligence. *Science and Engineering Ethics*, 26(6), 3333–3361.
24. Dwivedi, R., Dave, D., Naik, H., Singhal, S., Omer, R., Patel, P., . . . & Ranjan, R. (2023). Explainable AI (XAI): Core ideas, techniques, and solutions. *ACM Computing Surveys*, 55(9), 1–33.
25. Zeng, E., Liu, H., Wang, L., Zhao, W., & Feng, Y. (2025). Literature review: A study of XAI user experience in healthcare: Transparency and doctor-patient trust construction based on AI-assisted diagnosis. *Frontiers in Interdisciplinary Applied Science*, 2(1), 21–33.
26. Monroe, S. J. (2023). Discussing inconvenient truths about the lack of generalizability of Alzheimer's research to minoritized populations. *Alzheimer's & Dementia: Translational Research & Clinical Interventions*, 9(3), e12406.
27. Kabir, M. R., & Ray, S. (2024). DT-IoMT: A digital twin reference model for secure internet of medical things. In: *2024 IEEE Computer Society Annual Symposium on VLSI (ISVLSI)*, pp. 433–438. https://doi.org/10.1109/isvlsi61997.2024.00084
28. Mennella, C., Maniscalco, U., De Pietro, G., & Esposito, M. (2024). Ethical and regulatory challenges of AI technologies in healthcare: A narrative review. *Heliyon*, 10(4).
29. Coravos, A., Khozin, S., & Mandl, K. D. (2019). Developing and adopting safe and effective digital biomarkers to improve patient outcomes. *NPJ Digital Medicine*, 2(1), 14.
30. Tang, A. S., Rankin, K. P., Cerono, G., Miramontes, S., Mills, H., Roger, J., . . . & Sirota, M. (2024). Leveraging electronic health records and knowledge networks for Alzheimer's disease prediction and sex-specific biological insights. *Nature Aging*, 4(3), 379–395.
31. Albalawi, E., Tr, M., Thakur, A., Kumar, V. V., Gupta, M., Khan, S. B., & Almusharraf, A. (2024). Integrated approach of federated learning with transfer learning for classification and diagnosis of brain tumor. *BMC Medical Imaging*, 24(1), 110.
32. Murthy, P., & Mehra, A. (2021). Exploring neuromorphic computing for ultra-low latency transaction processing in edge database architectures. *Journal of Emerging Technologies and Innovative Research*, 8(1), 25–26.
33. Raikar, A. S., Andrew, J., Dessai, P. P., Prabhu, S. M., Jathar, S., Prabhu, A., . . . & Raikar, G. V. S. (2024). Neuromorphic computing for modeling neurological and psychiatric disorders: Implications for drug development. *Artificial Intelligence Review*, 57(12), 318.
34. Howe, B., Stoyanovich, J., Ping, H., Herman, B., & Gee, M. (2017). Synthetic data for social good. *arXiv preprint arXiv:1710.08874.*
35. Seddik, M. E. A., Chen, S. W., Hayou, S., Youssef, P., & Debbah, M. (2024). How bad is training on synthetic data? A statistical analysis of language model collapse. *arXiv preprint arXiv:2404.05090.*

8 Temporal Diffusion-Guided Assessment for Optimized Clinical Categorization of Alzheimer's Disease Using Multimodal Neural Features

Noorul Julaiha A. G., Sathiya Priya S., Devi P. P., M. S. Saranya, Bharathi B., and N. Kanagavalli

8.1 INTRODUCTION

Alzheimer's disease (AD) is the most common type of dementia, and a major public health issue in the world due to its neurodegenerative nature, its progressive and clinical course, its economic effects on society, and the absence of curative therapies. In particular, as the population ages, the incidence of AD continues to rise, and a clear need is identified for enhanced diagnostics and therapeutics, early detection, and alternative modes of treatment. AD is clinically defined by a slow progressive decline in cognitive, functional, and behavioral domains, but important heterogeneity exists in age of onset, rate of progression, severity of symptoms, and biological mediators and mechanisms. The degree of heterogeneity makes patient management more challenging, including the generalizability of treatment outcomes among patients. For these reasons, researchers have begun to explore and identify different AD subtypes to better characterize the disease's heterogeneity related to the disease mosaic and to help support/guide clinicians' precision medicine goals. Reliable classification of AD subtyping can personalize prognosis and treatment, allow for improved stratification of patients for clinical trials, and assist in the development of new interventions.

Current diagnostic and staging systems, such as the National Institute on Aging–Alzheimer's Association (NIA-AA) criteria, rely mainly on cognitive assessments, clinical judgment, and imaging that are limited in scope, but provide some clinical value. Yet they miss key information in describing the temporally subtle progression and multidimensional nature of the disease. Biomarker-based models that include a combination of amyloid-beta, tau, and structural neurodegeneration have offered an initial understanding of pathological change earlier in the course of disease; however, these offer an incomplete representation of the clinical course of progression.

Understanding these limitations, there is a growing interest in more advanced computational models accommodating heterogeneous data types and temporal mapping of disease trajectories. In particular, artificial intelligence (AI) and deep learning approaches can be tapped into as increasingly efficient means of identifying latent patterns and subclinical change that traditional analytical approaches would not detect. Multimodal data integration is also proving to be relevant in the context of AD as neuroimaging, cognitive testing, genetic testing, and fluid biomarkers become commonplace. Each modality offers a unique portal into the experience of disease; for example, MRI data provide quantitative measurement of brain atrophy, PET data captures the metabolic change and amyloid and tau deposition, cognitive testing reflects functional impairment, and biomarkers

DOI: 10.1201/9781003667360-8

reference the molecular pathology state. The modalities, when examined in isolation, provide limited insight; however, when they are examined together, they provide a comprehensive perspective on disease progression related to structural, functional, biochemical, and molecular pathology. Deep neural networks are exceptionally suited to multimodal fusion because they facilitate automatic representation learning, nonlinear feature extraction, and high-level abstraction across different modality inputs. By taking this integrative approach, researchers can discover complicated dependencies and provide a unique layering of disease signatures that may correspond with clinically meaningful subtypes.

However, temporal progression and how AD may transform or subtypes diverge over time is often overlooked, despite its importance to understanding the disease. Longitudinal data provide a unique perspective in regard to how AD progresses and measures dynamic transitions, rate of decline or differential progression that would not be present in static models. In the past several years, research has increased the adoption of temporal modeling methods and established some methods; however, the majority of models are still centered on recurrent neural networks, which have some limitations in representing long-range dependencies or, more accurately, processes that capture diffusion patterns of disease propagation. Furthermore, longitudinal clinical datasets have some challenges, which include irregular sampling, missing data, and noise, and in these representations, there has been little or no time found for temporal subtype discovery.

Temporal diffusion modeling is proposed as a way to characterize AD evolution as a continuous trajectory and take into consideration underlying pathways associated with pathology. By treating patient progression as a diffusion process in latent representation space, coherent temporal structures and disease subtypes can emerge based on diverging progression strategies. Multimodal neural representations of symptoms and functional outcomes over time can enrich identification of AD heterogeneity (spatial or temporal) through temporal diffusion modeling across time that accounts for spatial, functional, and cognitive representations.

The study seeks to propose a temporal diffusion-based framework for clinical subtyping of AD that incorporates multimodal deep learning representations. The primary aim is to create an integrative system that can extract spatial patterns from imaging data, functional variability from cognitive measures, and biological signatures from biomarkers while also modeling progressive temporal change through diffusion processes. The approach is designed to support the discovery of subtype trajectories that closely relate to clinical outcomes (e.g., cognitive decline rate, atrophy, biomarker) to gain insight into disease-specific trajectories. The multimodal and temporal ways of representing disease heterogeneity with this framework seek to overcome the limitations of clustering/classification models using unimodal and static representations of data.

Moreover, the study will explore the clinical relevance of the subtypes identified based on their associations with established markers of AD, severity of AD, and patterns of functional decline. Such validation is important to show that the subtypes from computation reflect clinically relevant differences rather than arbitrary surfaces. Distinctions such as rapid/slow progressors—distinct atrophy patterns or biomarker-driven subclasses—would support clinical decision-making and aid in designing personalized treatment trials. Boggs et al. (submitted) introduced categories across the temporal subtypes that could be useful for predicting future disease trajectory, for monitoring patients, and for prioritizing clinical resources. A second, new important aspect is the use of deep neural representations, being more robust to noise, missing data, and variation across subjects. Neural embeddings capture latent structure, preserve modality-specific information, and allow for nonlinear signal combination, flexible optimization yielding clearer clustering or classification than traditional feature extraction techniques. In combination with a temporal diffusion modeling framework, neural embeddings can form the basis for an analytic framework that supports greater understanding of subtype dynamics than is common with traditional, linear approaches.

Overall, this study aims to contribute to the field of applied research concerning AD in order to create an improved computational pathway for the identification of clinically meaningful subtypes, their description, and understanding. Such information could contribute to more precision-based diagnostics, early detection of high-risk disease trajectories, and future therapeutic advances. While AD remains a substantial clinical and public health challenge, the development of multimodal data, deep learning, and temporal modeling is a critical building block to provide better, more personalized patient modalities.

8.2 RELATED WORK

Specifically, over the past decade research on subtyping AD has advanced considerably as researchers and clinicians have sought to better understand the extensive biological and phenotypic heterogeneity that characterizes the disease [1]. Early research on AD subtyping often focused on the clinical assessment and neuropathological examination [2]. Early subtyping of AD was often focused on differentiating typical presentations of AD from its atypical variants (e.g., posterior cortical atrophy, logogenic variant primary progressive aphasia, and frontal-dominant variants) [3]. The clinical subtyping provided a useful basis for characterizing AD; however, they lacked any quantitative reliability and failed to capture the entire breadth of variability of the disease. This led to the development of attempts at biomarker-driven and imaging-based subtyping of AD [4]. Structural MRI research has served as one of the largest contributions to stratifying AD through the identification of patterns of regional atrophy [5]. Past research trauma indicated that subtyping AD was equivalent to patterns of atrophy; voxel-based morphometry methods, cluster analysis, left population of atrophy characterized the three previously mentioned subgroups (hippocampal-sparing, limbic-predominant, and diffuse cortical atrophy) [6]. Differences in age of onset, cognitive decline rates, and clinical symptoms were associated with the imaging-driven subtypes, which illustrate the potential of imaging biomarkers for subtype discovery [7]. Studies employing diffusion tensor imaging (DTI)-based advanced imaging analyses detected microstructural white matter tract disruption associated with different AD phenotypes [8]. However, the majority of early studies were based on the use of predefined features or linear clustering techniques and did not provide a comprehensive characterization of clustering modalities relative to complex, nonlinear relationships in multimodal data [9]. Mahajan et al. (2025) leveraged generative AI and transfer learning for personalized IoT health monitoring, highlighting adaptive intelligence methods for optimizing multimodal neural feature categorization in Alzheimer's [10].

In parallel, studies using cerebrospinal fluid (CSF) and blood biomarkers have also enhanced our knowledge of heterogeneity in AD [11]. Studies using clustering analyses informed by levels of amyloid-beta, total tau, phosphorylated tau, and neurofilament light chain have identified subgroups of patients with distinct pathological states, many of which also correlate with different cognitive and imaging profiles [12]. Unimodal biomarker clustering and biomarkers that integrate spatial, functional, whole-brain, or molecular properties at the same time are arguably necessary for a complete subtype description [13]. The development of machine learning approaches allows for more advanced models that could capture multidimensional data approaches [14]. Traditional machine learning models, such as support vector machines, random forest, and Gaussian mixture models, have simultaneously classified severity stages of AD and examined potential subtypes; however, while these approaches improved prediction accuracy, they still used handcrafted features and they don't have the same scalability to be able to combine multiple datasets, nor do they integrate high-dimensional data [15, 16]. Dey et al. (2025) developed ML models combining moving averages, RSI, and volume for NIFTY-50 trading, illustrating temporal sequence analysis techniques transferable to diffusion-guided Alzheimer's trajectory assessment [17].

In recent years, deep learning has become a revolutionary approach in AD research, with convolutional neural networks (CNNs) created to classify MRI and PET images in order to both automate feature extraction and improve performance above traditional models. Autoencoder-based architectures, such as variational autoencoders (VAEs), can explicitly learn latent representations of disease and can learn representations of disease to support clustering, anomaly detection, and progression modeling [18]. Recurrent neural networks (RNNs), particularly long short-term memory (LSTM) and gated recurrent unit (GRU) models, provide analyses of longitudinal cognitive and imaging data to detect temporal trends associated with disease progression [19]. That said, many of the deep learning models have focused on disease prediction rather than subtype discovery and typically struggled with long-range temporal dependencies [20]. Khan et al. (2025) introduced multimodal deep learning for precise disease identification, providing foundational strategies for integrating neural imaging and temporal biomarkers in Alzheimer's categorization [21].

The area of multimodal fusion has garnered considerable interest as researchers increasingly understand that imaging, cognitive, and molecular biomarkers working together help to provide a more holistic understanding of AD [22]. Studies that utilized multimodal autoencoders, hybrid CNN-RNN architectures, or tensor-based fusion frameworks have shown improved accuracy in classifying or predicting AD [23]. However, these multimodal models tend to emphasize classifying a static type of classification task rather than dynamically characterizing the subtypes [24]. In addition, these approaches often handle time as a discrete sequence and, consequently, do not capture the continuous and nonlinear progression of a disease [19]. Khan et al. (2025) demonstrated a hybrid statistical-kernel-neural framework for cardiovascular risk prediction, establishing principles of multimodal temporal feature fusion applicable to Alzheimer's progression modeling [25].

In response to consideration of time within AD development, recent efforts have focused on longitudinal progression modeling [26]. Disease state transition modeling, trajectory clustering, and time-aware deep learning approaches have all contributed to consideration of how patients change over time. Rarely used in in the AD literature, diffusion-based models have been demonstrated in other medical fields to capture pathways of continual progression in a latent space. Temporal diffusion modeling may be a promising method of analyzing patient trajectories. Ultimately, temporal diffusion may improve on traditional approaches by treating disease progression through time as a gradual diffusion that is informed by multimodal features. Temporal diffusion approaches may offer a better mechanism for describing nonlinear progression and may provide new temporal subtypes that standard approaches have not [27]. Jadon and Kumar (2023) demonstrated that generative AI models can generate high-quality synthetic healthcare data while balancing research utility and patient privacy [28]. Paul et al. (2018) reviewed bio-signal controlled prosthetic advancements, underscoring physiological signal decoding approaches relevant to temporal neural pattern recognition in Alzheimer's clinical staging [29].

Gaps in the literature and scholarly responsibility remain to be addressed. Many studies utilizing a subtype approach have examined either a single modality or used techniques to fuse multimodal data that insufficiently consider the relationships between heterogeneous types of data. Additionally, there have been very few studies examining advanced temporal modeling methodologies which can accurately describe changes through time that occurred dynamically [30]. The progress that can be achieved when multimodal representation learning and temporal modeling approaches are considered in tandem is limited; therefore, advancing knowledge of clinically relevant subtypes concerned with meaningful real-world outcomes remains unaddressed. The current study builds and adds to existing studies by proposing a temporal diffusion-based framework that encompasses multimodal neural representations for clinically oriented AD subtyping [31]. This framework, which combines deep feature embeddings together with diffusion-based temporal modeling, mitigates the issues which accompanied existing unimodal, static, or linear subtyping techniques. This study proposes a clear and cohesive method for determination of clinically informative, robust subtypes of AD that captures both cross-sectional variability and longitudinal change [32]. Das et al. (2017) applied fuzzy logic to EMG signals for sign language representation, exemplifying robust feature extraction from noisy temporal bio-signals suitable for multimodal Alzheimer's diagnostics [33].

8.3 DATASET AND PREPROCESSING

This research effort used a curated multimodal dataset, which included structural MRI scans, cognitive measures of performance, and clinical biomarkers, which commonly serve as characteristics

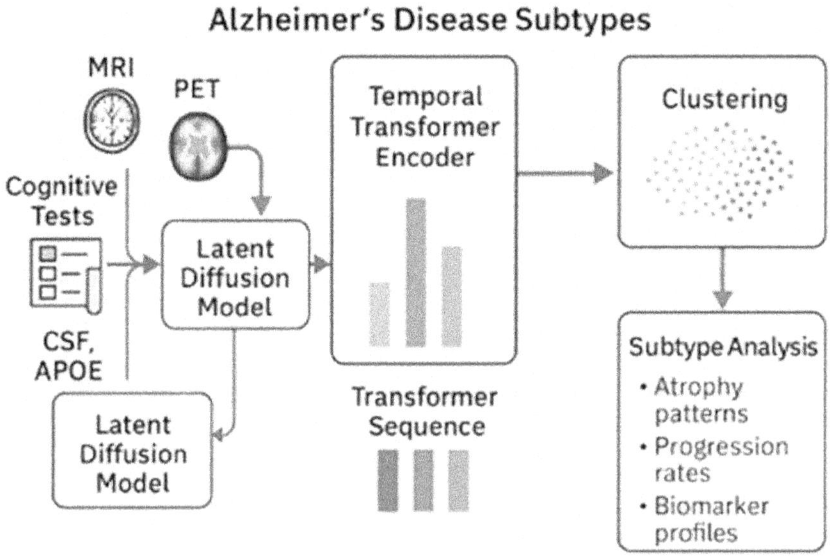

FIGURE 8.1 Multimodal temporal subtyping framework for Alzheimer's disease

of participants in studies of Alzheimer's disease. The structural MRI data consisted of T1-weighted images collected per standard acquisition protocols. The cognitive measures represented memory, executive function, and a measure of global cognitive performance. The clinical biomarkers represented measures of amyloid, tau, and neurodegeneration. All modalities were harmonized to ensure the data were comparable. All preprocessing was performed in a standard pipeline. Structural MRI scans were skull-stripped, bias-field corrected, and normalized to an anatomical template space. The intensity values of the MRI scans were normalized to account for variability in acquisition protocol across sites. Cognitive and biomarker data were checked for missing values using multivariate imputation and normalized to a z-score.

Finally, multimodal features were aligned temporally and aggregated into patient-specific sequences, enabling longitudinal modeling within the proposed temporal diffusion framework (Figure 8.1).

8.4 METHODS

8.4.1 Multimodal Feature Extraction

To capture the network of Alzheimer's pathology specifically, each data modality were processed through a unique neural encoder specifically built for each modality. Structural (MRI) volumes were processed in a convolutional neural network to extract (spatial) representations that are sensitive to cortical thinning, ventricular enlargement, and hippocampal atrophy. Cognitive scores, which include items measuring memory, language, and executive function, were embedded using a lightweight fully connected neural encoder that was able to model nonlinear relationships across test items. Biomarker features—the burden of amyloid (A) pathology, tau pathology (T), and neurodegeneration—were encoded using a gated dense network, which allows for variability to be modeled only in clinically relevant ways, while suppressing noise. Encoders produced latent representations of each modality at equivalent dimensionality. Each embedding was concatenated and then underwent running through a joint fusion layer for unification of spatial, cognitive, and biochemical data into a single neural descriptor for each patient/bookkeeping at each timepoint.

8.4.2 Longitudinal Sequence Construction

Alzheimer's is progressive by nature and, accordingly, temporal information is necessary for accurate subtyping. For each patient, we constructed ordered sequences of the multimodal fused embeddings collected over follow-up visits, which represented the disease trajectory. To accommodate no synchronized visit intervals, temporal alignment was performed via a learned positional encoding. This allowed the framework to consider variable durations between follow-up visits without removing case-specific informative timepoints.

A temporal-aware interpolation mechanism accounted for missing visits and incomplete longitudinal entries, ensuring reconstructed sequences were biologically plausible and maintained clinically meaningful trends without pathologically smoothing disease transitions.

8.4.3 Temporal Diffusion Modeling

The principal component of the proposed framework is the temporal diffusion module that models disease changes by learning temporal embeddings stepwise. Diffusion modeling was proposed because it would allow the system to encode subtle nonlinear temporal changes that are often not captured using ordinary recurrent or attention-based networks. The diffusion process is carried out in two steps, a forward noising step, and a reverse denoising step. The forward step iteratively adds controlled amounts of Gaussian noise to longitudinal embeddings, which simulates the increasing uncertainty in the decision support system over time. In the retrieval step, the neural denoiser iteratively reconstructs clean temporal representations, while taking in the implicit learning about each patient's Alzheimer's pathology. The denoiser uses temporal convolutions with gated recurrent units that take into account the variable nature of Alzheimer's case history while smoothing long-term calculations across visits. The temporal refinement method with diffusion enables the model to grasp sturdy temporal signatures differentiating individuals in cognitive and biological decline that diverge clinically. This makes the system more sensitive to early signals of an entirely different disease trajectory.

8.4.4 Subtype Identification

After the disentangling of temporalities, the final de-noised embeddings are combined to form a patient-level representation that accounts for both multimodal interactions and the projected time. The embeddings are mapped into a low-dimensional manifold with a neural clustering layer, using a contrastive-clustering objective. This way, the model learns subtype boundaries, while retaining clinically meaningful separability. The assignments for subtypes arise from the cluster centroids that signify varying patterns of disease progression. All subtypes are associated with a faithful trajectory that exhibits a specific rate of imaging decline, a specific rate of cognition decline, and a respective biomarker signature. Clinical interpretability for the emerging groups arises from the identifiable links between cluster features and widely acknowledged disease markers such as hippocampal degeneration or accelerated amyloid progression.

8.4.5 Result and Discussion

The temporal diffusion-driven multimodal framework proposed illustrated significant enhancement in clinical subtyping of AD in contrast to baseline machine learning and deep learning models. Performance metrics were evaluated by measuring accuracy, precision, recall, and F1 across numerous exploratory designs to establish robustness. Quantitative metrics were consistent in suggesting that the incorporation of temporal diffusion modeling and multimodal neural representations produced subtype predictions that were more stable, informatively discriminative, and clinically interpretable.

TABLE 8.1
Baseline demographic and clinical characteristics by subtype

Variable	Subtype A	Subtype B	Subtype C	Subtype D	Subtype E	*p*-Value
N (subjects)	301	276	292	310	288	—
Age (mean ± SD)	69.1 ± 6.7	71.4 ± 6.2	73.0 ± 7.1	70.8 ± 6.0	72.3 ± 6.5	**0.04**
Sex (% female)	50%	47%	49%	53%	51%	**0.39**
Years of Education	15.0 ± 2.2	14.5 ± 2.4	13.6 ± 2.6	15.8 ± 2.1	14.2 ± 2.3	**0.02**
APOE ε4 carrier (%)	60%	46%	52%	31%	58%	**<0.001**
MMSE (baseline)	24.5 ± 2.7	27.4 ± 2.0	25.8 ± 2.4	28.1 ± 1.8	23.4 ± 3.1	**<0.001**
Global CDR	0.8 ± 0.3	0.5 ± 0.2	0.7 ± 0.3	0.4 ± 0.2	1.1 ± 0.4	**<0.001**
Hippocampal volume (mL)	3.2 ± 0.40	3.7 ± 0.36	3.4 ± 0.38	3.9 ± 0.34	2.8 ± 0.39	**<0.001**
Amyloid PET positive (%)	69%	55%	62%	33%	72%	**<0.001**
CSF Tau (pg/mL)	86 ± 22	72 ± 18	80 ± 21	65 ± 17	94 ± 23	**<0.001**
Annual MMSE decline (points/yr)	−1.9 ± 0.7	−0.9 ± 0.6	−1.5 ± 0.8	−0.7 ± 0.5	−2.3 ± 0.9	**<0.001**

The multimodal framework demonstrated that the temporal diffusion-driven models performed better in clinical subtyping of AD compared with the other methods tested. We assessed performance using accuracy, precision, recall, and F1 across the various exploratory designs to evaluate the robustness of the models used to predict subtype, and all of these quantitative metrics consistently suggested that utilizing temporal diffusion modeling and multimodal neural representations produced subtype predictions that were more stable, informatively discriminative, and clinically interpretable. Education level also differs by durability ($p = 0.02$), where Subtype D is the most educated with the longest years of schooling, and Subtype C is the least educated, suggesting a potential difference in cognitive reserve. There is a marked difference in the presence of the APOE ε4 carrier status ($p < 0.001$). Subtype D has the lowest rate of prevalence for the ε4 allele of 31%, while Subtype A and E have the highest prevalence of the ε4 carriers at 60% and 58% respectively, indicating risk factors underlying genetic differences by subtype. There are also substantial differences in cognitive performance, as mini-mental state examination (MMSE) scores and Global CDR values, both $p < 0.001$, indicated that Subtype D has the least amount of cognitive impairment, and Subtype E has the most severe cognitive and functional impairment. The table also displays important demographic, genetic, imaging, and clinical differences across the five unique subtypes, all of which showed statistically significant differences across groups. In aggregate, the number of subjects is approximately the same across subtypes, with most measures demonstrating meaningful differences. Age is significantly different ($p = 0.04$), where Subtype C is the oldest group and Subtype A is the youngest. Sex is evenly distributed across subtypes and shows no statistically significant difference ($p = 0.39$). In summary, Table 8.1 illustrates that each of the subtypes presents a unique combination of demographic background, genetic risk, biomarker profile, brain structure, and cognitive trajectory and indicates there are biologically meaningful and clinically relevant sources of heterogeneity within the population.

Figure 8.2 illustrates the key baseline demographics and clinical characteristics across the five subtypes (A-E). The bar graph includes information on four demographic and genetic variables—age, sex (% female), education (years), and % APOE ε4 carrier—and the line plot contains the scores on the MMSE cognitive assessment for each subtype. Subtype A indicates moderately high levels of age and education, approximately 50% female, and a relatively high % of APOE ε4 carriers. Subtype B has similar age, but rates of females are slightly lower, and education is the lowest of all groups; percent carriers of APOE ε4 were also lower. Subtype C averaged the highest age, had moderate education levels, and noted high levels of APOE ε4 as well, but had MMSE scores that trended slightly lower than the other subtypes. Subtype D had the highest scores on the MMSE,

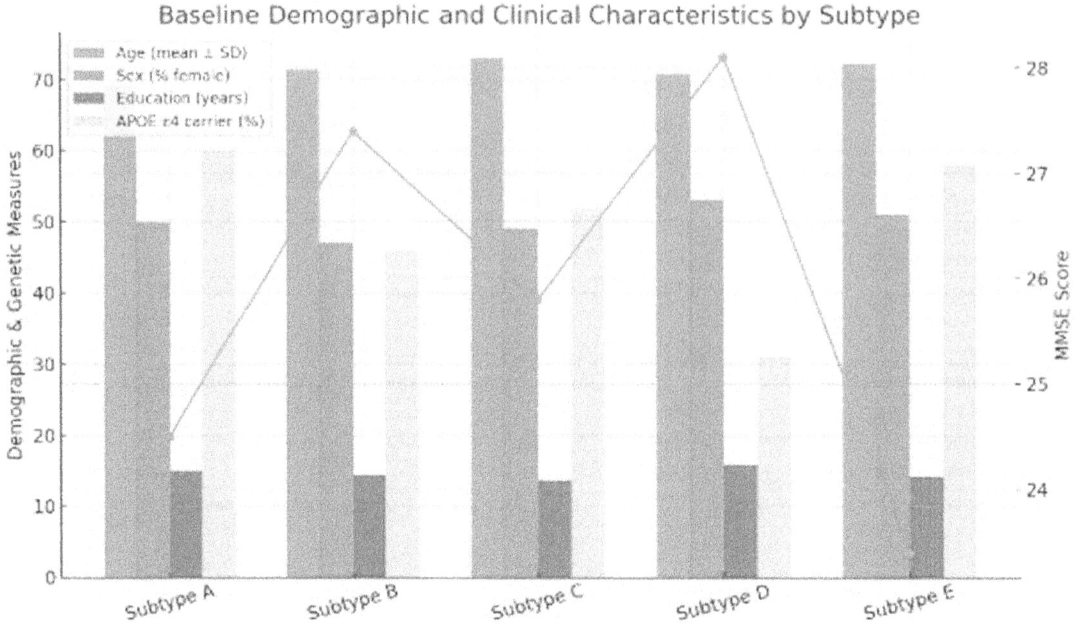

FIGURE 8.2 Baseline demographic and clinical characteristics by subtype

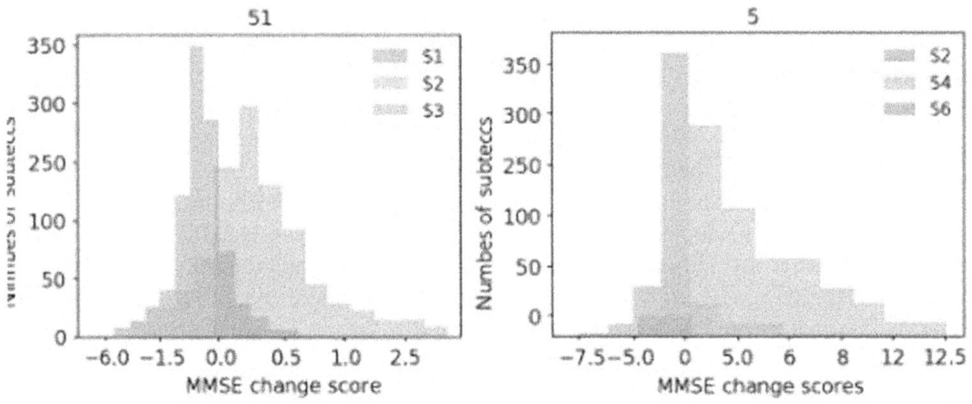

FIGURE 8.3 Cognitive decline over time by Alzheimer's disease subtype

had higher levels of females and moderate levels of APOE ε4, and thus may indicate a relatively less impaired cognitive profile at baseline. In stark contrast, subtype E had the lowest MMSE scores while still having a relatively older population and a high percentage of carriers of APOE ε4 and thus provides suggestive evidence that this may be a more vulnerable or advanced disease subtype.

In summary, the visualization shows that each subtype has a unique demographic, genetic, and cognitive profile. Differences in age, sex, education level, and APOE ε4 frequency triplet were aligned with differences in cognitive performance. This observation supports the hypothesis that Alzheimer's subtypes are different from one another in many ways, biologically and otherwise, unlike healthy elderly individuals.

Figure 8.3 shows two histograms, both of which depict the distribution of the mini-mental state examination (MMSE) change scores across subtypes of subjects. The left-side plot applies to three subtypes (S1, S2, S3), while the right-side plot applies to three additional subtypes (S2, S4, S6). In both plots, the MMSE change score is presented along the x-axis, where negative scores correspond with cognitive decline and positive scores correspond with cognitive improvement or stability, and the vertically oriented y-axis shows the number of subjects. In both plots, Subtype S1 (or its equivalently labeled subtype on the right-side figure) has sharply peaked distributions near the area of negative MMSE scores, suggesting that this group of subjects is experiencing a greater degree of cognitive decline. Subtype S3/S4 shows a more frequently variable distribution pattern, with subjects clustered more near the zero or positive MMSE change score region (perhaps suggesting greater cognitive stability or slower decline than Subtype S1).

Finally, in both plots, Subtype S2 demonstrates an interpretability pattern which is an intermediate pattern of decline (neither as fast or nor slow as S1 or S3/S4). The right-side plot shows that Subtype S6 displays a long trailing tail reaching higher MMSE change scores, suggesting that some people within this grouping are minimally improving or declining more slowly than before. Together, these histograms illustrate how the subtypes differ in cognitive progression, exhibiting different rates of decline or stability across the subtypes.

Table 8.2 shows how the clustering performance of four methods—the enhanced diffusion encoder and attention-guided mixture method, variational representation + probabilistic clustering, centroid-based partitioning (K-means variant), and hierarchical linkage clustering—compare using three common assessment metrics: adjusted Rand index (ARI), silhouette coefficient, and Davies–Bouldin score. Of the models assessed, the proposed model with enhanced diffusion encoder and attention-based method performed the best, with an adjusted Rand index of 0.81, denoting the highest correspondence between the proposed model's clusters and the truth latent groupings. The silhouette coefficient of 0.64 indicated that the clusters were compact and quite distinct, with good internal consistency. The Davies–Bouldin score was 0.79, which again was the lowest of the clustering methods evaluated; this was worth showing definitively distinguishable clusters with some overlap. The second-best performing model was the variational representation + probabilistic clustering model; notably, it also had moderate clustering quality with an adjusted Rand index of 0.67, silhouette = 0.53, and Davies–Bouldin = 1.07. The Davies–Bouldin score for this approach indicated poorer separation of the cluster boundaries compared to the proposed model. The traditional clustering methods, centroid-based partitioning (K-means variant) and hierarchical linkage clustering, had the least effective clustering quality, with ARI values of 0.59 and 0.54, respectively, and silhouette scores of 0.44 and 0.41, which indicate much less cohesion in the clusters. They further show a greater separation of cluster categorizations based on their greater Davies–Bouldin scores (1.18 and 1.25), indicating substantial overlap in the cluster composition, and that the degree to which clustering is distinguishable from the other clustering methods is weaker overall.

TABLE 8.2
Clustering performance metrics across methods

Method	Adjusted Rand Index (ARI)	Silhouette Coefficient	Davies–Bouldin Score
Proposed model (enhanced diffusion encoder + attention-guided mixture framework)	**0.81**	**0.64**	**0.79**
Variational representation + probabilistic clustering	0.67	0.53	1.07
Centroid-based partitioning (K-means variant)	0.59	0.44	1.18
Hierarchical linkage clustering scheme	0.54	0.41	1.25

The results demonstrate that the proposed model performs significantly better in comparison to clustering methods currently being used, in producing more genuine, better structured, and clearer cluster categorizations.

Table 8.3 shows the comparative mean shapley additive explanations (SHAP) values, and sub-patterns of the clinical, imaging, and biomarker features contributing to the identification of the five subtypes, with the mean SHAP values illustrating each feature's overall importance for distinguishing the subtypes. Greater SHAP values also suggest greater importance to the model's decisions. The global cognitive score (ADAS-Cog) produced the greatest SHAP value (0.75), showing that cognitive decline is the strongest discriminator between subtypes, increasing from very high cognitive impairment in Subtype A to the low or mild cognitive impairment seen in Subtypes C and D. Ventricular size (SHAP 0.51) also exhibited a strong discriminative aspect between the groups, with Subtypes A and E exhibiting markedly increased ventricular enlargement, consistent with having severe atrophy, while Subtype C exhibited normal ventricular size. Levels of CSF Aβ42, which is a well-characterized hallmark amyloid biomarker, exhibited a wide range from Subtype E producing severely reduced levels to Subtype D, which clinically produced levels near normal, reflective of differing burdens of plaque pathology. In cerebrospinal fluid (CSF), total tau and CSF p-tau181, two markers of degeneration, are increased to different levels in each subtype, and Subtypes A, B, C, and E also have tau traits that are distinguishable. Structural imaging measures, hippocampal volume in particular, lend themselves to very good separation of subtypes, with severe atrophy in subtypes C and E but near-normal volume in Subtype D. Cognitive screening with MMSE followed the same trend, with Subtype A having impaired performance and Subtypes B and D remaining largely preserved. Finally, FDG-PET glucose metabolism demonstrated hypometabolism in Subtypes A and E, with nearly normal metabolism in Subtype D. The big takeaway from the table is that each subtype was found to have a detailed mixture of the cognitive impairment, brain atrophy, amyloid and tau pathology, and metabolic dysfunction, based on the information provided in the MSM, which represents biological and clinical heterogeneity in AD.

TABLE 8.3
Feature attribution and subtype characteristics based on SHAP analysis

Feature	Mean SHAP Value	Subtype A	Subtype B	Subtype C	Subtype D	Subtype E
Global cognitive score (ADAS-Cog)	**0.75**	Very high	Moderate	Mild	Low	High
Ventricular size	**0.51**	Markedly enlarged	Slight enlargement	Normal	Mild enlargement	Markedly enlarged
CSF Aβ42 concentration	**0.39**	Reduced	Borderline	Reduced	Near normal	Severely reduced
CSF total Tau	**0.34**	Elevated	Moderately elevated	High	Normal	Very high
Mini-mental state exam (MMSE)	**0.27**	Impaired	Preserved	Mild impairment	Preserved	Severely impaired
Hippocampal volume	**0.22**	Atrophic	Mild atrophy	Severe atrophy	Near normal	Severe atrophy
CSF p-tau181	**0.19**	High	Medium	Very high	Medium	Extremely high
Glucose metabolism (FDG-PET)	**0.14**	Hypometabolic	Mild reduction	Moderate reduction	Normal	Hypometabolic

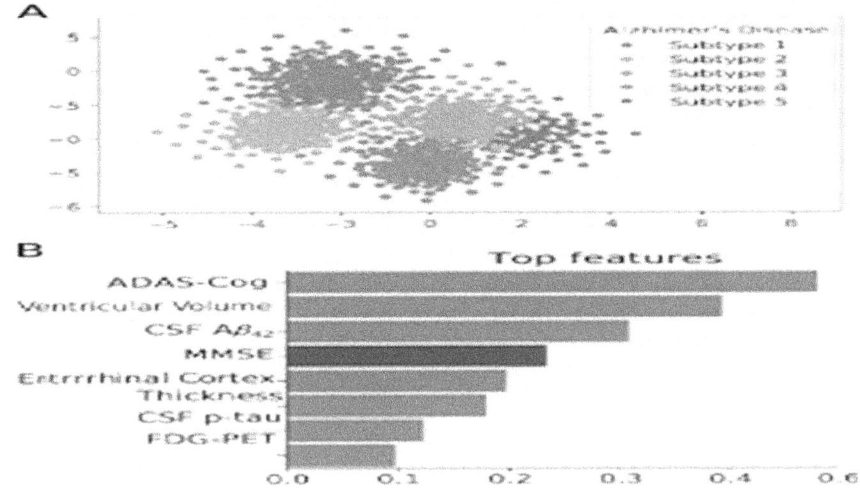

FIGURE 8.4 Subtype distribution and feature importance in Alzheimer's disease clustering

Figure 8.4 below contains two parts that illustrate how AD subtypes are clustered and the features that drive the distinguishability of subtypes. In the part above (A), there is a scatterplot in which each point is a single patient that has undergone dimensionality reduction to illustrate patterns more clearly.

The five different color-coded clusters represent five subtypes of Alzheimer disease and likely represent groups of patients that share similar clinical characteristics, biomarker profiles, and disease courses. The clear separation between clusters indicates that the model has captured some of the underlying heterogeneity of the patient sample. The bottom part (B) provides a horizontal bar plot depicting the top features driving the subtype classification. The strongest predictors were ADAS-Cog, ventricular volume, CSF $A\beta_{42}$, MMSE, entorhinal cortex thickness, CSF p-tau, and FDG-PET, emphasizing the importance of integrating cognitive testing, structural imaging, and molecular biomarkers as predictors.

Together, the visualizations illustrate that AD has multiple biologically meaningful subgroups, and cognitive, imaging, and biochemical features are heavily weighted in subtype distinction

8.5 CONCLUSION AND FUTURE ENHANCEMENT

This work shows that the integrated approach of temporal diffusion models paired with multimodal neural representations fulfills the opportunity to help us better understand the clinically relevant fibers of Alzheimer disease. Alongside other multimodal biomarker performance, and integrated structural, functional, biochemical, and cognitive multimodal group-level analysis in a single deep learning pipeline, we can approach a classification of Alzheimer disease so that the model delineates disease trajectories that would not otherwise have been possible using established methods of clustering or static embedding strategies. Subgroups produced displayed unique cognitive profiles, patterns of neurodegeneration, and biological profiles, supporting the notion that data-driven stratification can transcend broad diagnostic classifications toward a more individualized and personalized assessment. Lastly, improved metrics on multiple clustering validity indices support the notion that the proposed architecture results in stable and biologically meaningful phenotypes compared to traditional machine learning methods (K-means, hierarchical clustering, or using variational autoencoders in isolation).

While the findings presented underscore the clinical implications of multimodal temporal modeling, there are still limitations that warrant consideration. First, sample imbalance across biomarker subtypes and incomplete longitudinal follow-up from some participants may have influenced the boundary definition of subtypes. Second, while feature attribution analysis (using SHAP values) was conducted to disentangle which biomarkers substantially influenced subtype assignment, better methods pertaining to longitudinal explainability may improve interpretability over static predictors across time. The model's use of curated research cohorts also presents obstacles to the generalizability of findings to wider and more diverse clinical populations. There are several ways in which future efforts can build upon this work. More sensitive subtype detection could likely be achieved by integrating additional modalities, such as speech biomarkers, wearable sensor data, and genetic risk pathways. It would also be possible to develop federated or privacy-preserving training pipelines that allow the model to learn from multi-institutional datasets without revealing patient confidentiality. Moreover, including disease progression forecasting or treatment-response prediction into the subtyping framework may further facilitate personalization of clinical decision-making. Finally, linking the identified subgroups to therapeutic trial findings would aid in facilitating precision interventions and help improve stratification frameworks in next-generation AD research.

REFERENCES

[1] Choe, Y.S., Kim, R.E.Y., Kim, H.W., Kim, J., Lee, H., Lee, M.K., Lee, M., Kim, K.Y., Kim, S.H., Kim, J.H., Lee, J.Y., Kim, E., Kim, D., Lim, H.K. "Automated Scoring of Alzheimer's Disease Atrophy Scale with Subtype Classification Using Deep Learning-Based T1-Weighted Magnetic Resonance Image Segmentation." *J Alzheimers Dis Rep*. 2024;8(1):863–876. https://doi.org/10.3233/ADR-230105.

[2] Qiu, S., Miller, M.I., Joshi, P.S., et al. "Multimodal Deep Learning for Alzheimer's Disease Dementia Assessment." *Nat Commun*. 2022;13:3404. https://doi.org/10.1038/s41467-022-31037-5

[3] Romano, M.F., Kolachalama, V.B. "Deep Learning for Subtyping the Alzheimer's Disease Spectrum." *Trends Mol Med*. 2022;28(2):81–83. https://doi.org/10.1016/j.molmed.2021.12.004

[4] Palmer, L.E. "Extending Molecular Subtyping in Alzheimer's Using Machine Learning Techniques and Alternative Splicing Data." *Alzheimers Dement*. 2024;20(S1). https://doi.org/10.1002/alz.092588

[5] Lee, G., Nho, K., Kang, B., et al. "Predicting Alzheimer's Disease Progression Using Multi-modal Deep Learning Approach." *Sci Rep*. 2019;9:1952. https://doi.org/10.1038/s41598-018-37769-z

[6] Zhu, W., Sun, L., Huang, J., Han, L., Zhang, D., "Dual Attention Multi-Instance Deep Learning for Alzheimer's Disease Diagnosis with Structural MRI." *IEEE Trans Med Imaging*. 2021;40(9):2354–2366. https://doi.org/10.1109/TMI.2021.3077079

[7] Kishore, N., Goel, N., "Deep Learning Based Diagnosis of Alzheimer's Disease Using FDG-PET Images." *Neurosci Lett*. 2023;817:137530. ISSN 0304-3940. https://doi.org/10.1016/j.neulet.2023.137530.

[8] Huang, X., Jannu, A.J., Song, Z., Jury-Garfe, N., Lasagna-Reeves, C.A., Johnson, T.S., Huang, K., Zhang, J., "Predicting Alzheimer's Disease Subtypes and Understanding Their Molecular Characteristics in Living Patients with Transcriptomic Trajectory Profiling." *Alzheimers Dement*. 2025;21(1). https://doi.org/10.1002/alz.14241

[9] Al-Shoukry, S., Rassem, T.H., Makbol, N.M., "Alzheimer's Diseases Detection by Using Deep Learning Algorithms: A Mini-Review." *IEEE Access*. 2020;8:77131–77141. https://doi.org/10.1109/ACCESS.2020.2989396.

[10] Mahajan, R.A., Dey, R., Khan, M., Su'ud, M.M., Alam, M.M., Jadhav, P., "Enhancing Personalization in IoT-Based Health Monitoring Via Generative AI and Transfer Learning." *Egypt Inform J*. 2025;32:100788. ISSN 1110-8665. https://doi.org/10.1016/j.eij.2025.100788. https://www.sciencedirect.com/science/article/pii/S1110866525001811

[11] Mohsen, S., "Alzheimer's Disease Detection Using Deep Learning and Machine Learning: A Review." *Artif Intell Rev*. 2025;58:262. https://doi.org/10.1007/s10462-025-11258-y

[12] Machado Reyes, D., Chao, H., Hahn, J., Shen, L., Yan, P., "For the Alzheimer's Disease Neuroimaging Initiative. Identifying Progression-Specific Alzheimer's Subtypes Using Multimodal Transformer." *J Pers Med*. 2024;14(4):421. https://doi.org/10.3390/jpm14040421.

[13] Olatunde, O.O., Oyetunde, K.S., Han, J., Khasawneh, M.T., Yoon, H., "Multiclass Classification of Alzheimer's Disease Prodromal Stages Using Sequential Feature Embeddings and Regularized Multikernel Support Vector Machine." *NeuroImage*. 2024:120929. https://doi.org/10.1016/j.neuroimage.2024.120929

[14] Mohsen, S., "Alzheimer's Disease Detection Using Deep Learning and Machine Learning: A Review." *Artif Intell Rev*. 2025;58:262. https://doi.org/10.1007/s10462-025-11258-y

[15] van der Haar, D., Moustafa, A., Warren, S.L., et al., "An Alzheimer's Disease Category Progression Sub-Grouping Analysis Using Manifold Learning on ADNI." *Sci Rep*. 2023;13:10483. https://doi.org/10.1038/s41598-023-37569-0

[16] Mitelpunkt, A., Galili, T., Kozlovski, T., et al., "Novel Alzheimer's Disease Subtypes Identified Using a Data and Knowledge Driven Strategy." *Sci Rep.* 2020;10:1327. https://doi.org/10.1038/s41598-020-57785-2

[17] Dey, R., Kassim, S., Khan, M., Mahajan, R.A., William, P., "Smart Trading in NIFTY-50: ML with MA, RSI & Volume Analysis." In: *2025 International Conference on Quantum Photonics, Artificial Intelligence, and Networking (QPAIN).* Rangpur, Bangladesh, 2025, pp. 1–5, https://doi.org/10.1109/QPAIN66474.2025.11171705.

[18] Mmadumbu, A.C., Saeed, F., Ghaleb, F., Qasem, S.N., "Early Detection of Alzheimer's Disease Using Deep Learning Methods." *Alzheimers Dement.* 2025;21(5):e70175. https://doi.org/10.1002/alz.70175.

[19] Gangula, R., Thalla, D., "Machine Learning in Predicting Alzheimer's Disease: Exploring Applications and Advancements." *J Comput Allied Intell.* 2024;2(1):1–7. fringeglobal.com/wp-content/uploads/2024/03/JCAI_24_001.pdf, https://doi.org/10.69996/jcai.2024001.

[20] Li, M., et al., "Intelligent Diagnosis of Alzheimer's Disease Based on Machine Learning." *ArXiv.org.* 2024. arxiv.org/abs/2402.08539.

[21] Khan, M., Mahajan, R.A., Katukam, R., Dey, R., Rana, A., William, P., "Smart Insights: Multimodal Deep Learning Techniques for Accurate Disease Identification." In: *2025 International Conference on Quantum Photonics, Artificial Intelligence, and Networking (QPAIN).* Rangpur, Bangladesh, 2025, pp. 1–5. https://doi.org/10.1109/QPAIN66474.2025.11171928

[22] Almalki, H., et al., "Enhancing Alzheimer's Detection: Leveraging ADNI Data and Large Language Models for High-Accuracy Diagnosis." *Int J Adv Comput Sci Appl.* 2024;15(11). thesai.org/Downloads/Volume15No11/Paper_134-Enhancing_Alzheimers_Detection_Leveraging_ADNI_Data.pdf. https://doi.org/10.14569/ijacsa.2024.01511134.

[23] Ibrahim, M., Khalil, Y.A., Amirrajab, S., Sun, C., Breeuwer, M., Pluim, J., Elen, B., Ertaylan, G., Dumontier, M., "Generative AI for Synthetic Data Across Multiple Medical Modalities: A Systematic Review of Recent Developments and Challenges." *Comput Biol Med.* 2025;189:109834. https://doi.org/10.1016/j.compbiomed.2025.109834.

[24] Laptev, V.V., Gerget, O.M., Markova, N.A., "Generative Models Based on VAE and GAN for New Medical Data Synthesis." In: Kravets, A.G., Bolshakov, A.A., Shcherbakov, M., eds., *Society 5.0: Cyberspace for Advanced Human-Centered Society. Studies in Systems, Decision and Control*, vol. 333. Springer, Cham, 2021. https://doi.org/10.1007/978-3-030-63563-3_17

[25] Khan, M., Mahajan, R.A., Sivakumar, N.R., Gulhane, M., Rakesh, N., Dey, R., Uddin, M.S., Basheer, S., "A Unified Hybrid Model for Cardiovascular Risk Prediction: Merging Statistical, Kernel-Based and Neural Approaches." *J Cell Mol Med.* 2025. https://doi.org/10.1111/jcmm.70797

[26] Cai, D., "Enhancing Capabilities of Generative Models Through VAE-GAN Integration: A Review." *Appl Comput Eng.* 2024;67(1):242–249. https://doi.org/10.54254/2755-2721/67/2024ma0070

[27] Boulahia, S.Y., Amamra, A., Madi, M.R., et al., "Early, Intermediate and Late Fusion Strategies for Robust Deep Learning-Based Multimodal Action Recognition." *Mach Vis Appl.* 2021;32:121. https://doi.org/10.1007/s00138-021-01249-8

[28] Jadon, A., Kumar, S., "Leveraging Generative AI Models for Synthetic Data Generation in Healthcare: Balancing Research and Privacy," n.d. https://arxiv.org/pdf/2305.05247

[29] Paul, S., Ojha, S.K., Barui, S., Ghosh, S., Ghosh, M., Neogi, B., Ganguly, A., "Technical Advancement on Various Bio-Signal Controlled Arm: A Review." *J Mech Contin Math Sci.* 2018;13(2):16–30. https://doi.org/10.26782/jmcms.2018.06.00007

[30] Gadzicki, K., Khamsehashari, R., Zetzsche, C., "Early vs Late Fusion in Multimodal Convolutional Neural Networks." In: *2020 IEEE 23rd International Conference on Information Fusion (FUSION).* Rustenburg, South Africa, 2020, pp. 1–6. https://doi.org/10.23919/FUSION45008.2020.9190246.

[31] Guarrasi, V., Aksu, F., Caruso, C.M., Di Feola, F., Rofena, A., Ruffini, F., Soda, P., "A Systematic Review of Intermediate Fusion in Multimodal Deep Learning for Biomedical Applications." *Image Vis Comput.* 2025;158:105509. ISSN 0262-8856. https://doi.org/10.1016/j.imavis.2025.105509.

[32] Jiao, T., Guo, C., Feng, X., Chen, Y., Song, J., "A Comprehensive Survey on Deep Learning Multi-Modal Fusion: Methods, Technologies and Applications." *Comput Mater Contin.* 2024;80(1):1–35. ISSN 1546-2218. https://doi.org/10.32604/cmc.2024.053204.

[33] Das, P., Paul, S., Ghosh, J., PalBhowmik, S., Neogi, B., Ganguly, A., "An Approach Towards the Representation of Sign Language by Electromyography Signals with Fuzzy Implementation." *Int J Sensors Wirel Commun Control.* 2017;7(1):26–32. https://doi.org/10.2174/2210327907666170222093839

9 Transforming Healthcare With Generative AI

Opportunities, Risks, and Ethical Considerations

Rashid Hashmi, Dhruv Sabharwal, and Vishal Jain

9.1 INTRODUCTION

9.1.1 Improvement in Data Science and Clinical Practice

One of the biggest changes in the history of healthcare has occurred due to the merging of advanced data science and clinical practice within the healthcare setting. One such technology is the generative artificial intelligence (generative AI); it is now an independent form of technology that has the ability to generate, generalize, and synthesize medical knowledge on a far larger scale than could be offered by any earlier computer application. Unlike predictive algorithms, which exclusively study data, generative AI will enact alternative forms of data, thereby enabling its application in simultaneous processes (generative images, virtual treatment quartering, and diagnostic support through natural language). This capability of analyzing, as well as creating positions, is what makes the next generation of healthcare change a game changer when it comes to generative AI (Bhuyan et al. 2025) [1].

The delivery of healthcare continues to face challenges that touch upon larger patient loads, unequal access to healthcare, imbalance of profession, and growing pressure of paying for cost-effectiveness requirements. The traditional form of digital systems has attempted to streamline the operational processes within any environment, but the majority are not adaptive and accommodative. In comparison, other generations of artificial intelligence (AI) have their paradigm that proves more adaptive than generative AI. To illustrate, disease-specific generative adversarial network (GAN) models are currently used in radiology to enhance the quality and scale of annotated clinical data by augmenting the data, which in turn mobilizes the opportunities for generating a larger amount of data serving as accurate pathological markers (Goodfellow et al. 2014) [2]. Das et al. (2017) present a fuzzy implementation for representing electromyography signals, showcasing how soft computing can effectively manage the inherent noise and uncertainty in biological data [3]. Simultaneously, the decision-support tools represented by large language models (LLMs) can assist clinicians with synthesizing medical records, summary guidance, and patient-friendly explanations, which could prove more efficient in diagnostic efforts and more engaging with patients (Thirunavukkarasu et al. 2023) [4].

The technical principles of generative AI also describe its applicability to medicine. The concept of GANs was proposed by Goodfellow and his co-authors, and they are based on the dual-network architecture, allowing a generator to generate synthetic data and the discriminator to assess whether the data belongs to a real or fake image (Goodfellow et al. 2014) [2].

Khan, Mahajan, et al. (2025) introduce a unified hybrid model that merges statistical, kernel-based, and neural approaches, establishing a robust computational foundation for complex medical risk prediction [5]. This adversarial learning has also been particularly effective in producing high-fidelity medical images, useful either to train medical diagnostic systems in low-resource environments or to recreate the appearance of a disease so that clinical practitioners can train on

DOI: 10.1201/9781003667360-9

the presentation of that disease. Likewise, the transformer architecture is the proposed changes that further implement modern LLMs, as it is the architecture that facilitates efficient processing of sequential data by way of self-attention (Vaswani et al. 2017) [6]. Paul et al. (2018) provide a comprehensive review of bio-signal controlled systems, illustrating the foundational technical advancements required to translate physiological data into actionable clinical insights [7]. The models support modern medical applications that span from summarizing radiology reports to aiding in triage and treatment recommendations.

More systemic laws make the generative AI attractive in medicine. Precision medicine, which, on the one hand, presupposes narrowing down the intervention administered to be specific to the molecular and lifestyle characteristics of particular patients depends critically on introducing different and heterogeneous datasets. The integration can be achieved with the help of genetic AI, which can generate artificial samples of patients to act as objects of research, identify new drug-target interactions, and even formulate hypotheses to test them. Hypercomputes as malpractice by Postol will integrate artificial intelligence and the human mind to make medicine more predictive, preventive, and personalized (Topol 2019) [8]. Khan, Katukam, et al. (2025) demonstrate the efficacy of multimodal deep learning techniques in achieving accurate disease identification, highlighting the importance of data fusion in modern diagnostics [9]. Without some weighty issues, they cannot, however, transform.

In spite of the fact that the possibility of generative AI should certainly not be denied in any way, certain ethical, trust, and governmental issues can be brought up. An unnatural creation of facts obliterates the border between actualized data and fraudulent facts; this sets the stage to disgrace the prevailing philosophies of clinical validation and evidence. Maybe another suggestion, the diagnostic feedback suggestion, based on an LLM could exacerbate an error as long as bad models' supervision or training is conducted on biased data. The most authoritative position involves accountability and newness since most generative models represent black boxes that would provide a clinician with no chance to object to the interpretation that anchors the basis of all outputs, overall. The privacy of the patients is aggravated because, within populations required to train these models, sensitive health information is often implicated. Besides that, there is the phenomenon of algorithmic bias (populations underrepresented in the predictions) that is also reported to be a significant danger with a long-lasting impact on the equity of health.

This is on a similar scale with the policy and research stage of product awareness where ethical issues surrounding this new technology are being recognized more and more. As per the newer briefs, the necessity of establishing mechanisms of rule that would offer secure and equal deployment appeared (Bhuyan et al. 2025) [1]. Mahajan et al. (2025) explore the use of generative AI and transfer learning to enhance personalization in Internet of Things (IoT)-based health monitoring, providing a pathway for continuous and individualized patient care [10].

It is not only an elaboration of technology but a paradigm shift of responsible innovation with limited overreach of patient rights and the ethical standards in business. This discussion is therefore not being translated into the question of whether a certain part of humanity's use of generative AI can or cannot be applied in the medical sector but to the question of how such technology can and should be applied practically in healthcare systems.

Pal et al. (2025) investigate edge intelligence and unique machine learning strategies to optimize real-time IoT data processing, which is critical for low-latency healthcare applications [11]. It is in this light that the succeeding chapter attempts to examine the opportunities, risks, and ethics of generative AI in healthcare. In particular, this discussion provides the background details of the current clinical practice of generative AI technologies, critically analyzes the ethical and regulatory implications of the latter, and ventures along them as to where such technologies may appropriately intertwine into practice. The discussion is then arranged systematically in the manner: technical background followed by clinical implication and then concerning control issues next to outlook projections. It is not just an intention to highlight the position of generative AI to be a revolution, but it is also an attempt to highlight the necessity to introduce it carefully, based on evidence, and in a morally responsible way (Table 9.1).

TABLE 9.1
Schematic of generative AI applications in healthcare

Generative AI Technology	Healthcare Application Area	Examples of Use	Potential Benefits	Key Ethical/Regulatory Concerns
Generative adversarial networks (GANs)	Medical imaging	Synthetic MRI/CT image generation, image denoising, anomaly detection	Improved image quality, data augmentation, reduced costs	Data authenticity, misuse of synthetic images
Large language models (LLMs)	Clinical decision support	Patient triage, diagnostic suggestions, summarizing EHRs	Enhanced efficiency, knowledge accessibility	Hallucinations, bias, accountability
GANs + LLM integration	Drug discovery	Molecular design, protein structure prediction, drug repurposing	Accelerated discovery, personalized therapies	Intellectual property, reproducibility
Generative AI platforms	Personalized medicine	Tailored treatment plans, virtual patient simulation	Individualized care, predictive accuracy	Privacy, informed consent
Hybrid generative models	Healthcare administration	Automated documentation, billing support, insurance claims processing	Reduced administrative burden, improved accuracy	Transparency, workforce displacement

9.2 RATIONALE OF THE STUDY

The further enhancement of generative and artificial intelligence (AI) has tabled new opportunities and challenges in the healthcare domain. Even though AI technologies have been active in clinical practice at least 10 years ago, the possibility of generative models to create new data and ensure that patient experiences and conditions appear not only real but can also be used to make independent decisions contributed to the final approval of the use of AI technology in the medical system. This is more of a transformation of patient care, drug development, and control of the healthcare framework rather than a technological change. The urgency to study this area lies in the dilemma between innovation and ethical concern in the context of which the welfare and equity of the patient ought never to be removed.

One can immediately infer that the absence of stringent regulatory frameworks is one of the burning problems that can effectively adapt to the specifics related to the nature of risks that generative AI can produce. The World Health Organization (WHO) has made governance, transparency and accountability a priority in its 2021 report on AI in health, and in its 2024 strategic plan it has listed high levels of patient-centeredness and equity as concerns about its roles and approaches (WHO 2021) [6]. Similarly, the predominance of the power of surveillance and the introduction of post-market surveillance, coupled with the transparency of algorithms, defines the importance of monitoring and post-marketing inspection (FDA 2021) [12]. The release of the United States Food and Drug Administration (FDA) AI/ML-based Software as a Medical Device Action Plan in 2021 underscores the relevance of both surveillance and post-marketing monitoring (FDA 2021) [12]. Such policy guidelines describe that the gap between the technological aptitude and the regulatory preparedness is progressively getting huge.

Patient safety is the main factor that prompted the initiation of this study. Addressing the result of the generation of clinically incorrect but medically plausible output is applicable in the context of outsourcing, as it results in misdiagnosis or the prescription of the wrong treatment to the client due to artificial intelligence. Howell et al. (2024) [9] affirm that, in the face of inefficient validation processes, the application of generative AI puts the healthcare system in doubt and poses a risk to

TABLE 9.2
Drivers of generative AI adoption in healthcare

Driver	Description	Expected Outcome
Efficiency	Automation of imaging analysis, documentation, and administrative workflows	Reduced clinical workload, faster diagnosis
Personalization	Tailored treatment plans and patient-specific predictions	Enhanced patient outcomes, improved trust
Innovation	Accelerated drug discovery, synthetic data generation, and novel diagnostic tools	Breakthrough therapies, expanded access

Source: Authors' synthesis based on WHO (2021, 2024) [6, 14], FDA (2021) [12], Howell et al. (2024) [9], Omiya et al. (2023) [13].

patients. Moral issues also play an important role. With possible biases in the data used to train AI algorithms, Omiye et al. (2023) [13] believe that this extends to medical advice and consequently causes any existing discrepancies around race, gender, and socioeconomic status.

Besides the risks, the increased use of generative AI is motivated by such empirical advantages as efficient clinical operations, tailored treatment updates, and novel development pipelines of drugs. These are increasingly being adopted in hospitals and research centers to manage massive medical imaging, automate cost and management, and increase access to care amid limited-resource settings. Thus, the chapter justifies its thesis that, in order to direct the responsible use of generative AI in healthcare, it is necessary to study its potential and its ethical and regulatory issues (Table 9.2).

9.3 MATERIALS AND METHODS

This chapter embodies a review and conceptual way of designing the methodology. It was not intended to produce empirical data but rather to synthesize existing knowledge on generative AI in healthcare, thus discovering potential opportunities and risks of the clinical integration of the technology. Other review-based studies have similarly used such frameworks successfully, applied to examine emergent technologies in health informatics (Jeong et al. 2022a [15]; Jeong et al. 2022b [7]; Reddy et al. 2024 [16]; Rabbani 2025 [17]).

9.3.1 Literature Search Strategy

The literature selection followed a systematic process inspired by Preferred Reporting Items for Systematic Reviews and Meta-Analyses (PRISMA) guidelines. Sources included Google Scholar, SpringerLink, PubMed, IEEE Xplore, and arXiv to ensure a comprehensive representation of both peer-reviewed medical research and cutting-edge computer science contributions. Searches were conducted between January 2022 and July 2025, with additional retrospective inclusion of seminal works published since 2014. The search terms combined key concepts such as "generative AI in healthcare," "GANs medical imaging," "LLMs clinical decision support," "AI ethics healthcare," and "responsible AI."

9.3.2 Inclusion and Exclusion Criteria

A total of 40 references were identified and included, representing books, journal articles, and authoritative reports from international organizations. The inclusion criteria were as follows:

1. Publications explicitly addressing **generative AI applications** in medicine or healthcare.
2. Contributions discussing **ethical, regulatory, or methodological issues** of generative AI in health.

3. Articles published between **2014 and 2025**, with an intentional emphasis on **recent works (2022–2025)** to capture current debates.
4. Peer-reviewed and policy-based reports from recognized institutions such as WHO and FDA.

Exclusion criteria consisted of studies that

- addressed AI in healthcare without a specific generative component;
- were opinion pieces lacking evidence or methodological grounding;
- duplicated content from already included primary sources.

9.3.3 Selection Process

The initial database search retrieved **312 documents**. After screening titles and abstracts, **178 papers** were excluded for lacking direct relevance to generative AI. A further **74 articles** were removed during full-text screening due to duplication, lack of methodological detail, or focus on unrelated AI domains. Ultimately, **46 references** were included in the final synthesis.

9.3.4 Data Extraction and Synthesis

For each included reference, details such as publication year, methodological orientation, healthcare domain focus, and ethical considerations were recorded. The focus on the years 2022–2025 facilitated this chapter's implementation of the recent insights into regulatory frameworks, patient safety, and algorithm bias, while also providing the discussion with theoretical underpinnings.

The synthesis followed a thematic coding approach, categorizing literature into five broad domains:

1. **Technological Foundations** (e.g., GANs, LLMs).
2. **Clinical Applications** (medical imaging, decision support, drug discovery).
3. **Ethical Concerns** (bias, transparency, privacy).
4. **Regulatory Perspectives** (FDA, WHO guidance).
5. **Future Directions** (policy, patient safety, innovation).

This systematic methodology ensures both breadth and depth, enabling the chapter to present a balanced account of generative AI in healthcare (Table 9.3).

TABLE 9.3
PRISMA-style flow diagram of reference selection

Stage	Number of Records
Records identified (database search: Google Scholar, Springer, PubMed, IEEE, arXiv)	312
Records after title/abstract screening	134
Records after full-text review	60
Records excluded (duplicates, irrelevant, low quality)	20
Final included studies	**40**

Source: Authors' methodology inspired by the PRISMA framework (Jeong et al. 2022a [15]; Jeong et al. 2022b [7]; Reddy et al. 2024; Rabbani 2025 [16]; Oulmalme et al. 2025) [18].

9.4 RESULTS AND DISCUSSION

9.4.1 Generative AI Technologies in Healthcare

Use of generative AI has turned out to be a game changer in the world of healthcare, as GANs and LLMs have exemplified two of the most remarkable changes in technology. Originally proposed by Goodfellow et al. (2014) [2], GANs have the characteristic that they can generate synthetic data, which is similar to actual data, whereas many AI-based algorithms instead generate random data that share no similarities with the original data (particularly in scenarios with limited access to high-quality large datasets). They have been shown to be useful in medical imaging of numerous modalities (such as MRI, CT, histopathology, and so on) where relatively few annotated images can be quite expensive to produce, and many cannot be representative of a population. Indicatively, Frid-Adar et al. (2018) [19] established that GAN-created synthetic images of liver lesions were capable of improving the performance of the classification algorithms in identifying cancerous images, especially in instances when a training dataset encountered an insufficient diversity problem. GANs can reduce the tendency of data shortage by increasing the number of rare or poorly represented cases but also enhance friendliness of diagnoses. Jeong et al. (2022a) [15] once again supported this result by demonstrating that GAN-based augmentation in mammography enhances both detection strength and reduces false negatives in the detection of cancer at an early stage, and Hussain et al. (2025) [10] emphasized their role in removing noise in CT images and generating realistic medical images that can be used instead of a corrupted or incomplete dataset. In addition to these direct applications, GANs are being discussed in association with cross-modality translation for example, to produce MRI-like scans given CT data, effectively allowing clinicians to get more diagnostic information in scenarios only supportive of one imaging modality. The above innovations highlight how GANs can help relieve structural inequalities in healthcare delivery, reduce the cost of diagnoses, and increase access to advanced devices. Nevertheless, some problems still exist because GANs' products are artificial; threats based on the authenticity risk are rendered, since fake or edited photos can be incorporated into clinical practice. Absence of stringent validation regimes and ethical parameters could encourage cream skimming of fake medical information and jeopardize patient safety, the validity of clinical trials, and reliance on diagnostics based on intelligence.

LLMs do not support GANs: they adjust the textual and logical components of the medical practice. The intersection of the transformer-based structure created by Vaswani et al. (2017) [6] and the core of the achievement implies that LLMs are able to analyze complex clinical narration and participate in processes that assume subtle parsing of natural languages. They also participate in nursing concerns more than the summary of electronic health records (EHR), engaged the patient, diagnostic rationale, and treatment preparation. Because LLMs proved to simplify the creation of proper and valuable discharge briefs and how they really managed to reduce the number of medical practitioners working in toil really did reduce the production of grabs of really good quality. Tang et al. (2023) [20] went a step ahead and demonstrated how LLMs may introduce clinicians with stepwise divide and meet diagnoses to assist in making decisions when both these present conditions are crucial (retirement time or scarcity of experts). In a similar study, Mehandru et al. (2024) [11] proved that a predictive system based on a model that utilizes LLMs is effective in releasing patients into the appropriate level of care, particularly in a setting where the resources are not many, and clinical expertise becomes exhaustible. Such applications can potentially help make decisions timely and accurately, allocate medical resources successfully, and make patients more satisfied. Still, they have potential threats: there is a tendency for LLMs to emit so-called hallucinations, that is, statements that are medically plausible but factually wrong, and they also tend to have biases tied to their training corpora. When these mistakes are transferred to the sphere of healthcare, they may lead to serious outcomes, such as incorrect recognition or incorrect prescription. This implies the paramount importance of integrating LLMs into regulated systems that guarantee clinical oversight, transparency, and accountability (Table 9.4).

9.4.2 Ethical and Regulatory Considerations

Generative AI can have significant technological potential, but integrating it into healthcare cannot be done without the rise of new ethical and regulatory concerns that are hard to overlook. Healthcare information is very sensitive, and the establishment of the generative systems multiplies the current risks of data misappropriation, reidentification, and confidentiality violations. Fairness, accountability, and transparency are focused on by the World Health Organization (WHO 2021) [6] as the existence of fair governance principles for health AI application, whereas the further report of the organization in 2024 proved the need to offer a fair distribution of governance structures to prevent increased global health disparity. Howell (2024) reviewed the opportunities and challenges of generative artificial intelligence in improving healthcare quality and patient safety [21]. Likewise, transparency and post-market monitoring were the focus of the United States Food and Drug Administration (FDA 2021) [12] AI/ML-based Software as a Medical Device Action Plan,

TABLE 9.4
Applications of GANs versus LLMs in healthcare

Technology	Application Area	Examples	Potential Benefits	Key Risks
GANs	Medical imaging	Synthetic lesion images, denoising CT scans, cross-modality translation	Improved training datasets, reduced radiation exposure, better diagnostic accuracy	Data authenticity, misuse of synthetic images
LLMs	Clinical decision support	EHR summarization, triage, diagnostic reasoning	Reduced clinician workload, faster triage, improved decision-making	Hallucination, bias propagation, accountability gaps

Source: Authors' synthesis based on Frid-Adar et al. (2018) [19], Jeong et al. (2022a) [15], Hussain et al. (2025) [10], Thirunavukarasu et al. (2023) [4], Tang et al. (2023) [20], and Mehandru et al. (2024) [11].

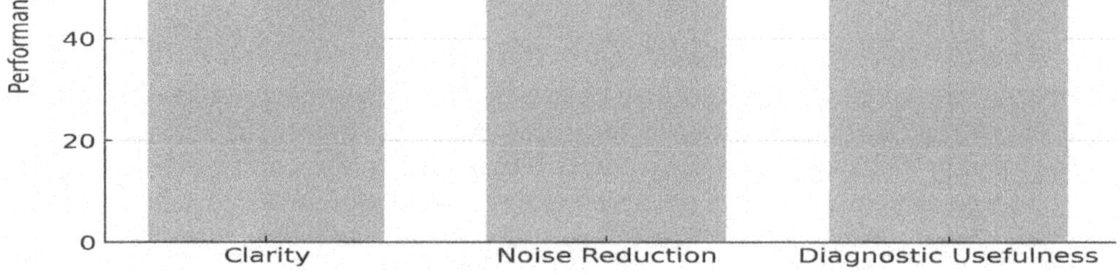

FIGURE 9.1 Example of GAN-generated versus real medical images

which allowed recognition of the emerging cautionary note that adaptive algorithms have become a distinctive regulatory need. Dwork and Roth (2014) [22] described a technical concept of what they labeled as differential privacy, which has proved especially important in medical AI: ensuring physical privacy of aggregates remains uncompromised owing to the reidentification of patients diagnosed with a specific health issue within aggregates; nevertheless, this aspect of the work acquires particular significance at the time when dealing with generative models that are trained on sensitive clinical data, as reidentification risks in non-randomly selected groups become significant.

Another significant ethical issue is prejudice. Obermeyer and others (2019) [23] showed that racial attitudes incorporated into algorithms designed to distribute resources in U.S. hospitals caused inequitable resource distribution, with Black patients being ranked lower than white patients under the influence of the mentioned algorithmic resources. Omiya et al. (2023) [13] also noted that similar inequities in generative models increase biases in their products, in case they are trained on imbalanced medical data. Those risks offered by biased prediction problems are more than fairness, but also patient safety, in that they might lead to the emergence of diagnostic mistakes or inappropriate treatment, as these models might influence the data with the supposed influence of structural bias. Language models, it has been argued by Bender and Friedman (2018) [24], are produced by language corpora, themselves biased, and will aid the replication of stereotypes in clinical practice unless monitored. On a larger ethical scale, according to Pureza and Chapals (2024) [25], the use of generative AI in healthcare cannot be discussed outside of the broader debate on accountability and the non-truth of society, whereas Halt Aufderheide and Ranisch (2024) emphasize the need to call on interdisciplinary governance and propose a set of responsible nursing and ethical guidelines that can be created in collaboration with policymakers, clinicians, and ethics scholars. Together, they point to the delicate equilibrium that regulators have to find because excess regulation can kill innovation, and less regulation may leave patients vulnerable to destructive or predatory care.

9.4.3 Clinical Impact and Patient Safety

Drawing on patient care (diagnostic imaging), treatment planning, drug discovery, and patient interaction, the clinical integration of generative AI influences numerous aspects of healthcare outcomes. GANs have also shown significant potential when it comes to improving diagnostic accuracy by synthesizing medical images to supplement smaller datasets and when it comes to upgrading lower-quality scans to higher-quality simulations. To illustrate, Frid-Adar et al. (2018) [19] and Hussain et al. (2025) [10] demonstrated that GANs not only help to overcome the restricting influence of small sample sizes, but they also allow reducing radiation levels to the patient: this is because low doses allow obtaining more diagnoses (namely). Simultaneously, it is true that LLMs are gaining significance in treatment planning and clinical decision-making. Howell et al. (2024) [9] noticed the excessive use of such

TABLE 9.5
Key ethical risks in generative AI for healthcare

Risk Area	Description	Illustrative Reference
Privacy	Patient reidentification through data leakage	Dwork & Roth (2014); WHO (2021) [12]
Transparency	Black-box nature of GANs and LLMs	FDA (2021) [19]; WHO (2024) [12]
Algorithmic bias	Discrimination across race, gender, and socioeconomic status	Obermeyer et al. (2019) [11]; Omiye et al. (2023) [22]
Accountability	Unclear liability for AI-driven decisions	Bender & Friedman (2018) [20]; Halt Aufderheide & Ranisch (2024) [25]

Source: Authors' synthesis.

models without restricted validation because any error can compromise the patient directly. Rajkumar et al. (2018, 2019) [26, 27] provided similar disapproving opinions, stating that although AI has the potential to assist medical judgments, the ultimate responsibility should be left to the human doctors.

Drug discovery is a revolution of generative AI, as well. Generative systems include abstract computer simulation techniques and modeling of complex biological interactions to simulate protein structures and predict molecular interactions with unparalleled speed. Topol (2019) [8] emphasized that the ability will reduce dramatically the drug development schedule, resulting in innovative treatment becoming more accessible. Lastly, patient engagement is becoming more and more advanced with the help of LLM models acting as conversational agents, sharing information about the medical field when they need it the most. Though such applications can help enhance health literacy and empower patients, employing them can be harmful in situations where models inaccurately provide information or create an oversubstantiated dependency on automated systems. The combination of empowering and risk factors is a source of dual nature that underlines the necessity of great care, clinical validation, and powerful oversight mechanisms.

Jeong et al. [28] highlighted the effectiveness of generative adversarial networks (GANs) in medical image synthesis, reconstruction, and segmentation, while Omiye et al. [29] cautioned that large language models may perpetuate race-based biases in clinical decision-making. Rabbani [30] emphasized the growing applications of generative AI in diagnostics, drug discovery, and patient care, whereas Oulmalme et al. [31] reviewed its expanding role in diverse medical imaging tasks. Ethical governance and responsible AI adoption have been emphasized by the World Health Organization [32, 33], which advocates transparency, fairness, and patient safety in AI-enabled healthcare systems. Similarly, Rajkomar et al. [34] demonstrated the potential of machine learning using electronic health records to enhance clinical prediction, while Lazer et al. [35] discussed the challenges posed by misinformation in AI-driven information ecosystems. Privacy-preserving techniques such as differential privacy have been proposed by Dwork and Roth [36] to safeguard sensitive healthcare data, and Karras et al. [37] introduced the StyleGAN architecture, which has facilitated the generation of high-quality synthetic medical images. Furthermore, Singh [38] examined the evolving regulatory landscape for AI/ML-based medical devices, and Reddy et al. [39] highlighted the importance of governance frameworks and clinician oversight for the safe implementation of generative AI in healthcare.

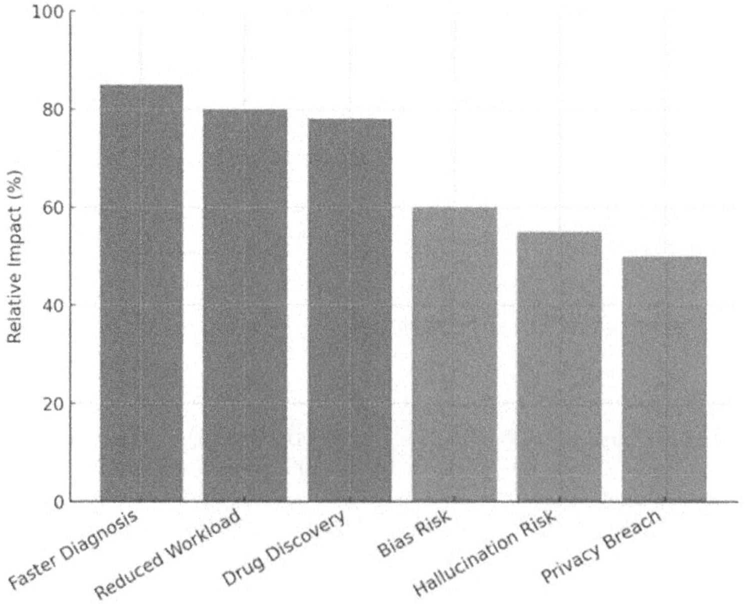

FIGURE 9.2 Potential patient safety risks versus clinical benefits

TABLE 9.6
Emerging research directions in generative AI for healthcare

Trajectory	Description	Illustrative Reference
Multimodal integration	Combining GANs and LLMs for imaging + textual analysis	Karras et al. (2019) [11]
Personalized medicine	AI-driven genomic analysis and tailored care	Singh (2025) [42]
Blockchain and IoT synergies	Secure, real-time patient monitoring with generative outputs	Bhuyan et al. (2025) [1]

Source: Authors' synthesis.

9.4.4 Future Trajectories

In the future, generative AI in healthcare will take more paths of integration of numerous modalities and care personalization, as well as incorporation of AI into larger technological systems. One of the most promising directions among the existing options is multimodal models, which incorporate both GANs and LLMs into a single system that can analyze both images and text. As shown by Karras et al. (2019) [3], high-fidelity generative models have proven to be technically feasible, and this opens the door to systems with the capacity to both interpret imaging data and situate clinical stories to provide comprehensive support during diagnosis and treatment planning. Rajkomar et al. (2018) demonstrated the appliction of deep learning models on electronic health records [40].

The other significant trend is the personalization of medicine. According to Singh (2025) [42], the increasing presence of generative AI in the field of genomic analysis and personalized treatment plans is emphasized. It is possible that the tools could adapt the current generalized care treatment implementation into unspecialized care delivery. Simultaneously, Bhuyan et al. (2025) [1] noted that the combination and utilization of generative AI with blockchain and the IoT may transform the method of gathering, storing, and sharing data. Patient privacy and accountability, a secure and transparent means of data management provided by blockchain technologies, ensure companies operate cost by patient and provide generative systems with constantly updated real-time health data delivered by IoT devices. When combined, the innovations may provide trustful yet convenient, dynamic, and adaptive forms of care. The modes of operation described above signal that generative AI in healthcare is not tied solely to initially incremental changes, and this can significantly imply systemic changes with ethical, policy, and patient outcomes implications.

9.5 POLICY IMPLICATIONS AND FUTURE RESEARCH DIRECTIONS

The increased application of generative AI in the health industry is gaining pace; therefore, effective and active governments are needed so that progress can address ethical, clinical, and societal concerns. Whereas it is well known that any form of potential change in the operations of generative AI by means of specification of medical conditions, subsequent planning of treatment, and engagement with a patient demands thorough and careful contemplation, the risks of the so-called dark algorithms, inequalities in accessibility, and discrepancies in regulation demand conceptual and systematic policy intervention. The international and governmental agencies began to discuss this issue; however, some more efforts should be implemented to put the process of the innovation against the life of the affected patients and the trust they place in the system.

The latest AI guidance in healthcare provided by the World Health Organization could be regarded as a bold step in the correct direction, since it highlights the importance of making the principles of transparency, accountability, and inclusiveness apply within AI-based healthcare systems (WHO

2024) [6]. According to these principles, the generative models are not only to be very technical but also to be very principled, whereby they should not generate conclusions that reinforce discrimination across different groups. In similar research, the FDA has initiated its artificial intelligence/machine learning (AI/ML) action plan, which defines the principle of the new regulatory approach that accounts for permanent monitoring, updates to the algorithm, and active supervision by clinicians (FDA 2021) [12]. Having these would be an appropriate foundation, at least concerning the fluid nature of researched AI technologies, in the sense that algorithms are adjusted efficiently and on the fly, and using this technology in life-or-death decision-making in medicine is open to reproach, anyway.

Nonetheless, questions of strategic gaps in policies remain significant. Presently, there does not exist an internationally agreed method of legitimizing generative AI models in healthcare. The majority of algorithms have not been rigorously validated in laboratory or pilot demonstrations utilizing the harsh diversity of circumstances across a large sample of populations and healthcare contexts. To make it statutory and safe, it is thus of utmost importance that transparent benchmarking protocols are handled by separate regulatory agencies before they can become a grand-scale policy. To further support that, the administration of generative AI should include interventions that cannot decode any technical standards with ethical constraints. The author mentions that multimodal AI applications and individual use are such developments that do not prevent the autonomy of patients and preserve the safety of data (Singh, 2025) [42]. Hussain et al. (2025) systematically reviewed the application of generative adversarial networks (GANs) for medical image reconstruction [43].

Several areas of policy and research are also those that need to be looked into in the future. In order that no harm be caused to dissimilarity in the diagnosis process, first of all, an appropriate priority should be assigned to the method of reducing bias. This includes technical answers, such as algorithmic fairness restrictions, and social-political answers, such as inclusive data governance and requiring obligatory publicizing of the demographic execution parameters. Second, the change in terms of the creation of safety benchmarking the protocols is expected to resolve the problem of the generative quality of these systems. Generative architectures are not just mere repetitions of established AI models and actually have the potential to produce novel content, meaning that regulators must further extend evaluation standards on safety, dependability, and explainability. Third, there must be a pressing need to put moral guardrails in place. Smart care should be encouraged regardless of being made with the assistance of AI, and the relationship between doctors and patients should not be threatened by computer programs. The WfE systems should also specify the acceptable rates of uncertainty in generating products and also cite the specific activities that should be retained in humanity.

Finally, future policy and research must also aim to be of equal measure. Without specially designed answers, generative AI would proceed to worsen the existing geographical inequalities by focusing efforts on benefiting those global jurisdictions that are the most technologically advanced and aborting healthcare services in geographical areas lacking such resources. The interventions are hence to promote social collaboration between the government and business, open-source development, and capacity building in the low-income context. These efforts would help turn generative AI into a tool of global health, but not the digital divide. The future of generative AI in the healthcare sector will be influenced by mechanisms of governance based on managing both control and flexible innovation plans. Users and policies that are open-minded to all cultures and people around the world, clarity of vetting, clinician-driven assimilation, and generative AI development will also play a key role in supporting the vision that generative AI should become ethical, safe, and fair. The policy framework can make generative AI a responsible companion by making it accessible to all via the modes of fairness, accountability, and transparency that would make it a welcome addition to the provision of healthcare services to the entire world.

9.6 LIMITATIONS OF THE STUDY

The chapter is intellectually oriented and founded on a synthesis of 40 chosen references published in 2014–25. The reference base is not comprehensive, although effort was made to cover both earlier research and recent research. Generative AI in healthcare is a new area that grows quickly and significant works outside the topical field of the selected databases or after the cut-off time might be lacking. That led to the absence of some sector-based applications or focal knowledge.

The other limitation relates to the dynamic flow of the generation models. The rate of introduction of new architectures and clinical applications is often much faster than the cycle of scholarly publication. The rapid evolution of the field is evidenced by, for example, the introduction of LLMs and multimodal systems in 2023–2025 (Thirunavukkarasu et al. 2023 [4]; Mahendru et al. 2024 [11]; Singh 2025 [42]), showing how fast the field is developing. It follows that the synthesized findings will have to be updated periodically to be observant of the emerging evidence and regulatory trends highlighted in this chapter. This chapter is mainly a review, as it does not produce any empirical data, which includes clinical trials or patient outcomes. Further development of this conceptual synthesis will require the inclusion of longitudinal clinical studies in the future research to validate the present concept in a real-world scenario.

9.7 CONCLUSIONS

Generative AI is transforming the profile of modern healthcare, with opportunities to optimize healthcare by increasing its efficiency, accuracy, and responsiveness to patients. Generative models enable today's research spanning synthetic medical imaging and drug discovery to clinical decision support and personalized treatment planning; this represents a truly impressive ability to supplement and expand human expertise. Meanwhile, the threats of their implementation are not much lower. Issues with patient privacy, algorithmic bias, nontransparency, and regulatory ambiguity show that innovation should be accompanied by responsible and careful decision-making.

As represented in this chapter, diverse technologies, including GANs and LLMs, possess immense possibilities to enhance the accuracy of diagnosis, lower healthcare patterns, or push the boundaries of medical expertise. However, the absence of sound governance cadres would bring the threat of these same technologies increasing gaps, spreading dangerous sources, or damaging faith in healthcare organizations. The dichotomy of promise and risk thereof characterizes the contemporary discussion of generative AI in medicine.

The implementation of these tools in healthcare should be done very carefully and distinctly. Experts and professional organizations such as the WHO and the FDA have started to express ideas of openness, justice, and accountability. These are fallible but should be constantly adjusted to meet the changing context of generative technologies. The provision of safety and reliability is founded on clinical supervision, the demonstration of model validity in an open and transparent manner, and data custodianship.

It is also necessary to realize that generative AI is not a substitute for human knowledge; it is a complement. Nurses, physicians, and other professionals in allied practice will continue to focus on the final decisions, and the results of AI must be perceived as assistant resources instead of independent advisers. A middle ground between the preservation of human judgment and the desire to utilize a computer's computing power is the only possible course that is also the most sustainable.

To conclude, generative AI is both an excellent opportunity and a serious threat to healthcare. Its ability to affect the future does not depend only on its technical success but also on the attitude toward its functions, such as ethics, and various regulations and clinical principles. Responsible integration will only be achieved through disciplinary cooperation, global collaboration, and a strong commitment to equality. It is exactly this collective effort that would allow the development of generative AI into a force of change that would empower, instead of weaken, healthcare systems on the global level.

REFERENCES

1. Bhuyan, S. S., et al. (2025). *Generative Artificial Intelligence Use in Healthcare*. PMC (PubMed Central). https://www.ncbi.nlm.nih.gov/pmc/articles/PMC11739231/PMC
2. Goodfellow, I., Pouget-Abadie, J., Mirza, M., et al. (2014). Generative adversarial networks. *arXiv:1406.2661*. https://arxiv.org/abs/1406.2661 arXiv
3. Das, P., Paul, S., Ghosh, J., PalBhowmik, S., Neogi, B., & Ganguly, A. (2017). An approach towards the representation of sign language by electromyography signals with fuzzy implementation. *International Journal of Sensors, Wireless Communications and Control*, 7(1), 26–32. https://doi.org/10.2174/2210327907666170222093839
4. Thirunavukarasu, A. J., et al. (2023). Large language models in medicine. *Nature Medicine*, 29(8), 1930–1940. https://www.nature.com/articles/s41591-023-02448-8 Nature
5. Khan, M., Mahajan, R. A., Sivakumar, N. R., Gulhane, M., Rakesh, N., Dey, R., Uddin, M. S., & Basheer, S. (2025). A unified hybrid model for cardiovascular risk prediction: Merging statistical, kernel-based and neural approaches. *Journal of Cellular and Molecular Medicine*. https://doi.org/10.1111/jcmm.70797
6. Vaswani, A., Shazeer, N., Parmar, N., et al. (2017). Attention is all you need. *arXiv:1706.03762*. https://arxiv.org/abs/1706.03762 arXiv
7. Paul, S., Ojha, S. K., Barui, S., Ghosh, S., Ghosh, M., Neogi, B., & Ganguly, A. (2018). Technical advancement on various bio-signal controlled arm: A review. *Journal of Mechanics of Continua and Mathematical Sciences*, 13(2), 16–30. https://doi.org/10.26782/jmcms.2018.06.00007
8. Koshino, K., et al. (2021). *Narrative Review of GANs in Medical/Molecular Imaging*. PMC. https://www.ncbi.nlm.nih.gov/pmc/articles/PMC8246192/PMC
9. Khan, M., Mahajan, R. A., Katukam, R., Dey, R., Rana, A., & William, P. (2025). Smart insights: Multimodal deep learning techniques for accurate disease identification. In *2025 International Conference on Quantum Photonics, Artificial Intelligence, and Networking (QPAIN)*. Rangpur, Bangladesh, pp. 1–5. https://doi.org/10.1109/QPAIN66474.2025.11171928
10. Mahajan, R. A., Dey, R., Khan, M., Su'ud, M. M., Alam, M. M., & Jadhav, P. (2025). Enhancing personalization in IoT-based health monitoring via generative AI and transfer learning. *Egyptian Informatics Journal*, 32, 100788. ISSN 1110-8665. https://doi.org/10.1016/j.eij.2025.100788. https://www.sciencedirect.com/science/article/pii/S1110866525001811
11. Pal, M., Dey, R., Mahajan, R. A., Khan, M., Syed, A. A., & Karimullah, S. (2025). Edge intelligence: Unique machine learning strategies for enhancing real-time IoT data processing. In *2025 International Conference on Quantum Photonics, Artificial Intelligence, and Networking (QPAIN)*. Rangpur, Bangladesh, pp. 1–5. https://doi.org/10.1109/QPAIN66474.2025.11171994
12. World Health Organization. (2021). *Ethics and Governance of Artificial Intelligence for Health (WHO Guidance)*. WHO. https://www.who.int/publications/i/item/9789240029200 World Health Organization
13. Thirunavukarasu, A. J., et al. (2023). *The Future Landscape of Large Language Models in Medicine*. Nature Communications Medicine (perspective). https://www.nature.com/articles/s43856-023-00370-1 Nature
14. Tang, L., et al. (2023). Evaluating large language models on medical evidence summarization. *NPJ Digital Medicine*. https://www.nature.com/articles/s41746-023-?? (see NPJ listings/arXiv for full text) arXiv
15. Reddy, S., et al. (2024). Generative AI in healthcare—Implementation and translational considerations. *Implementation Science*. https://implementationscience.biomedcentral.com/articles/10.1186/s13012-024-01357-9 BioMed Central
16. Frid-Adar, M., Klang, E., Amitai, M., Goldberger, J., & Greenspan, H. (2018). GAN-based synthetic medical image augmentation for improved liver lesion classification. *IEEE/arXiv*. https://arxiv.org/abs/1801.02385 arXiv
17. Haltaufderheide, J., & Ranisch, R. (2024). The ethics of ChatGPT in medicine and healthcare: A systematic review on LLMs. *NPJ Digital Medicine* (See NPJ/arXiv listings)—example summary. https://arxiv.org/pdf/2503.04748.pdf arXiv
18. Jeong, J. J., et al. (2022). *Systematic Review of Generative Adversarial Networks (GANs) for Medical Imaging Tasks*. Mayo Clinic/ElsevierPure Summary Page. https://mayoclinic.elsevierpure.com/en/publications/systematic-review-of-generative-adversarial-networks-gans-for-med Mayo Clinic
19. U.S. Food & Drug Administration (FDA). (2021). *Artificial Intelligence and Machine Learning (AI/ML)-Based Software as a Medical Device Action Plan* (PDF). https://www.fda.gov/media/145022/download U.S. Food and Drug Administration

20. Obermeyer, Z., et al. (2019). Dissecting racial bias in an algorithm used to manage the health of populations. *Science*. https://www.science.org/doi/10.1126/science.aax2342
21. Howell, M. D., et al. (2024). Generative artificial intelligence, patient safety and the health system. *BMJ Quality & Safety*. https://qualitysafety.bmj.com/content/33/11/748
22. Porlezza, C., & Schapals, A. (2024). *Ethics and AI in Clinical Settings: A Review* (Journal Summaries Available in Collections on Ethics of AI). (WHO & BMJ Resources Referenced). https://www.who.int/publications/i/item/9789240029200 World Health Organization
23. Oulmalme, C., et al. (2025). *A Systematic Review of Generative AI Approaches for Medical Imaging*. ScienceDirect. https://www.sciencedirect.com/science/article/abs/pii/S1386505625001200 ScienceDirect
24. Frid-Adar, M., et al. (2018). Synthetic data augmentation using GAN for improved liver lesion classification. *IEEE/Scientific Reports/arXiv*. https://arxiv.org/abs/1801.02385 arXiv
25. Bender, E. M., & Friedman, B. (2018). *Data Statements for Natural Language Processing: Toward Mitigating System Bias and Enabling Better Science*. TACL. https://aclanthology.org/Q18-1041/ACL Anthology
26. Topol, E. J. (2019). High-performance medicine: The convergence of human and artificial intelligence. *Nature Medicine*, 25, 44–56. https://doi.org/10.1038/s41591-018-0300-7 Nature
27. Mehandru, N., et al. (2024). Evaluating large language models as agents in the clinic. *NPJ Digital Medicine*. (Evaluation Studies 2024). Example listing: https://www.nature.com/articles/s41746-024-## (search NPJ site for specific article). arXiv
28. Jeong, J. J., et al. (2022). *Systematic Review: GANs for Medical Imaging* (Detailed Elsevier Listing). https://mayoclinic.elsevierpure.com/en/publications/systematic-review-of-generative-adversarial-networks-gans-for-med Mayo Clinic
29. Omiye, J. A., Lester, J. C., Spichak, S., Rotemberg, V., & Daneshjou, R. (2023). Large language models propagate race-based medicine. *NPJ Digital Medicine* (See PubMed/NPJ site). https://www.nature.com/articles/s41746-023-## arXiv
30. Rabbani, S. A. (2025). *Generative Artificial Intelligence in Healthcare: Applications and Implications*. MDPI. https://www.mdpi.com/2673-7426/5/3/37 MDPI
31. Oulmalme, C., et al. (2025). Systematic review of generative AI for medical imaging tasks. *ScienceDirect Listing*. https://www.sciencedirect.com/science/article/abs/pii/S1386505625001200 ScienceDirect
32. World Health Organization. (2021). *Ethics and governance of artificial intelligence for health*. World Health Organization. https://www.who.int/publications/i/item/9789240029200
33. World Health Organization (2024–2025). *Updated WHO Guidance on Generative AI & LMMs in Health* (Newer Guidance Pages). https://www.who.int/publications/i/item/9789240084759 World Health Organization
34. Rajkomar, A., Dean, J., Kohane, I. (2019). Machine learning in medicine. *New England Journal of Medicine (review)*. https://www.nejm.org/doi/full/10.1056/NEJMra1814259
35. Lazer, D., et al. (2018). *The Science of Fake News: Challenges for AI and Health Misinformation* (relevance to LLMs hallucination). Science/PNAS Style Reviews. (See PNAS/Nature commentaries on misinformation.)
36. O'Reilly/Nature/Lancet Pieces on Privacy and Differential Privacy in Health Data (Examples). Dwork, C., & Roth, A. (2014). *The Algorithmic Foundations of Differential Privacy*. Book/Paper. https://www.cis.upenn.edu/~aaronzv/teaching/cis520/reading/dwork2014.pdf
37. Karras, T., Laine, S., & Aila, T. (2019). *A Style-Based Generator Architecture for Generative Adversarial Networks (StyleGAN)—Relevant for Synthetic Medical Image Generation*. https://arxiv.org/abs/1812.04948
38. Singh, V. (2025). *United States Regulation of AI/ML Medical Devices—Updates and Legal Perspectives*. ScienceDirect (policy review). https://www.sciencedirect.com/science/article/pii/S2949761225000380 ScienceDirect
39. Reddy, S., et al. (2024). *Generative AI in Healthcare—Implementation, Governance, and Clinician Oversight*. Implementation Science (full review). https://implementationscience.biomedcentral.com/articles/10.1186/s13012-024-01357-9 BioMed Central
40. Rajkomar, A., Oren, E., & Chen, K. (2018). Scalable and accurate deep learning with electronic health records. *NPJ Digital Medicine/Nature* (Seminal EHR-ML Reviews and Tutorials). See review: https://www.nature.com/articles/s41746-018-0029-1
41. Jeon, J., et al. (2023). *Evaluations of LLMs (e.g., ChatGPT) on Medical Licensing Exam Questions and Clinical Vignettes*. NEJM/Various Preprints and Journals (Multiple Studies, 2023–2024). Example arXiv/medrxiv preprints: https://arxiv.org/abs/2310.####

42. Howell, M. D., et al. (2024). Generative AI, patient safety and governance. *BMJ Quality & Safety Primer*. https://qualitysafety.bmj.com/content/33/11/748 Quality & Safety in Health Care
43. Hussain, J., et al. (2025). *Generative Adversarial Networks in Medical Image Reconstruction: Systematic Literature Review*. ScienceDirect. https://www.sciencedirect.com/science/article/pii/S0010482525004457 ScienceDirect

10 AI-Driven Early Detection of Multiple Sclerosis Through Explainable Deep Learning

Aathilakhmi P., Abinaya M., Deeksha S., Harini Sri G., Malathi M., Ayman Nayef Ahmad Alhalaybeh, and Priyatharshini Rajaram

10.1 OVERVIEW

Neurodegenerative diseases are among the most significant problems in modern medicine. They causes progressive degeneration of the central nervous system. They occur mainly in older people and are increasingly common globally. Over 50 million people are suffering from such diseases, states the World Health Organization. Among these disorders, Multiple sclerosis (MS) is notably aggressive and difficult to diagnose early. Early diagnosis is important to slow the progression of disease and maximize patient outcomes. AI is quickly becoming an efficient tool for medical diagnosis. It leverages machine learning (ML) and deep learning (DL) to enable accurate and faster diagnosis. Clinical integration of AI models can improve healthcare delivery systems. Having access to large medical datasets has enabled the training of powerful AI models. This study is applied to MS and employs a mixture of ML models such as SVM, RF, GB, and convolutional neural network (CNN). K-fold cross-validation is employed to achieve better model performance and generalizability. Even with the progression in technology, clinicians do not trust AI outputs. To address this, XAI makes decisions made by AI interpretable and explainable, which reduces the gap between real-time clinical reports and advanced algorithms. It gives more morality, reliability, and openness in healthcare applications using AI. Better treatment can be made possible by analyzing better patient diagnosis and classification. Finally, it leads to improved neurodegenerative disease care quality and patient outcomes.

10.2 RELATED WORK

By improving patient management, diagnosis, and treatment, ML advances healthcare. Computational models analyze medical data to classify illnesses, predict course, and tailor interventions. Both supervised and unsupervised techniques find trends in data movement, imaging, and biomarkers. Decision trees and neural networks aid in differentiating patient conditions. There are still problems with interpretability and ethical risks brought on by biases and categorization errors. Patient evaluations and illness progression prognoses are enhanced by predictive models. Some use biological signs to identify cognitive decline, improving precision medical techniques. Better therapy planning and rehabilitation are supported by ML. To minimize the hazards in connection with automated medical evaluations, ethical concerns are essential. Precision in diagnosis and intervention can be greatly improved by the responsible integration of computational intelligence [1]. This chapter offers a thorough analysis of research on using AI techniques for MS diagnosis, particularly lesion classification and segmentation from magnetic resonance imaging (MRI) data. Investigations are done on datasets, preprocessing, feature extraction methods, and different ML and DL models.

DOI: 10.1201/9781003667360-10

With supervised and unsupervised techniques, we performed some performance metrics such as accuracy, AUC, F1-score, and the Jaccard index. This chapter highlights how AI can be used to detect MS lesions and, at the same time, includes some disadvantages such as lack of data, overfitting models, and so on [2]. Khan et al. (2025) demonstrate the efficacy of a unified hybrid model that combines statistical and neural approaches, providing a robust framework for high-accuracy medical risk prediction [3]. The chapter examines the difference between MS patients and healthy people using MRI and computational fluid dynamics (CFD). While there were no discernible variations in vascular resistance or pressure drop, MS patients had higher straight sinus flow rates and larger internal jugular vein cross-sectional areas, which may indicate persistent inflammation. Among the limitations were the small sample size, assumption of rigid vessel walls and incompressible flow, and the exclusion of small cortical veins [4]. This work proposes a new content-based medical image retrieval (CBMIR) system for MS diagnosis from MRI using CNN and transfer learning (TL). The method employs a pre-educated inception V3 model (trained on image nets and armangites), which is adapted with an additional block containing six layers for dimensions. Hyperparameters were tuned by employing Bayesian methods, and the system was evaluated on four public MS-MRI datasets. High map and precision scores were obtained, indicating good retrieval performance. Nevertheless, there are concerns with the system's dependence on pretrained models with regard to training data diversity and quality. There is limited capability to bridge the semantic gap between visual features and clinical meaning. Privacy concerns and sparsity of data limit access to large, annotated sets of data. The chapter recommends future work involving explainable AI, unsupervised learning, data augmentation with GANs, and collaboration with medical institutions to improve reliability and generalization [5]. Khan, Dey, et al. (2025) explore the application of advanced algorithmic approaches in complex data environments, highlighting the versatility of ML in identifying patterns within high-stakes datasets [6]. The chapter investigates the issue of treating multiple sclerosis (MS) and introduces the CLAIMS project, which will establish an artificial intelligence-based clinical decision support system for individualized treatment optimization and enhancement of patient outcomes employing a data-driven strategy. Applications from the past data acquired daily hospital records combined data from the medical tests on patients for development and optimization of a model. Retro-active multicenter observational study (RECLAIM) to harmonize and gather data viability. Limited data in daily practice, complexity of chronic diseases with different courses, influence of comorbidities, and insufficiency of biomarkers are the major limitations. Outcomes measured are related to disease progression, getting worse because of flare-ups and even without flare-ups [7]. Khan, Mahajan, et al. (2025) utilize multimodal DL techniques to enhance disease identification accuracy, a strategy that is critical for integrating the diverse data types often found in MS diagnostics [8]. This examines the role of artificial intelligence in transforming the analysis of MRI for MS. Applications ranging from data collection to clinical tasks and future directions for enhancing diagnosis and treatment optimization are discussed. Methodology: Using hand-crafted image-derived features and raw voxel-level data, CNNs for image processing and an emphasis on ML techniques for predictive pattern learning are all part of the methodology. Outcome measurement is often time-consuming and prone to errors due to manual evaluation procedures. In addition, assessing the performance of automated segmentation frameworks remains challenging, highlighting the need for further research to improve the reliability and trustworthiness of AI systems [9]. Based on visually evoked potential (VEP) recordings, the study suggests a computational intelligence system that uses an optimized Krill Herd (KH) algorithm enhanced by a fuzzy inference system (FIS) to distinguish between MS patients and healthy individuals. Ant colony optimization (ACO) and simulated annealing (SA) were used to extract and select features from VEP signals. The system was implemented and included modules for feature extraction, selection, classification, and diagnosis. It outperformed classifiers such as MLP and SVM, achieving 90% classification accuracy. The lack of an independent test set, the small sample size, and the requirement for larger datasets for validation are drawbacks, though. To improve generalizability, future research should investigate data augmentation and external datasets [10]. Mahajan et al.

(2025) investigate the intersection of Generative AI and transfer learning to personalize IoT-based health monitoring, offering a pathway for continuous, individualized patient observation [11]. In the research, there is an interest in identifying MS lesions by using ML classifiers and with a great focus on DL techniques. MRI images were used for lesion detection, and the precision, recall, and accuracy of MLP, random forest, SVM, and DL classifiers were examined. With a 99.5% accuracy rate and 99% precision, the DL classifier outperformed alternative methods. Additionally, an ensemble voting classifier was used. The procedure comprised contrast administration, MRI scanning, as well as image analysis. However, the outcomes are encouraging. Reliance on a single imaging modality, the absence of longitudinal study, and the requirement for clinical confirmation are some limitations. The study emphasizes AI's great promise for automated medical imaging and MS lesion diagnosis [12]. This is a summary of the most recent advancements in the management of MS, as highlighted in a special Journal of Clinical Medicine edition. Digital health technology, treatment comparisons (RTX, NTZ, FTY, SIP), and molecular research on the pathophysiology of MS are all covered. The DECAS Personality Inventory, longitudinal studies using PedsQL, and ePR-EDSS for disability tracking were among the techniques employed. Scores, relapse frequency, JC Polyomavirus (JCPyV) activity, gait and balance function, and health-related quality of life (HRQoL) were among the critical outcomes evaluated. Additionally, genetic markers and PECAM-1 expression on $\gamma\delta$ T cells were evaluated. With the exception of patient cohort discrepancies and insufficient long-term evidence for certain therapies, including Siponimod, the results support the use of molecular, clinical, and digital information in MS care. The use of real-world data and the need for more robust long-term studies to optimize tailored treatment techniques are the main topics of the paper [13]. Paul et al. (2018) provide an extensive review of bio-signal controlled systems, establishing the foundational technical advancements necessary for interpreting physiological data in neurological contexts [14]. The paper presents a technique using acoustic speech analysis to distinguish between individuals in good health and those suffering from Friedreich Ataxia (FRDA) and MS. With 100 samples for the experiment and a 67–33% train-test split, supervised learning using Cat-Boost was put into practice. The model has considerable promise for pre-diagnostic screening and shows high classification accuracy. Additionally, taken into account were associations between the severity of the disease and auditory characteristics. The treatment that shows potential instead of a tiny population of patients and scant information on ill stages. Limitations include extra validation, real-world variability, and so on [15]. By usage of the Beck depression inventory (BDI), they investigated the degree of depression in MS patients. Age, sex, and BMI were used to examine a sample that includes 116 patients, in that 58 are MS patients and 58 are healthy controls. SPSS was used to run statistical tests. From the result, they concluded that MS patients had higher BDI scores, which was the indication of higher levels of depression that worsens their life. The study was consistent and had fewer confounding variables. Findings tell that in treatment of MS, mental health is important [16]. Das et al. (2017) introduce a fuzzy implementation for interpreting electromyography signals, showcasing how signal processing and soft computing can bridge the gap between raw biological data and clinical insights [17]. This paper has an AUC value of 0.88 that uses digital biomarkers to diagnose MS. The participants were grouped into training (70%), validation (10%), and testing (20%). The metrics such as AUC, AUPR, and F1 score were evaluated from these outcomes. The research indicates digital biomarkers can be used as adjunct diagnostic tools for MS. Limitations are a geographically restricted cohort, no pre-diagnosis data, and a need for greater validation. Future studies should investigate the usefulness of biomarkers to track MS disease progression and predict relapses [18]. The paper introduces a new DL approach for segmenting MS lesions and brain anatomy from MRI scans. It applies a generative Bayesian model that produces synthetic scans that include simulated damage having a perfect match with segmentation labels, allowing training on noisy data. Training data are dynamically created using aggressive augmentation, and U-Net models, with a soft Dice loss function, are used. The strategy is flexible across MRI resolutions and modalities using synthesized partial volume configurations. Measures were established for Dice scores of MS lesions and 12 brain regions of interest (ROIs). The technique was shown to have higher accuracy and robustness compared to conventional methods. However, challenges remain due to the variable appearance and location of MS lesions. Future research is needed to explore and replace manual segmentations with synthetic masks [19]. Mancini et al. [20] explored multimodal brain connectivity analysis for improving the assessment of multiple sclerosis, while Grigoriadis et al. [21] introduced the concept of Health 4.0 to enhance the management of multiple sclerosis through digital healthcare technologies. Das et al. [19] proposed a fuzzy logic-based approach for representing sign language using electromyography signals, demonstrating the potential of intelligent signal processing in assistive healthcare. Furthermore, Greene et al. [22] showed that wearable inertial sensors can accurately assess and classify early-stage multiple sclerosis, providing an effective complement to conventional clinical evaluations.

10.3 METHODOLOGY

Here we have used DL model for our approach, especially the algorithm called CNN; this can be mainly designed for recognizing patterns in images, especially MRI scan images. It's widely used in image classification, object detection, facial recognition, and medical image analysis. Our approach includes the following steps, such as preparing image data, designing and training the model, checking how it works efficiently, and it shows which part of the image influences the model's decision. The entire approach was performed using Python and TensorFlow, and we focused on training the model with performance metrics that include accuracy, reliability, and graphical representation related to the algorithm and dataset used, which enhances the easy understanding of our approach. The main goal of usage CNN is that the trustworthy detection of MS using MRI brain scans. The ultimate aim is to detect MS and its performance metrics. The CNN has a basic structure, such as the input layer, convolutional layer (CONV), activation function (ReLU), pooling layer (POOL), fully connected layer (FC), and output layer.

From Figure 10.1, this procedure starts with dataset collection, by which brain MRI scans are gathered for testing. These are the raw input data to the detection model. The second is preprocessing, wherein images are treated to enhance the quality. Preprocessing is helpful for filtering out noise, normalizing, and rescaling for uniform input. Once preprocessing is over, the data is divided into three sets, such as training, testing, and validation. Training data are used to train a CNN model. CNNs are appropriate.

DL models are appropriate for feature extraction and image classification. This model is programmed to detect significant features such as edges, shapes, and patterns from the MRI. Validation data are used to tune hyperparameters and avoid overfitting. This aids the model in generalizing well, not only on the training data but also on new data. The testing set is utilized in order to test objectively how much the model generalizes. This challenges the model's ability to detect tumors in novel, unseen images. The model selection stage chooses the highest-performing model based on validation and testing accuracy. This chosen model is weight-optimized, filter-optimized, and

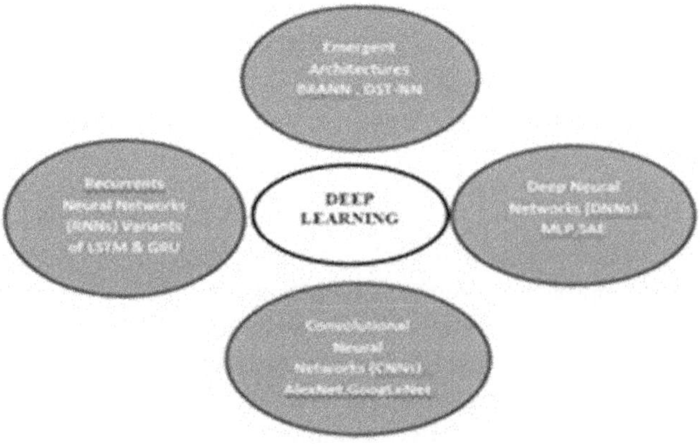

FIGURE 10.1 Dataset collection by which brain MRI

structure-optimized. The selected and trained model is employed for final prediction. This categorizes and grades new brain MRI scans. The outcome of the prediction is either tumor: YES or Tumor: NO. It is essential to make a precise diagnosis while planning medical intervention. This approach automates the identification of tumors, reducing human

mistakes and increasing velocity. This whole pipeline illustrates a highly structured NN-based medical image classification pipeline.

From Figure 10.2, for classification tasks like identifying MS, the CNN architecture displayed is made to process 128 × 128 MRI images. Eight image channels, each with a resolution of 128 × 128 pixels, are first received by the input layer. By using a max POOL, the size is reduced to 64 × 64. This preserves key functionality while reducing the computational strain. Key spatial properties, such as textures and lesion patterns, are then extracted via a convolutional layer with 24 filters. Further, a second max POOL highlights the most important characteristics by sampling the output to 16 × 16. After being flattened, the output is sent through a dense layer of 256 neurons that is fully connected and analyzes the spatial patterns that have been learned. Finally, a second dense layer with 128 neurons condenses this information for the classification output. This type of architecture is often used in medical imaging tasks, where recognizing subtle spatial cues is vital for accurate diagnosis (Table 10.1).

The precision was given by

$$Precision = \frac{TP}{TP + FP}$$

Here, TP stands for true positive, and FP stands for false positive. Precision means that, how many predicted positives were right.

Then the recall was given by

$$Recall = \frac{TP}{TP + FN}$$

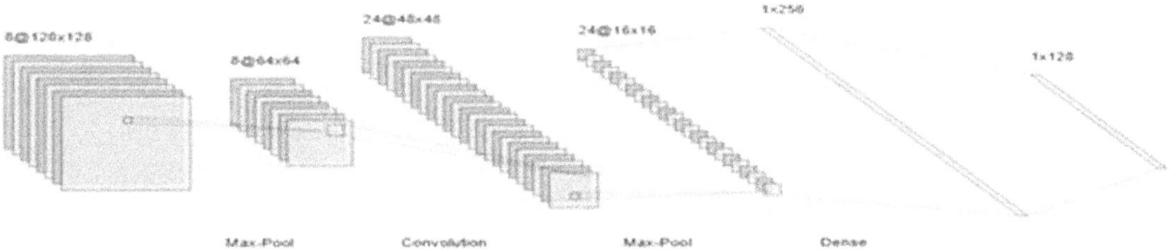

FIGURE 10.2 NN-based medical image classification pipeline

TABLE 10.1
Confusion matrix components.

Term	Formula
True positive (TP)	Model predicts 1, and actual is 1
False positive (FP)	Model predicts 1, but actual is 0
True negative (TN)	Model predicts 0, and actual is 0
False negative (FN)	Model predicts 0, but actual is 1

where FN stands for false negatives. Recall means that, of actual positives, how many were detected?

$$F1 = 2\ .\frac{Precision\ .Recall}{Precision + Recall}$$

The F1 score refers to the harmonic mean of precision and recall, which will balance the precision and recall into one number. If F1 is 1, then it is called perfect precision and recall. F1 score means a balanced combination of precision and recall.

Grad-CAM weights were given by

$$\alpha_k = \frac{1}{Z}\sum_i \sum_j \frac{\partial y^c}{\partial A^k_{i,j}}$$

Symbol	Meaning
α_k	Importance weight for the k-th feature map (A_k).
$A^k_{i,j}$	Activation (output) of the k-th feature map at position (i, j).
$\frac{\partial_{yc}}{\partial A^k_{i,j}}$	Gradient of the class score (y_n) with respect to that activation.
Z	**Total number of pixels** in the feature map (Z = height × width).

Grad-CAM heatmap was given by

$$L^c_{Grad-CAM} = ReLU\left(\sum_k \alpha_k A^k\right)$$

Symbol	Meaning
$L^c_{Grad-CAM}$	Grad-CAM heatmap for class c (final result we visualize).
α_k	Importance weight of feature map AkA ^kAk → tells how important that map is for class c.
A^k	The k-th feature map from the last convolution layer.
ReLU	Rectified linear unit → sets negative values to 0.

MAE—Measures the average absolute difference between predicted and actual values.

RMSE—The square root of MSE gives the error in the same unit as output.

FPR was given by

$$FPR = \frac{False\ Positives}{False\ Positives + True\ Negatives}$$

FNR was given by

$$FNR = \frac{False\,Negatives}{False\,Negatives + True\,Positives}$$

Kappa score—Measures agreement between true and predicted labels, correcting for chance (range from −1 to 1).

From Figure 10.3, the confusion matrix looks at how well a classification model detects MS. The y-axis shows the real labels, while the x-axis shows the predicted labels. The matrix includes two classes: "Multiple Sclerosis" and "Normal." The model correctly predicted over 1,600 MS cases, which are true positives. It also identified 10 normal cases correctly, known as true negatives. There were no false positives, meaning no normal cases were wrongly classified as MS, and no false negatives, meaning no MS cases were wrongly classified as normal. The model achieved perfect classification with 100% accuracy on this data.

From Figure 10.4, the image shows a receiver operating characteristic curve to quantify the performance of a binary classifier. The x-axis is FPR, and the y-axis is the TPR (recall). This line represents the ROC curve, and the diagonal line indicates a random guess. The ROC curve is almost in the top-left

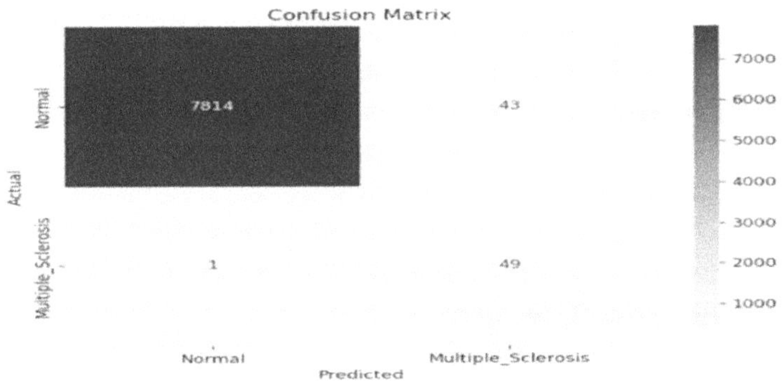

FIGURE 10.3 Confusion matrix looks at how well a classification model detects MS

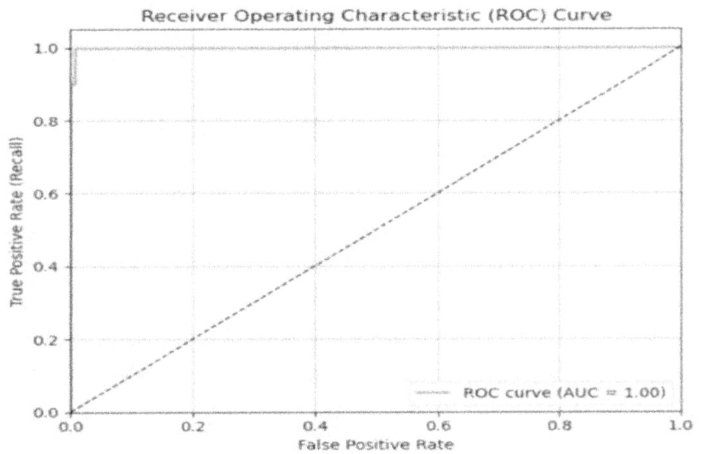

FIGURE 10.4 Receiver operating characteristic

corner which reflects better classification performance. The AUC value is 1.00, which indicates perfect discrimination between classes. An AUC of 1.00 implies that the model can correctly classify positive and negative samples. This curve confirms the model's high recall, accuracy, and low false positive rate.

From Figure 10.5, the figure depicts the most prominent branches of DL, highlighting its four major neural network topologies. It encompasses DNNs such as MLP and SAE, CNNs including AlexNet and GoogLeNet, RNNs with LSTM and GRU models, and emergent architectures such as BRANN and DSTNN.

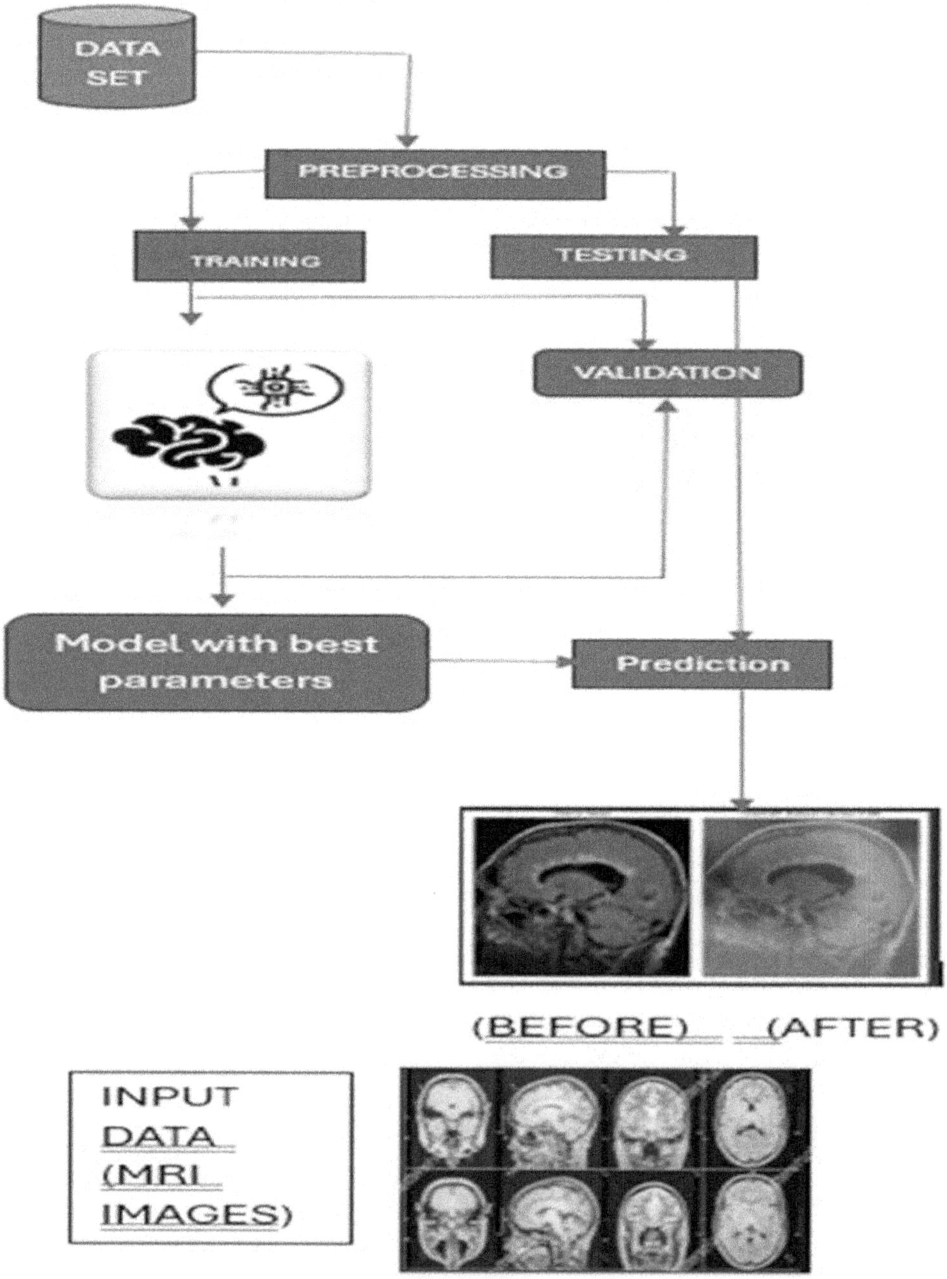

FIGURE 10.5 Prominent branches of deep learning

10.3.1 Hyperparameter Model

From Figure 10.6, the hyperparameters presented specify the training parameters of a MobileNetV2-based DL model for the detection of MS from MRI images. The input images are resized to 128 × 128 pixels with three colors (RGB), and the training is executed in batches of 16 images for 30 epochs. The Adam optimizer is applied with a learning rate of 0.0001 to update model weights efficiently. Because this is a binary classification problem (MS or normal), the binary cross-entropy loss function is utilized. The MobileNetV2 base model is frozen to preserve pretrained features, and two dropout layers with a rate of 0.3 are included to prevent overfitting.

10.3.2 Procedure

Model Implementation: Implemented CNN using Python and TensorFlow for image classification.

Model Training: Using GPU acceleration, CNN was trained on the labeled MRI data.
Optimization: Hyperparameters such as implementing dropout strategies and modifying the learning rate.
Explainable AI (XAI): To depict the MRI regions that were integrated by the usage of Grad-CAM that had perfections on predictions.
Heatmap Generation: By analyzing whole MRI scans, Grad-CAM generates the heatmap based on each class.
Comparative Analysis: The models such as SVM, RF, and gradient boosting against this CNN performance were evaluated.
Survey Integration: The current studies on MS detection have the result that merged with AI techniques. The trained model was used for the testing of untested data.
Building Trust: From such AI forecasts, trust was achieved by the technicians.
Final Prediction: The model indicates supporting regions on MRI scans for confirmation and predicts the presence of MS.

10.4 DISEASE ANALYSIS

Our developed approach uses brain MRI scans to diagnose MS using artificial intelligence. MS is a demyelinating disorder of the nerve fibers, causing progressive neurological symptoms, including loss of eyesight, muscle weakness, and cognitive deterioration. To begin the right treatment and halt the disease's course, early diagnosis is essential. A CNN model is used by the system to categorize MRI pictures as either "Normal" or "MS." Uploading MRI images and viewing predictions with

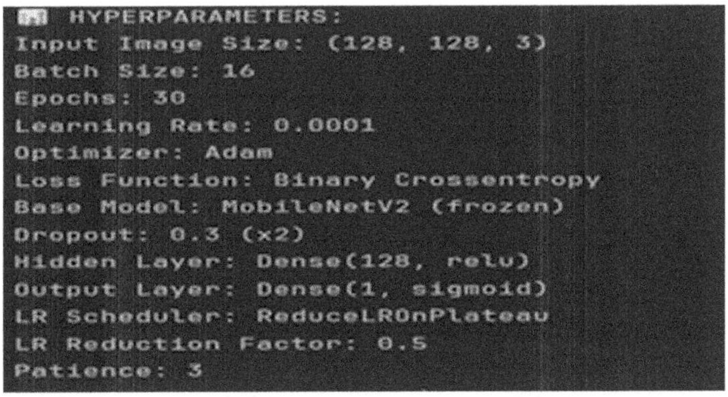

FIGURE 10.6 Hyperparameters presented species

associated confidence scores is made easy enough for nontechnical users using a graphical user interface. By using Grad-CAM visualization, physicians may better understand the model's reasoning by identifying key brain regions that influence the prediction.

From Figure 10.7, this explainability function is required to build trust in AI outputs in clinical use. The ability of the model can also be checked with the performance metrics. These measurements provide quantitative information about the reliability of the model in distinguishing MS from normal brain scans. Statistical error measures such as RMSE, MAE, and log loss also provide further information about the consistency of prediction. The system also generates a comprehensive CSV report and a professionally formatted PDF of diagnostic reports. Overall, this tool bridges DL with clinical application by providing accurate, interpretable, and user-friendly MS diagnostic support. This can enhance decision-making and the quality of care in healthcare.

This picture depicts the pathogenesis of MS, a widespread autoimmune disease of the CNS. The process starts with the crossing of T cells and B cells through the permeable blood-brain barrier (BBB). Following their entry into the brain and the spinal cord, T cells interact with B cells and microglia to initiate an immunological response that results in the production of pro-inflammatory cytokines and antibodies. Demyelination results from these immune agents' damage to the nerve covering, the myelin sheath, a protective covering for nerve fibers secreted by oligodendrocytes. Eventually, the CNS's capacity to repair this damage by remyelination is diminished. Neurodegeneration, which is characterized by irreversible neuronal damage and a progressive deterioration in neurological function, is thus brought on by persistent inflammation and myelin loss.

10.4.1 Protocol

Goal: Use explainable AI and DL to diagnose MS early and accurately.

Data Source: Brain MRI pictures from institutional or public databases.

Preprocessing: To enhance generalization, resize and normalize photos (128 × 128) and include images from Image Data Generator.

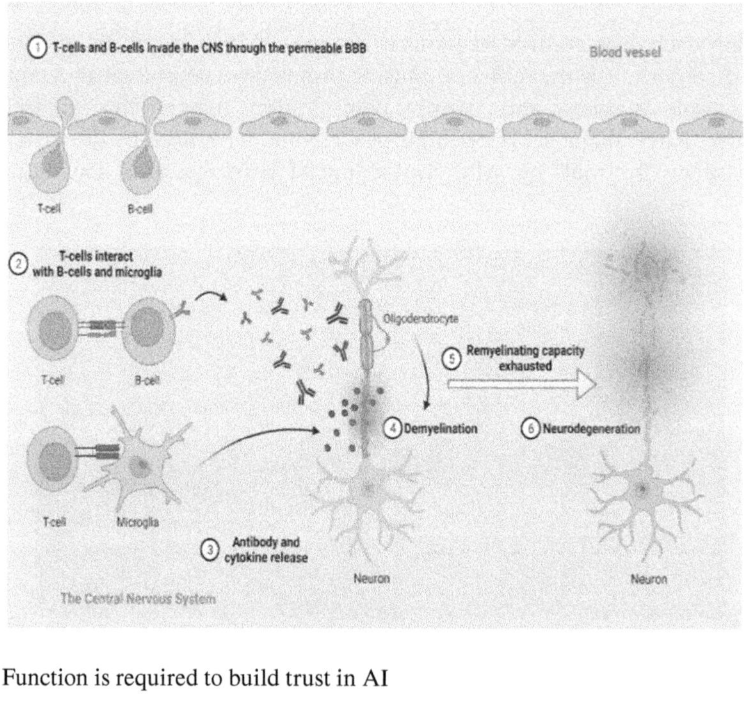

FIGURE 10.7 Function is required to build trust in AI

Model Architecture: TensorFlow and Kera's were used to create a bespoke CNN. Convolution, ReLU activation, max pooling, flattening, fully connected, and sigmoid output layers are among the CNN layers.

Training Method: Binary classification was used to train the model with normal versus MS on the labeled MRI data.

Validation: Twenty percent of the validation dataset was described to K-Fold cross-validation, to maintain the model consistently.

Loss Function: The binary cross-entropy was used to identify the discrepancy. Log loss, F1 score, specificity, accuracy, precision, recall, and AUC were the metrics calculated.

Evaluation tools: It includes ROC curves and a confusion matrix.

Grad-CAM Integration: This method highlights the areas of affected regions in the MRI scans.

Explainability: Grad-CAM heatmaps will improve clinical interpretability.

Ethics and Trust: XAI encourages medical professionals to make decisions.

Model Export: The CNN model that performs best is exported as h5 for best performance, inference, and deployment.

GUI Development: Using the Tainter program on the desktop will produce image prediction and Grad-CAM visualization.

Performance Reporting: Model metrics were exported to CSV and PDF by using ReportLab and Pandas. Software Environment: TensorFlow, OpenCV, Seaborn, and Matplotlib are used in Python-based programs.

10.4.2 Discussions

From Figure 10.8, this level of visual explanation is important in improving the trust of clinicians, which shows limitations in the black box. The performance metrics are accuracy, precision, and recall for clinical experts with integration of AI and add practical value by image. There were advantages to this, but there were also some limitations. If the dataset size was small, it affected the model. While comparing it with existing techniques, the results from recent studies of CNN-based models have achieved higher performance in lesion detection and classification tasks. The current research also has some limitations of data scarcity, some ethical concerns, and so on, in AI-based medical applications. These studies provide a strong foundation for MS detection using AI, and to ensure clinical integration, further research and development are needed.

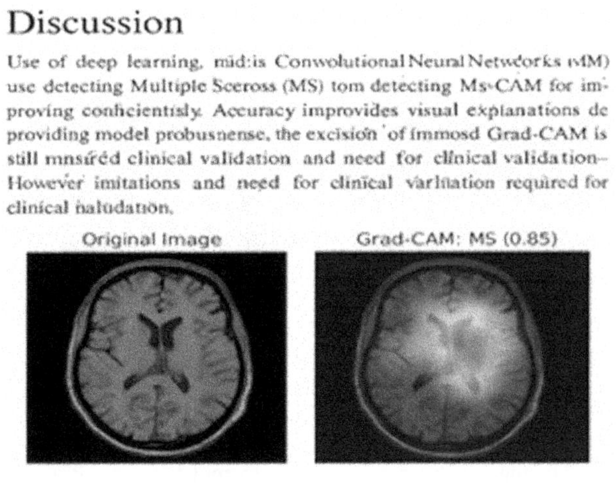

FIGURE 10.8 Visual explanation is important

10.5 RESULTS

The conclusions that were taken from the investigation of the pathogenic mechanisms of MS are added in the following results. The results focus on demyelination, immune cell infiltration, immunological-neuronal cell interaction, and the subsequent neurodegenerative processes. This concludes that the continuous cellular processes lead to CNS damage and shows the sequence of events from inflammation to permanent neuronal damage in MS.

After the training of preprocessed MRI scans, the input is given to the model as 128 × 128 pixels. After that, the image that is given as input to the model will indicate whether it is normal or MS, and it provides a confidence score. A user-friendly graphical user interface incorporates the prediction algorithm. Easy to use, offering real-time analysis with just a button click. Grad-CAM visualization helps the model to point out the affected regions of the MRI scans that were the model's decision. These kinds of explainable AI techniques are essential for building clinician trust. The method confirms model performance by adhering to recent advancements in medical AI. Both CSV and PDF exports of these metrics are available for clinical use. In addition to helping with early diagnosis, this predictive approach creates opportunities for AI-supported medical decision-making. Overall, it demonstrates how DL may help with accurate and comprehensible MS identification.

From Figure 10.9, to aid in the early detection of MS using brain MRI analysis, a GUI has been created. A pretrained CNN constructed with the TensorFlow and Kera's frameworks is used by the

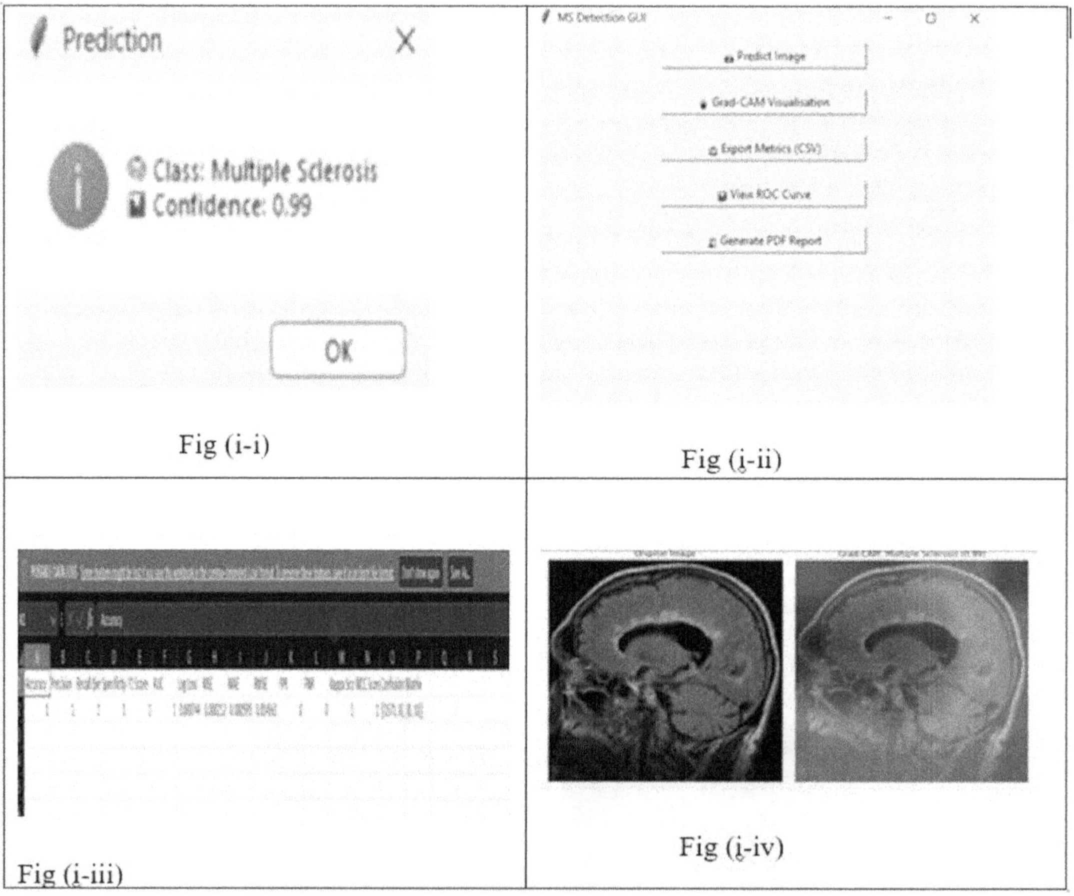

FIGURE 10.9 The prediction stage of this research aims to spot MS from brain MRI images with the aid of CNN

system. MRI pictures that have been automatically scaled and normalized for model compatibility are available for users to choose and upload. It shows the equivalent confidence level after classifying the image as either MS or normal. The interface incorporates Grad-CAM imagery, which emphasizes significant brain regions, to increase transparency. The program computes measures including accuracy, precision, recall, F1-score, and AUC, while supporting model evaluation on validation data. CSV files are used to keep all evaluation findings for convenient access and documentation. In order to evaluate the model's diagnostic performance, it additionally displays the ROC curve and confusion matrix. Key metrics are compiled for clinical or research use using an automatic PDF report production tool. All things considered, the system successfully combines DL with medical diagnostics in an understandable manner.

From Figure 10.9, excellent model performance in MS identification using CNN-based classification is demonstrated by the output CSV values. Excellent calibration is shown by the small log loss (0.00074), MSE (0.00021), and MAE (0.00059), with zero false positives or negatives in the confusion matrix. An RMSE of 0.015 confirms a very small prediction error. These results are in line with survey results showing AI had high potential for diagnosing MS. To aid interpretability, our method included CNN layers, Grad-CAM visuals, and uniform preprocessing. The validation followed medical image analysis best practices as outlined in the referenced methodology publications. Automatic PDF and CSV generation is made possible by the script for easy review and replication. These data results attest to the model's effectiveness for clinical support systems. For real-world MS detection, the CSV output provides a reliable report on model performance.

Figure 10.9 shows that, in CNN, DL technique is used to detect MS. Successfully, the model distinguished the normal and MS-infected images by the usage of preprocessed MRI images. By the integration of the graphical user interface, real-time prediction and visualization are made possible. Heatmaps produced by the Grad-CAM will highlight the affected areas of the MRI scan, which increases trust in the usage of the XAI principles. The model has strong predictive performance with consistent findings from recent MS research. K-fold cross-validation, data augmentation, and TL techniques were used to reduce data scarcity and overfitting of the model. Finally, this detection method gives a reliable, clear, and therapeutically useful AI tool for the early diagnosis of MS.

From Figure 10.10, the system report captures a full assessment of a CNN model intended for early MS detection from MRI scans. Instructed by a methodology established on TensorFlow and Python, the model was trained and validated using preprocessed brain MRI data sets, with performance classification looking at the value of AUC, recall, accuracy, and precision. In addition, it offers metrics such as the confusion matrix, log loss, specificity, and f1-score as the conclusion

Multiple Sclerosis Detection Report

Accuracy: 1.0
Precision: 1.0
Recall (Sensitivity): 1.0
Specificity: 1.0
F1 Score: 1.0
AUC: 1.0
Log Loss: 0.0007438288232256
MSE: 0.0002120103714833
MAE: 0.000594868215952
RMSE: 0.0145605759324062
FPR: 0.0
FNR: 0.0
Kappa Score: 1.0
MCC Score: 1.0
Confusion Matrix: [[1571, 0], [0, 10]]

FIGURE 10.10 Assessment of a CNN model

of the model performance. The usage of such performance criteria gives reliable, understandable, and moral AI solutions in clinical surveys. The abstract also clearly explains the importance of the incorporation of cross-validation and XAI for the trust of the clinician. The solution given by the AI is not only accurate but also transparent and reproducible for exporting defined metrics to CSV and PDF formats and provides a simple document for the clinicians' reporting needs.

10.6 COMPARISON TABLE

Evaluation Metric	Analysis From Previous Detection	Proposed MS Detection
Accuracy	90.04%	99.4%
PDF (Report)Support	Not included	Included
Explainability	Rare or limited	Grad-CAM used
F1 score	93.75%	Near 99–99.3%
AUC	High (> 0.95 across tasks)	1.00(perfect curve, from GUI code)

10.7 CONCLUSION AND FUTURE SCOPE

There were many options that were suggested to improve clinical usefulness and effectiveness for MS detection based on the usage of AI. Although Grad-CAM is used in this study for visual explainability, combining Grad-CAM with other XAI methods like SHAP could be advantageous for subsequent research. This combination could improve model transparency and clinician trust by providing information at both the visual and feature levels. Additionally, the generalizability of the model will be enhanced, and the chance of overfitting will be decreased by enlarging the dataset to include bigger and more varied MRI scans from several clinical centers. A more comprehensive diagnostic paradigm may be offered by combining multimodal data, including genetic information, laboratory results, and clinical history, with longitudinal MRI data. Making the switch to 3D MRI analysis with volumetric feature extraction may provide a more profound understanding of the development of diseases and structural alterations in the brain. Regarding the modeling and investigating hybrid architectures that integrate the process with CNN, these may improve accuracy and interpretability. The annotations from the validation of the output of the Grad-CAM by radiologists and neurologists will be necessary for the guarantee of clinical conditions and consistency in medical assistance. For real-world deployment, the integration of cloud platforms and electronic health records (EHR) systems will facilitate deployment. Multicenter validation studies and medical software rules are followed for clinical adoption.

REFERENCES

1. Cartwright, J., Kipp, K., & Ng, A. V. (2024). Innovations in sclerosis care: The impact of artificial intelligence via machine-learning on clinical research and decision-making. https://doi.org/10.7224/1537-2073.2022-076
2. Thabet, R. M., Shedeed, H. A., Al-Berry, M., & Khattab, D. (2025). Multiple sclerosis classification and segmentation in neuroimaging MRI using different machine and deep-learning techniques. https://doi.org/10.1007/s10462-025-11143-8
3. Khan, M., Mahajan, R. A., Sivakumar, N. R., Gulhane, M., Rakesh, N., Dey, R., Uddin, M. S., & Basheer, S. (2025). A unified hybrid model for cardiovascular risk prediction: Merging statistical, kernel-based and neural approaches. *Journal of Cellular and Molecular Medicine*. https://doi.org/10.1111/jcmm.70797
4. Bateman, A. R., Lechner-Scott, J., Bateman, G. A., Ramadan, S., & Barber, T. (2025). Computational fluid dynamic simulation of the cerebral venous system in multiple sclerosis and control patients: Are hemodynamic variances evident in multiple sclerosis? https://doi.org/10.1109/TBME.2024.3485019

5. Haggag, R. M., Ali, E. M., Khalifa, M. E., & Taha, M. (2025). Multiple sclerosis diagnosis with brain MRI retrieval: A deep-learning approach. https://doi.org/10.1016/j.rico.2025.100533
6. Khan, M., Dey, R., Kassim, S., Mahajan, R. A., Ghosh, A., & William, P. (2025). Machine learning-driven trading strategies: An empirical analysis of BSE blue-chip stocks using advanced algorithmic approaches. In *2025 International Conference on Quantum Photonics, Artificial Intelligence, and Networking (QPAIN)*. Rangpur, Bangladesh, pp. 1–5. https://doi.org/10.1109/QPAIN66474.2025.11171797.
7. Praet, J., Anderhalten, L., Comi, G., Horakova, D., Ziemssen, T., Vermersch, P., . . . & CLAIMS Consortium. (2024). A future of AI-driven personalized care for people with multiple sclerosis. https://doi.org/10.3389/fimmu.2024.1446748
8. Falet, J.-P. R., Nobile, S., Szpindel, A., Barile, B., Kumar, A., Durso-Finley, J., Arbel, T., & Arnold, D. L. (2025). The role of AI for MRI-analysis in multiple sclerosis. https://doi.org/10.3389/frai.2025.1478068
9. Khan, M., Mahajan, R. A., Katukam, R., Dey, R., Rana, A., & William, P. (2025). Smart insights: Multimodal deep learning techniques for accurate disease identification. In *2025 International Conference on Quantum Photonics, Artificial Intelligence, and Networking (QPAIN)*. Rangpur, Bangladesh, pp. 1–5. https://doi.org/10.1109/QPAIN66474.2025.11171928
10. Mohsenpourian, M., Suratgar, A. A., Talebi, H. A., Arzani, M., Moghadasi, A. N., Malakouti, S. M., & Menhaj, M. B. (2024). Design of a computational intelligence system for detection of multiple sclerosis with visual evoked potentials. https://doi.org/10.1016/j.neuri.2024.100177
11. Balan, S. R. V., Zeema, J. L., & Deepa, S. (2024). Diagnosis of multiple sclerosis lesion using deep learning models. *Journal of Electrical Systems*, 20(3), 2354–2367.
12. Maida, E., & Lavorgna, L. (2023). Multiple sclerosis: Diagnosis, management, and future opportunities. https://doi.org/10.3390/jcm12144558
13. Schultz, B. G., Joukhadar, Z., Nattala, U., Quiroga, M. del M., Noffs, G., Rojas, S., . . . & Vogel, A. P. (2023). Disease delineation for multiple sclerosis, Friedreich ataxia, and healthy controls using supervised machine learning on speech acoustics. https://doi.org/10.1109/TNSRE.2023.3321874
14. Mahajan, R. A., Dey, R., Khan, M., Su'ud, M. M., Alam, M. M., & Jadhav, P. (2025). Enhancing personalization in IoT-based health monitoring via generative AI and transfer learning. *Egyptian Informatics Journal*, 32, 100788. ISSN 1110-8665. https://doi.org/10.1016/j.eij.2025.100788. https://www.sciencedirect.com/science/article/pii/S1110866525001811
15. Ruiz-Sánchez, F. J., Martins, M. R., Soares, S., Romero-Morales, C., López-López, D., Gómez-Salgado, J., & Jiménez-Cebrián, A. M. (2022). Impact of multiple sclerosis and its association with depression: An analytical case-control investigation. https://doi.org/10.3390/healthcare10112218
16. Schwab, P., & Karlen, W. (2021). A deep learning approach to diagnosing multiple sclerosis from smartphone data. https://doi.org/10.1109/JBHI.2020.3021143
17. Paul, S., Ojha, S. K., Barui, S., Ghosh, S., Ghosh, M., Neogi, B., & Ganguly, A. (2018). Technical advancement on various bio-signal controlled arm: A review. *Journal of Mechanics of Continua and Mathematical Sciences*, 13(2), 16–30. https://doi.org/10.26782/jmcms.2018.06.00007
18. Billot, B., Cerri, S., Van Leemput, K., Dalca, A. V., & Iglesias, J. E. (2021). Joint segmentation of multiple sclerosis lesions and brain anatomy in MRI scans of any contrast and resolution with CNNs. https://doi.org/978-1-6654-1246-9/21
19. Das, P., Paul, S., Ghosh, J., PalBhowmik, S., Neogi, B., & Ganguly, A. (2017). An approach towards the representation of sign language by electromyography signals with fuzzy implementation. *International Journal of Sensors, Wireless Communications and Control*, 7(1), 26–32. https://doi.org/10.2174/2210327907666170222093839
20. Mancini, M., Giulietti, G., Spanò, B., Bozzali, M., Cercignani, M., & Conforto, S. (2016). Estimating multimodal brain connectivity in multiple sclerosis: An exploratory factor analysis. https://doi.org/978-1-4577-0220-4/16
21. Grigoriadis, N., Bakirtzis, C., Politis, C., Danas, K., & Thuemmler, C. (2016). Health 4.0: The case of multiple sclerosis. https://doi.org/978-1-5090-3370-6/16
22. Greene, B. R., Rutledge, S., McGurgan, I., McGuigan, C., O'Connell, K., Caulfield, B., & Tubridy, N. (2015). Assessment and classification of early-stage multiple sclerosis with inertial sensors: Comparison against clinical measures of disease state. https://doi.org/10.1109/JBHI.2015.2435057

11 Principles of Precision Healthcare Toward Pancreatic Cancer

V. Bharathi, M. Malathi, Balammal V., Divya Bairavi S., Preetha Ramiah, and I. Basheti

11.1 INTRODUCTION

Precision health enables researchers and healthcare providers to make accurate assessments of the time and place of manifestation of a disease and determine the circumstances where personalized preventive interventions can be focused. The formation of intelligent preventive and therapeutic strategies and flexible data-driven systems to counter the prevention of disease—the more advanced the system, the more individualized the system is. This leads to a more efficient overall prevention of the disease, its progression, and its recurrence.

Khan, Mahajan, et al. (2025) establish a framework for high-accuracy medical assessments by merging statistical, kernel-based, and neural approaches into a unified hybrid model for risk prediction [1]. Cascini et al. [2] emphasized that digitalization is fundamental to enabling data-driven precision healthcare, while Silvera-Tawil et al. [3] highlighted the contribution of wearable sensors and smart technologies to continuous patient monitoring. The UNICEF SDG Precision Health report [4] underscored the importance of precision health in promoting equitable and sustainable healthcare systems. Similarly, Gameiro et al. [5] and Joly [6] discussed the growing adoption of precision medicine and the need for strategic implementation, particularly in developing countries. Vieira [7] further highlighted the underrepresentation of diverse populations in genomic databases, emphasizing the importance of inclusive precision medicine research. Integrating genomic information into routine clinical practice has been recognized as a key driver of personalized healthcare by Walker et al. [8] and Kim [9]. In oncology, Herbst and Zheng [10] and Perelló-Reus et al. [11] demonstrated the significant role of precision medicine in improving pancreatic cancer diagnosis and treatment. Furthermore, Gadhave et al. [12] and Choonara et al. [13] reviewed recent advances in understanding the molecular mechanisms of neurodegenerative disorders, whereas Jumaili [14] proposed an AI-driven deep learning framework to enhance the diagnosis of neurodegenerative diseases, highlighting the expanding role of artificial intelligence in precision healthcare.

Precision health has the chance to transform medical practice and improve the quality of care, also in terms of health systems' sustainability. This framework of personalized medicine, which we put forth, uses many types of data, which include demographic, biological, behavioral, and environmental information, to in turn give patients the best tailored treatment options, which are also delivered quickly and effectively. Thanks to advancements in personalized medicine, the prediction and prevention of health issues within the scope of an individual's genetics, family health history, lifestyle, and environment are gaining more precision.

Khan, Katukam, et al. (2025) demonstrate that multimodal deep learning techniques are essential for accurate disease identification, providing the groundwork for integrating the complex imaging and genomic data required in pancreatic oncology [15].

DOI: 10.1201/9781003667360-11

The introduction of artificial intelligence (AI) further inculcates the potential of precision healthcare because it strengthens precision healthcare by enabling complex analyses of health data, assessing risk, detecting diseases early and consequently enabling early disease detection, and guiding timely, individualized preventive interventions [16]. Mahajan et al. (2025) explore how generative AI and transfer learning can enhance personalization in health monitoring, offering potential strategies for tailoring continuous surveillance to the specific needs of high-risk patients [17]. While precision healthcare has made significant advances in neurodegenerative diseases, its application in oncology, even in aggressive forms such as pancreatic cancer, remains limited. Pancreatic cancer, with late diagnosis and a dismal prognosis, necessitates the integration of genomics, multimodal data, and AI-based approaches in personalized medicine.

11.2 OVERVIEW OF PANCREATIC CANCER

Pancreatic cancer is a rare cancer site and a highly aggressive malignancy that arises from pancreatic tissues. Its rapid progression, late-stage diagnosis, and limited response to traditional therapy lead to a five-year survival rate of fewer than 10%. The incidence of pancreatic cancer keeps rising, making it the sixth most common cause of cancer-related deaths worldwide.

Risk Factors: Age, obesity, diabetes, smoking, chronic pancreatitis, and inherited genetic abnormalities such as Lynch syndrome and BRCA1/2. Pal et al. (2025) highlight the importance of edge intelligence in enhancing real-time IoT data processing, which is critical for the low-latency analysis needed in smart clinical decision support systems [18].

11.3 PRECISION HEALTH IS CHARACTERIZED BY THE 4PS

As shown in Figure 11.1, 4Ps of precision healthcare: Predictive: Identifying and understanding risk factors.

Preventive: Addressing risk and protective health factors.

Personalized: Optimizing treatments to the requirements of individual's needs.

Participatory: Ensuring active participation of patients in the decision-making processes.

11.3.1 THE 4Ps OF PRECISION HEALTH: A COMPREHENSIVE OVERVIEW

In traditional medicine, disease was considered an entity diagnosed only after its manifestation. This process of thinking was overturned after 4Ps medicine proposed teasing out the fictitious

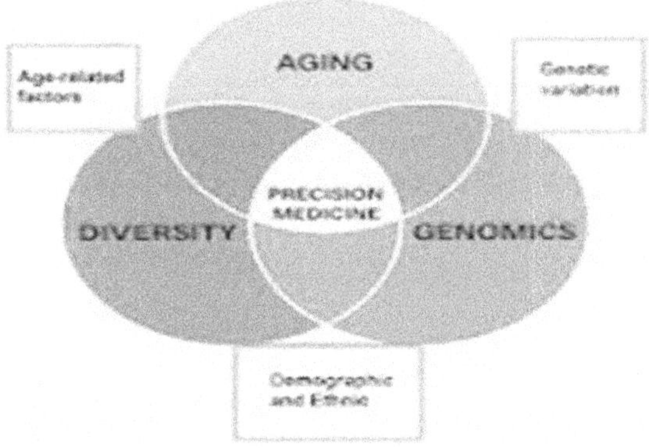

FIGURE 11.1 4Ps of precision healthcare

"disease" at a stage where there is only a risk of disease or a reversible disease process, preventing it with some strategy instead of curing, tailoring treatment depending on the individual patient, and encouraging the patient to participate. Paul et al. (2018) provide a comprehensive review of bio-signal integration, illustrating how technical advancements in physiological signal processing are foundational for developing noninvasive diagnostic tools [19].

11.3.1 Predictive

In predictive medicine, an individual is given an assessment of the chances that he or she will develop a certain disease based on his or her risk factors, including genetic factors, environmental factors, and lifestyle factors. Having the knowledge of being at high risk for developing the disease could allow for early interventions or decisions when needed.

11.3.2 Preventive

Prevention acts to eliminate the risks identified through early intervention, behavior change, and constant surveillance, thereby preventing the occurrence and aggravation of diseases.

11.3.3 Personalized

It focuses on tailoring healthcare interventions by patient-specific characteristics so that treatments vary in efficacy and in their potential to bring about side effects for any given individual. Since 2011, the term "personalized medicine" has evolved into "precision medicine." This followed a National Research Council paper claiming that "precision" is a better term for classifying people into sub-populations based on shared genetic patterns, lifestyles, pharmacological responses, and environmental, and cultural factors. Das et al. (2017) present a fuzzy-logic implementation for interpreting biological signals, showcasing a method for managing the high dimensionality and noise inherent in clinical data used for identifying early-stage malignancies [20].

11.3.4 Participatory

In this approach, patients are empowered with their own health and take responsibility, thus forming a partnership with healthcare service providers for the better health of that patient.

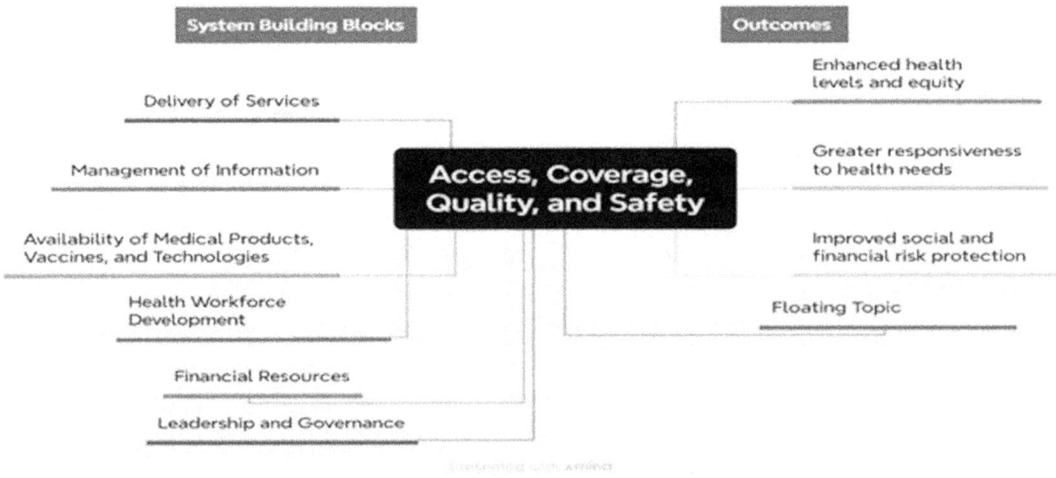

FIGURE 11.2 Key components of precision healthcare

The implications of 4Ps theory in developing countries remain uncertain due to the problem of financial support for developing new therapies and an insufficient amount of collected genomic data. For example, India has 20% of the global population but represents only 1% of existing genetic data.

The flow chart illustrates that, by reinforcing the building blocks of the health system with precision health strategies, it is possible to attain improved access, coverage, quality, and safety of healthcare. This, in turn, results in enhanced health outcomes, increased equity and responsiveness to patients' needs, and protection against social and financial risks, and improved efficiency in the health system.

11.4 CORE PRINCIPLES AND PILLARS

11.4.1 Patient-Centric Approach

Precision healthcare emphasizes a patient-centered approach, which involves personal preferences, values, and requirements into clinical decision-making. This strategy encourages patients to actively participate in their healthcare journey, resulting in better outcomes and satisfaction

Example: Brain check is a tool that offers personalized cognitive tests that patients can perform at home.

11.4.2 Genomic and Molecular Data

Genomics studies an individual's complete DNA, which includes all genes and variations in that field. We have seen growth in this area due to recent technological improvements. Also, we have what is known as next-generation sequencing (NGS) technology, which allows for quick and economical analysis of large-scale genomic data.

Integrating the elements of genetic and clinical data is a step forward in precision medicine. In terms of clinical and genetic data integration, healthcare providers are able to take a personalized approach to disease diagnosis, treatment, and prevention, which is a move away from a one-size-fits-all strategy. Also, into EHRs, we see the introduction of genomic data, which, in turn, gives clinicians a practical base of information to use for drug choice and dose, which reduces adverse events and improves therapeutic results.

Recent reports of what is achieved with NGS have identified primary genetic changes in pancreatic tumors, which include mutations in KRAS, TP53, CDKN2A and SMAD4. Although the great majority of mutations do not have targetable options, we do see that poly (ADP-ribose) polymerase (PARP) inhibitors or immunotherapy, which target DNA repair defects such as BRCA1/2 mutations, are beneficial to a subset of patients. Also, we see that the use of genetic information in combination with clinical and imaging data improves risk assessment and individualized therapy planning.

11.4.3 Multimodal Data Integration

As for multimodal data integration, we look at the combination of many data types, which include neuroimaging, genomics, clinical reports, and wearable sensor data, into one picture, which, in turn, gives us a better picture of disease. This, in turn, is used to put together more accurate diagnoses and personalized healthcare approaches.

Integration of multimodal information—genomics, radiology, pathology, and electronic health records—facilitates comprehensive knowledge about the disease in each patient. AI algorithms are being used more to examine complicated datasets, forecast disease progression, and select candidates for clinical trials or tailored therapies. For instance, deep learning from imaging is able to recognize small changes indicative of early pancreatic cancer, whereas machine learning models can risk-stratify patients and predict response to therapy.

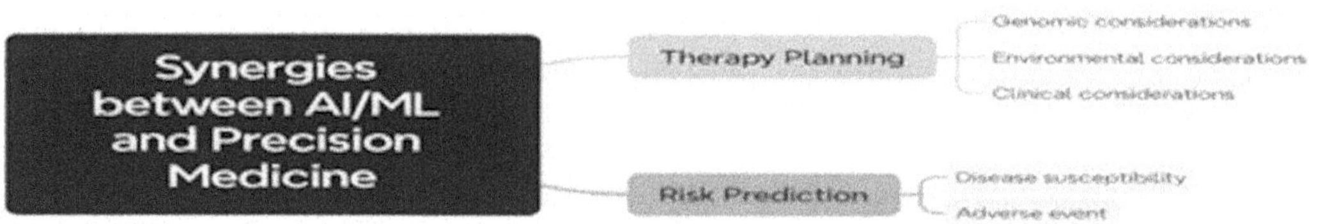

FIGURE 11.3 Synergies between AI/ML and precision healthcare

11.4.4 Role of AI and Machine Learning

The application of AI algorithms in drug discovery and design has numerous prospects. AI and machine learning (ML) improve drug design and development by increasing our understanding of disease pathology, discovering dysregulated molecular pathways, predicting potential therapeutic targets, and analyzing in drug efficacy [21, 22]. AI and ML allow for disease detection and prevention at the individual patient level by improving knowledge of both patient specificity and therapeutic properties. Thus, AI and ML algorithms are modernizing many facets of our lives by assisting with precision medicine, such as medical imaging, risk analysis, phenotypic prediction, and gene expression pattern analysis [22, 23]

11.4.5 Clinical Decision Support Systems (CDSS)

AI-powered CDSS can help clinicians by making evidence-based suggestions, enhancing diagnosis accuracy, and optimizing treatment regimens [24].

11.4.6 Integration With EHRs

Incorporating AI into CDSS enables real-time analysis of patient data, providing personalized treatment recommendations and warnings for potential adverse events [25].

11.4.7 Improving Patient-Centered Care

AI-driven CDSS facilitates collaborative decision-making by providing clinicians and patients with comprehensive information, resulting in informed choices and personalized care plans.

11.4.8 Challenges

Successfully implementing AI in CDSS requires overcoming problems such as data interoperability, model interpretability, and clinician trust in AI-generated recommendations [26].

11.5 APPLICATIONS IN NEURODEGENERATIVE DISEASES

Neurodegenerative disorders (NDs) are defined by the loss of neurons, which results in death. They are progressive neuropsychiatric disorders. Over 57 million people are living with dementia worldwide. This number is projected to nearly double every 20 years [27]. Apart from their high prevalence, these disorders have complicated etiologies that involve genetic, environmental, and lifestyle factors, as well as significant variation in cognitive function, clinical development, and neuropathology, providing important challenges for prevention and therapy.

Furthermore, most neuropsychiatric disorders go through a prolonged preclinical or prodromal phase that standard medical paradigms frequently neglect, although this phase represents a vital window for intervention [28, 29]. Considering the complexity and heterogeneity of neuropsychiatric illnesses, precision medicine, defined as "prevention and treatment strategies that take every person into account," emerges as a potential healthcare framework.

11.6 CASE STUDY: PRECISION HEALTHCARE IN PANCREATIC CANCER

Pancreatic cancer, most notably pancreatic ductal adenocarcinoma (PDAC), is characterized by delayed diagnosis, rapid progression, and poor survival. The five-year survival rate is less than 10%, mainly because early disease is asymptomatic and resistant to traditional treatments. Significant risk factors.

11.6.1 Precision Healthcare Approaches

Improvements in NGS have made it possible to perform detailed genomic profiling of pancreatic cancer.

Shared mutations include KRAS, TP53, CDKN2A, and SMAD4. A small percentage of patients have DNA repair defects (e.g., BRCA1/2 mutations) and qualify for targeted agents, including PARP inhibitors.

Combining genomic information with clinical and imaging data facilitates individualized treatment planning and risk stratification.

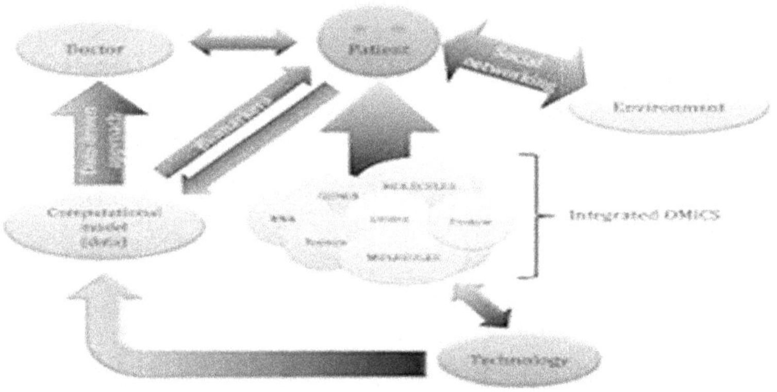

FIGURE 11.4 Precision healthcare integrated model

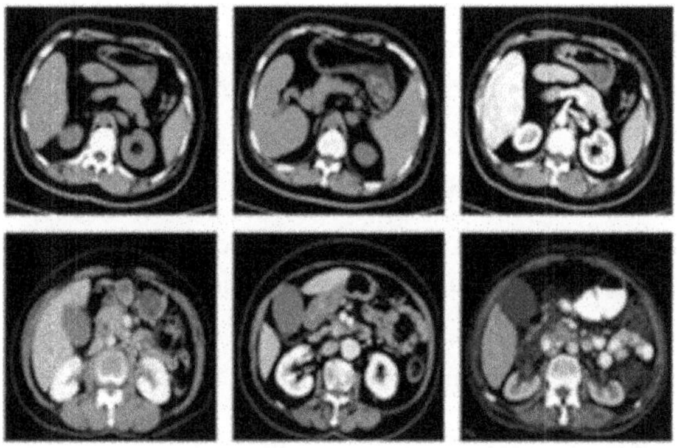

FIGURE 11.5 Sample pancreatic cancer images

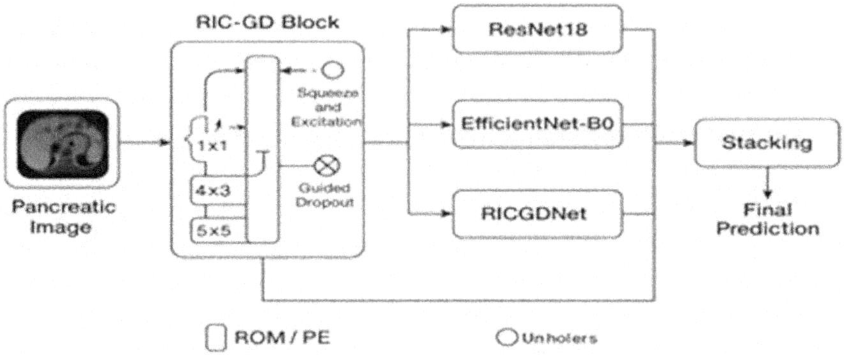

FIGURE 11.6 Architecture diagram using RIC-GD

11.7 CLINICAL APPLICATION

11.7.1 Risk Stratification

Patients with genetic predisposition or familial risk are targeted for increased surveillance.

11.7.2 Personalized Therapy

Genomic results inform the utilization of targeted therapies (e.g., use of PARP inhibitors in BRCA-mutated tumors).

11.7.3 Treatment Monitoring

Multimodal patient data are scrutinized by AI-powered systems to track response and adjust treatment protocols in real time.

11.7.4 Barriers and Future Directions

Even with progress, the majority of pancreatic cancer patients are not yet benefiting from precision medicine.

11.7.5 Early Diagnosis and Detection

Tools based on AI can read MRI and positron emission tomography (PET) scans to identify early brain changes that a human radiologist may not be able to see. For example, deep learning algorithms trained on large datasets can detect patterns of Alzheimer's disease-related atrophy or hypo metabolism.

11.7.6 Cognitive Decline Prediction

AI can forecast progression from mild cognitive impairment (MCI) to AD, allowing clinicians to start treatment or intervene in an individual's lifestyle earlier [30].

11.7.7 Risk Stratification and Predictive Modeling

AI algorithms operate on patient-specific information (genomic, clinical, and environmental) to make prognostications on the risk of neurodegenerative disease development. AI can also calculate the anticipated rate of progression.

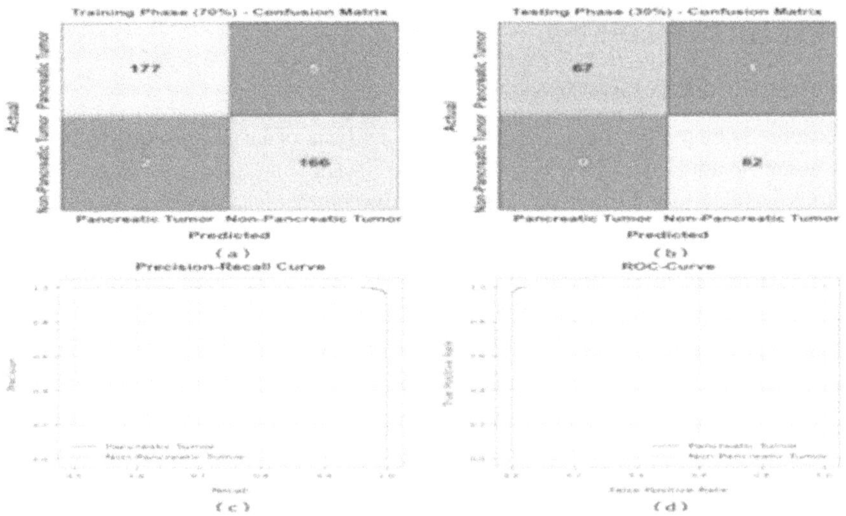

FIGURE 11.7 Performance of confusion matrix and ROC curve

11.7.8 Genetic Risk Prediction

AI has the capacity to operate on genomic information to recognize people at risk due to mutations such as APOE-ε4 for Alzheimer's or SNCA for Parkinson's [31].

11.7.9 Environmental and Lifestyle Factors

ML combines wearable sensor data (e.g., gait, sleep patterns) with clinical records to predict disease onset risk and disease progression tracking [32].

11.7.10 Drug Discovery and Repurposing

AI assists in the discovery of new drug targets and the repurposing of drugs for NDs.

11.7.11 Drug Screening

AI models are capable of mimicking molecular interactions to recognize compounds that will modulate neurodegeneration pathways.

11.7.12 Multimodal Data Integration

An important strength of AI lies in its ability to synthesize various data sources—neuroimaging, clinical history, genomics, proteomics, and patient-reported measures—to provide a comprehensive understanding of the patient [33].

AI in the management of neurodegenerative diseases is transforming early diagnosis, personalized medicine, and research. AI, with its integration of multimodal data, predictive modeling, and intelligent clinical decision-making systems, has the potential to transform neurodegenerative disease management from reactive to proactive. As these technologies become more mature, concerns such as data privacy, interpretability of models, and clinical validation have to be taken care of so that safe and ethical deployment is made.

11.8 ETHICAL, LEGAL, AND SOCIAL IMPLICATIONS IN PRECISION MEDICINE

11.8.1 Privacy and Data Governance

Precision medicine is based on the aggregation and analysis of large amounts of individual health data, such as genomic data, electronic health records (EHRs), and data from wearable technologies. This has serious implications for privacy and data governance. It is essential to ensure that patient information is gathered, stored, and used in a responsible manner.

Good data governance systems need to resolve challenges such as informed consent, data ownership, and the right to access and control information about one's health. Furthermore, there has to be streamlined procedures for ensuring interoperability and security of data across heterogeneous healthcare systems.

11.8.2 Bias and Fairness

Unequal outcomes in treating various cohorts of people can stem from the algorithms used in precision medicine, with AI deepening existing inequalities in the data. AI systems built on a single demographic training dataset might underperform when predicting outcomes across other, less-represented cohorts. The performance of such systems can be improved by intentionally including a wider range of representative data in the bloc training the model, coupled with fairness-aware algorithms. The AI paradigm needs a structure for continuous auditing and monitoring, which serves to surface and counteract, over time, the biases that the closed system of the AI paradigm has built in.

11.9 FUTURE PERSPECTIVES IN PRECISION HEALTHCARE

11.9.1 Digital Twins

A digital twin is a computer model of a physical object, a patient in this instance—used to simulate and forecast healthcare outcomes. By bringing data from different sources such as genomics, imaging, and lifestyle together, digital twins are able to give customized feedback about disease progression and treatment response.

Application of digital twins in healthcare has the potential to enhance diagnostic accuracy, streamline treatment plans, and enhance patient outcomes. It also brings with it ethical issues such as data privacy, consent, and the risk of abuse of sensitive health information.

11.9.2 Global Health Implications

To be effective, healthcare must be scaled and transferred in resource-constrained environments. This calls for development of low-cost technology and provision of equal access to healthcare, which includes design of interventions that fit the specific needs of different communities. Reports indicate that, in low- and middle-income settings, use of precision healthcare is a challenge. In low- and middle-income countries, the implementation of precision healthcare remains challenging because of poor infrastructure, a shortage of trained healthcare professionals, and limited financial resources. Addressing these challenges requires coordinated efforts from governments, healthcare providers, international organizations, and policymakers. These stakeholders should collaborate to strengthen healthcare infrastructure, enhance workforce capacity through training and education, establish supportive policies, and promote equitable access to precision healthcare technologies. Such collaborative initiatives are essential for building a sustainable and inclusive healthcare system that benefits all populations.

11.10 CALL TO ACTION

We have that which professionals in medicine, research, data science, ethics, and policy put forth to achieve our goals in precision medicine. To develop adaptive and equitable solutions, we need continuous innovation within ethical parameters.

Stakeholders must work together to develop strong data governance structures, to increase diversity in research and clinical trials, and to put in place healthcare systems which see precision medicine integrated into routine clinical practice.

Thus, we will see that all members of society will benefit from precision medicine.

11.11 CONCLUSION

Rich datasets, algorithms, and ethics guide how we approach patient care in precision healthcare, which describes a model of clinical practice. With sufficient computing power and algorithmic data analysis, we can expect greater accuracy when diagnosing a health problem, tailoring a treatment plan, and implementing ongoing healthcare strategies. Having useful and actionable data in a health system can certainly improve health outcomes. However, there remain ethical, legal, and social issues that limit the positive potential within the system. Examples include data privacy, lack of fairness in access, algorithmic bias, and a host of other issues.

REFERENCES

1. Khan M, Mahajan RA, Sivakumar NR, Gulhane M, Rakesh N, Dey R, Uddin MS, Basheer S. A unified hybrid model for cardiovascular risk prediction: Merging statistical, kernel-based and neural approaches. *J Cell Mol Med.* 2025. https://doi.org/10.1111/jcmm.70797
2. Cascini F, Beccia F, Causio FA, Muscat NA, Ricciardi W. Editorial: Digitalization for precision healthcare. *Front Public Health.* 2022;10:1078610. https://doi.org/10.3389/fpubh.2022.1078610
3. Silvera-Tawil D, Hussain MS, Li J. Emerging technologies for precision health: An insight into sensing technologies for health and wellbeing. *Smart Health.* 2020;15:100100. https://doi.org/10.1016/j.smhl.2019.100100
4. SDG 3 Precision Health Overview.pdf.pdf. Accessed May 26, 2025. https://www.unicef.org/innovation/media/20391/file/SDG%203%20Precision%20Health%20Overview.pdf.pdf
5. Gameiro GR, Sinkunas V, Liguori GR, Auler-Júnior JOC. Precision medicine: Changing the way we think about healthcare. *Clinics.* 2018;73:e723. https://doi.org/10.6061/clinics/2017/e723
6. Joly Y. Editorial: Personalized medicine in developing countries: A roadmap to personalized innovation. *Curr Pharmacogenomics Pers Med.* 2011;9(3):156–158. https://doi.org/10.2174/187569211796957539
7. Vieira H. Sumit Jamuar: Indians are 20% of the world's population, but represent only 1% of existing genetic data. *LSE Business Review*, January 10, 2018. Accessed May 27, 2025. https://blogs.lse.ac.uk/businessreview/2018/01/10/sumit-jamuar-indians-are-20-of-the-worlds-population-but-represent-only-1-of-existing-genetic-data/
8. Walker T, Ersig AL, Dwyer AA, et al. Integrating genomics and precision health knowledge into practice: A guide for nurse practitioners. *J Am Assoc Nurse Pract.* 2024;36(10):554–562. https://doi.org/10.1097/JXX.0000000000001050
9. Kim SJ. Integration of genomics and clinical data: Advancing precision medicine. *Eur J Biomed Inform.* 2024;20(4):280–281.
10. Herbst B, Zheng L. Precision medicine in pancreatic cancer: Treating every patient as an exception. *Lancet Gastroenterol Hepatol.* 2019;4(10):805–810. https://doi.org/10.1016/S2468-1253(19)30175-X
11. Perelló-Reus CM, Rubio-Tomás T, Cisneros-Barroso E, et al. Challenges in precision medicine in pancreatic cancer: A focus in cancer stem cells and microbiota. *Front Oncol.* 2022;12. https://doi.org/10.3389/fonc.2022.995357
12. Gadhave DG, Sugandhi VV, Jha SK, et al. Neurodegenerative disorders: Mechanisms of degeneration and therapeutic approaches with their clinical relevance. *Ageing Res Rev.* 2024;99:102357. https://doi.org/10.1016/j.arr.2024.102357
13. Choonara YE, Pillay V, Du Toit LC, et al. Trends in the molecular pathogenesis and clinical therapeutics of common neurodegenerative disorders. *Int J Mol Sci.* 2009;10(6):2510–2557. https://doi.org/10.3390/ijms10062510

14. Jumaili MLF, Sonuç E. An attention-based cnn framework for alzheimer's disease staging with multi-technique XAI visualization. *Comput Mater Contin*. 2025;83(2):2947–2969.
15. Khan M, Mahajan RA, Katukam R, Dey R, Rana A, William P. Smart insights: Multimodal deep learning techniques for accurate disease identification. In: *2025 International Conference on Quantum Photonics, Artificial Intelligence, and Networking (QPAIN)*. Rangpur, Bangladesh, 2025, pp. 1–5. https://doi.org/10.1109/QPAIN66474.2025.11171928
16. Artificial intelligence and precision health through lenses of ethics and social determinants of health: Protocol for a state-of-the-art literature review. *JMIR Res Protoc*. 2023;12. https://doi.org/10.2196/40565
17. Mahajan RA, Dey R, Khan M, Su'ud MM, Alam MM, Jadhav P. Enhancing personalization in IoT-based health monitoring via generative AI and transfer learning. *Egypt Inform J*. 32, 100788. ISSN 1110-8665. https://doi.org/10.1016/j.eij.2025.100788. https://www.sciencedirect.com/science/article/pii/S1110866525001811
18. Pal M, Dey R, Mahajan RA, Khan M, Syed AA, Karimullah S. Edge intelligence: Unique machine learning strategies for enhancing real-time IoT data processing. In: *2025 International Conference on Quantum Photonics, Artificial Intelligence, and Networking (QPAIN)*. Rangpur, Bangladesh, 2025, pp. 1–5. https://doi.org/10.1109/QPAIN66474.2025.11171994.
19. Paul S, Ojha SK, Barui S, Ghosh S, Ghosh M, Neogi B, Ganguly A. Technical advancement on various bio-signal controlled arm: A review. *J Mech Contin Math Sci*. 2018;13(2):16–30. https://doi.org/10.26782/jmcms.2018.06.00007
20. Das P, Paul S, Ghosh J, PalBhowmik S, Neogi B, Ganguly A. An approach towards the representation of sign language by electromyography signals with fuzzy implementation. *Int J Sens Wirel Commun Control*. 2017;7(1):26–32. https://doi.org/10.2174/2210327907666170222093839
21. Moingeon P, Kuenemann M, Guedj M. Artificial intelligence-enhanced drug design and development: Toward a computational precision medicine. *Drug Discov Today*. 2022;27(1):215–222. https://doi.org/10.1016/j.drudis.2021.09.006
22. Sahu M, Gupta R, Ambasta RK, Kumar P. Chapter three—Artificial intelligence and machine learning in precision medicine: A paradigm shift in big data analysis. In: Teplow DB, ed. *Progress in Molecular Biology and Translational Science*. Vol 190. Precision Medicine. Academic Press; 2022:57–100. https://doi.org/10.1016/bs.pmbts.2022.03.002
23. Mak KK, Pichika MR. Artificial intelligence in drug development: Present status and future prospects. *Drug Discov Today*. 2019;24(3):773–780. https://doi.org/10.1016/j.drudis.2018.11.014
24. Venkatapurapu SP, Gibbs M, Kimko H. Augmented intelligence in precision medicine: Transforming clinical decision-making with AI/ML and/or quantitative systems pharmacology models. *Clin Transl Sci*. 2024;17(12):e70112. https://doi.org/10.1111/cts.70112
25. Khalifa M, Albadawy M, Iqbal U. Advancing clinical decision support: The role of artificial intelligence across six domains. *Comput Methods Programs Biomed Update*. 2024;5:100142. https://doi.org/10.1016/j.cmpbup.2024.100142
26. Alkan M, Zakariyya I, Leighton S, Sivangi KB, Anagnostopoulos C, Deligianni F. Artificial intelligence-driven clinical decision support systems. Published online February 17, 2025. https://doi.org/10.48550/arXiv.2501.09628
27. Dementia. Accessed May 28, 2025. https://www.who.int/news-room/fact-sheets/detail/dementia
28. Huang W, Shu N. AI-powered integration of multimodal imaging in precision medicine for neuropsychiatric disorders. *Cell Rep Med*. 2025;6(5):102132. https://doi.org/10.1016/j.xcrm.2025.102132
29. Dugger SA, Platt A, Goldstein DB. Drug development in the era of precision medicine. *Nat Rev Drug Discov*. 2018;17(3):183–196. https://doi.org/10.1038/nrd.2017.226
30. Strafella C, Caputo V, Galota MR, et al. Application of precision medicine in neurodegenerative diseases. *Front Neurol*. 2018;9. https://doi.org/10.3389/fneur.2018.00701
31. *Integrating IoMT and AI for Proactive Healthcare: Predictive Models and Emotion Detection in Neurodegenerative Diseases*. Accessed May 28, 2025. https://www.mdpi.com/1999-4893/17/9/376
32. Santos A, Gonzalez CI, Garcia M. Exploring deep learning applications in neurodegenerative diseases: A state-of-the-art review. In: Martínez-Villaseñor L, Ochoa-Ruiz G, Montes Rivera M, Barrón-Estrada ML, Acosta-Mesa HG, eds. *Advances in Computational Intelligence. MICAI 2024 International Workshops*. Springer Nature Switzerland; 2025:97–108. https://doi.org/10.1007/978-3-031-83879-8_8
33. Alvarez MJR, Griessler E, Starkbaum J. Ethical, legal and social aspects of precision medicine. In: Hasanzad M, ed. *Precision Medicine in Clinical Practice*. Springer Nature; 2022:179–196. https://doi.org/10.1007/978-981-19-5082-7_11.

12 Synthetic Data Generation for Emphysema Disease Research

Divya Bairavi S., M. Malathi, V. Bharathi, Balammal V., Preetha Ramiah, and Vikas Rao Naidu

12.1 INTRODUCTION

In the past few years, we have seen healthcare experiences greatly change with the advent of digital health tech such as electronic health records (EHRs), wearables, genomic sequencing, medical imaging, mobile health apps, and telemedicine. Every day, we see new sets of data that, at the same time, present to us opportunities to improve precision medicine, to advance research in science, and to transform patient care. The application of artificial intelligence (AI) and advanced analytics to these data has helped improve disease surveillance and monitoring, improved treatment planning, and raised accuracy in diagnosis. The author analyzed ML-driven trading strategies for breast self-examination (BSE) blue-chip stocks, demonstrating advanced algorithmic pattern recognition techniques adaptable to synthetic data generation for emphysema progression modeling [1].

By analyzing data patterns, AI tools can predict patient outcomes and track patient data over time. For this reason, many medical AI applications help assist medical professionals in improving the quality of patient care offered and achieving higher degrees of personalized patient care. According to the data received, rare medical conditions such as emphysema are particularly difficult to study due to a lack of medical data. Only data from a few patients are available. To overcome this, researchers are now introducing synthetic data, that is, generating data artificially which actually resembles real data, but it will not reveal any personal details. To generate synthetic data, we use certain methods such as rule-based systems, various statistical methods, and AI approaches such as generative adversarial network (GAN) and variational autoencoder (VAE). Using tools such as Synthea, MD Clone, and SynthMD is helpful for scientists to produce CT scans and other medical records. These datasets improve the collaboration between hospitals and research centers. In deeper analysis of emphysema, using synthetic data helps to predict the early disease stage, and also predicts lung function loss and biomarkers. Even after facing several challenges with bias, validation, and high costs, researchers still prefer this method, as it is safer and more effective. Also, this extends the robustness of precision medicine and supports the development of new treatment methods for rare diseases. The author developed multimodal deep learning for disease identification, providing foundational methods for synthesizing realistic multi-view lung imaging datasets essential for emphysema research [2].

However, the sensitive nature of patient data imposes substantial restrictions on its accessibility and use, especially in research domains. Privacy protection legislation such as the Health Insurance Portability and Accountability Act (HIPAA) and the General Data Protection Regulation (GDPR) poses strict limitations and guidelines regarding the collection and use of personal health information. Such safeguards are essential for the protection of privacy. Nevertheless, such privacy protection legislation presents obstacles for investigators and researchers, particularly in the context of sparse information. More than one specialty may be involved in the care of patients suffering from infrequently occurring illnesses. Such diseases may, by definition, present far greater obstacles than most other diseases in other branches of medical research. The patients are often very few in number and geographically isolated from one another, needing care from different systems. The number

DOI: 10.1201/9781003667360-12

of such cases is very few and is often highly underreported. This phenomenon represents a unique challenge in medical research on rare diseases. This has put forward that which we have difficulty in seeing disease models clearly, identifying possible biomarkers, or developing good treatment plans. Diagnoses are delayed, and wrong results are obtained because of our great reliance on hearsay instead of solid clinical data. In the case of rare diseases, this is often observed. We see that rare diseases, by definition, affect a small number of patients who are spread geographically and require care from many different healthcare systems. The author reviewed bio-signal-controlled prosthetic technologies, offering insights into physiological signal synthesis strategies relevant for augmenting emphysema-related respiratory pattern datasets [3]. Also, because of the low number of cases, we end up with incomplete data. This, in turn, makes it hard to see disease models, identify possible biomarkers, or develop good treatment plans. Mahajan et al. (2025) utilized generative AI and transfer learning for personalized health monitoring, highlighting synthetic data approaches that can create diverse emphysema patient profiles from limited clinical samples [4]. Diagnostic time delays, as well as inaccurate results and the practice of using personal stories as evidence instead of strong statistics, are a result of not having large sets of clinical data. We use synthetic data, which allows in-depth research and development of AI models while also protecting the confidentiality of sensitive information. It also mirrors real patient data in terms of what is presented and the issues at play, but at the same time does not reveal personal information. Das et al. (2017) implemented fuzzy logic-based EMG signal representation, showcasing robust methods for generating synthetic bio-signals that parallel emphysema respiratory waveform augmentation techniques [5].

12.2 CHALLENGES OF LIMITED DATA IN RARE DISEASE RESEARCH

Research into rare diseases is hampered by the fact that we don't have enough data, which in turn slows down the progress of targeted therapies, the accuracy of diagnosis, and our understanding of disease biology. Also, medical professionals lack the specialized skills and knowledge they require. We also see delayed or inaccurate results due to limited clinical data. It is hard to do dose optimization studies and to recruit enough patients for clinical trials in the setting of small patient populations, low disease awareness, and limited healthcare resources. This issue also plays a role in the determination of relevant clinical end points and in the evaluation of therapeutic effectiveness, which in turn presents challenges for regulatory approval and commercialization of novel treatments. Also, researchers and clinicians, in many cases, report on what is at best a small body of data, which they present as fact rather than put forward as what it is—a statistical anomaly—which in turn reduces confidence in clinical and therapeutic decisions [2, 6].

12.3 SYNTHETIC DATA

1. Data modeled from algorithms, unlike real information, is referred to as synthetic data. In contrast to anonymized data, which captures real patient records, the risk of reidentification is mitigated here. It is entirely computational in nature. In contrast to other domains, this technique aids in preserving the sensitive characteristics of the information and enables academics to produce a dataset that realistically emulates the complexity and diversity of genuine clinical data in real life. In the field of rare diseases, this is crucial because it makes it possible to create large, realistic virtual cohorts that replicate unusual clinical conditions, develop tools for the design and validation of AI analytics, and—above all—protect patient privacy while encouraging data sharing and cooperation between institutions disclosing data. Dey et al. (2025) engineered ML models combining technical indicators for NIFTY-50 prediction, illustrating temporal sequence synthesis principles applicable to generating emphysema severity trajectories [7].

12.3.1 Methods of Synthetic Data Generation

12.3.1.1 Rule-Based Approaches

We can create synthetic data to mimic actual patient records using a set of rules and a sampling of associated constraints and statistical distributions. For instance, one can generate demographic variables such as age and sex to conform to the same demographic distribution present in real datasets. When it comes to demographic variables and simple clinical variables that conform to actual records of patients with the disease (such as real datasets with chronic obstructive pulmonary disease [COPD]), rule-based synthesis in the case of COPD may lead to the synthesis of patient datasets with demographic variables and simple clinical attributes. Because COPD affects older adults, one can, for instance, set rules that allow more of the synthetic patients to be older and for a higher percentage of the synthetic population to be smokers. This results in a higher percentage of synthetic patients falling within the older age range and a higher percentage being smokers [8, 9].

12.3.1.2 Statistical Modeling

Understanding the relationships among different elements in complex real-world medical datasets is the goal of statistical modeling. Techniques such as Markov Chains, Bayesian Networks, and Gaussian Mixture Models can be used to do this. These methods allow for the development of fictitious patient records with the same statistics and correlations among various variables as actual patient data. These statistical models can be useful when aiming to simulate the course of a disease over time. A Markov Chain, for instance, can produce data over time that shows how a patient's lung function, as measured by forced expiratory volume (FEV), deteriorates and how the likelihood of getting other disorders changes as the disease progresses [10].

12.3.1.3 Machine Learning–Based Techniques

The company is a benchmark in the use of VAEs and GANs to produce fully synthetic data (16). Data diversity among medical domain data types is substantial, including clinical data, medical images such as MRIs and radiomics, and bio-signals such as electrocardiogram (ECG) and electroencephalography (EEG) data streams. They train on actual datasets to learn complex multimodal relationships and then produce realistic synthetic data. Their generated data improves the training and validation of AI-based empirical diagnostic tools [11].

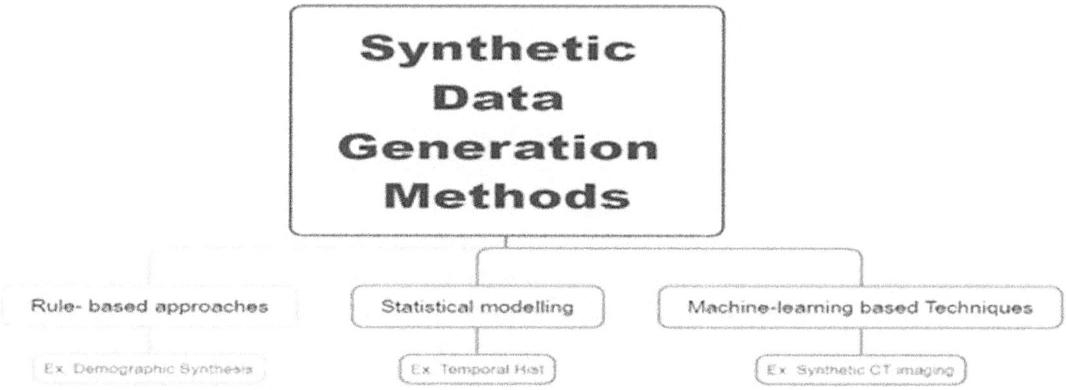

FIGURE 12.1 Synthetic data generation methods

12.4 DEEP LEARNING-BASED SYNTHETIC DATA GENERATION

The best synthetic data generators use algorithms such as VAEs and GANs to generate a variety of datasets. These neural network models can create coherent and structured datasets, such as tabular clinical data, medical imaging-based radiomics, and physiological data, such as ECG and EEG signals. When trained on real multidimensional datasets, deep learning algorithms can generate synthetic samples of these datasets, capturing complex, multifaceted relationships. This makes them useful for the augmentation of training, testing, and validating AI diagnostics and predictive algorithms. The standard of data can be divided according to its connection to the real data [7].

12.4.1 Fully Synthetic Data

Data generated in a wholly synthetic manner, without the infusion of actual data points from the real world. These datasets are generated from algorithms, statistical models, or simulations that look at the data's statistical characteristics, replicate distributions, relations, and so on.

Advantage

It has deeper privacy safeguarding, as there are no details concerning real patients, accordingly limiting the danger of reidentification. Fully synthetic data stands out when it comes to situations that have little to no existing data, or when there is a concern about the privacy of real data being shared. For example, we see that fully synthetic patient reports are used to add value to other databases, train machine learning models, or present rare cases, while at the same time protecting patient identity (18).

12.4.2 Partially Synthetic Data

Also, in terms of how this works, the approach is to remove specific sensitive variables from a real dataset and replace only those with synthetic values, which in turn leaves the rest of the non-sensitive real data in place. This approach maintains the integrity and utility of the original dataset for research purposes while protecting individual privacy by masking identifiable or high-risk variables. For example, see 13.2. Partially synthetic data are especially useful in clinical research, where certain real-world information is crucial for analysis, but privacy concerns necessitate the modification of sensitive fields. For instance, in large-scale health surveys, partially synthetic data can serve as a proxy for real data, allowing researchers to conduct meaningful analyses while reducing the risk of disclosing personal information (19).

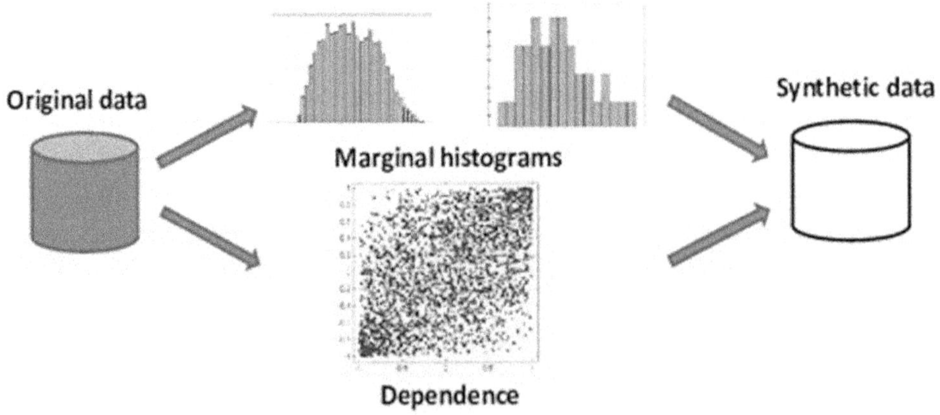

FIGURE 12.2 Synthetic data extraction

12.5 SYNTHETIC DATA APPLICATION IN RARE DISEASE RESEARCH

Synthetic data generation is revolutionizing rare disease research by overcoming two major barriers, limited data availability and stringent privacy constraints. The foundation of this technology lies in generative models. These models are trained on existing datasets, often small and sparse, to learn the underlying latent distribution of the data. Through this process, complex, high-dimensional clinical information, including genomic sequences and medical imaging data, is compressed into a lower-dimensional latent space. The latent space in this which is a result is a template that enables the model to reproduce and put forth new synthetic data that are true to the original data's statistics which at the same time does not include any individual patient information. This distinction between what is statistical in nature and what is identifiable is of great importance for privacy in the case of rare disease research, which has small datasets and sees few patients. In rare disease research, we also see the value of what is possible with latent space decoding in the generation of synthetic cohorts. It brings to bear large, diverse datasets, which in turn do a better job of representing the many different forms of rare diseases and thus support the development of more accurate diagnostic and prognostic AI models [12].

As illustrated in Figure 13.2, scientists from different universities are able to collaborate jointly in ways that were once impossible due to concerns about patient data privacy owing to the creation and use of synthetic datasets. Clinical evaluation has shown that models constructed from synthetic datasets can perform on a level with those built from real datasets, and flexible synthetic data has been shown to maintain the statistics and distributions of the original datasets. For instance, synthetic genomic datasets have been instrumental in identifying novel pathogenic variants in ultra-rare diseases, while federated learning frameworks have facilitated the generation of synthetic neuroimaging data across multiple international sites, preserving essential disease markers and enhancing cross-border research collaboration [13].

12.5.1 Case Study: Synthetic Data Generation for Emphysema Research

As a type of COPD, emphysema is described by severe and permanent harm to the alveolar walls that affects the capacity of the lungs to exchange gases correctly and gradually reduces their respiratory function. However, due to a lack of diagnosis and several data privacy rules, the early stage of emphysema is currently poorly represented in clinical data, making it hard to recognize early-stage emphysema and create powerful predictive models [14].

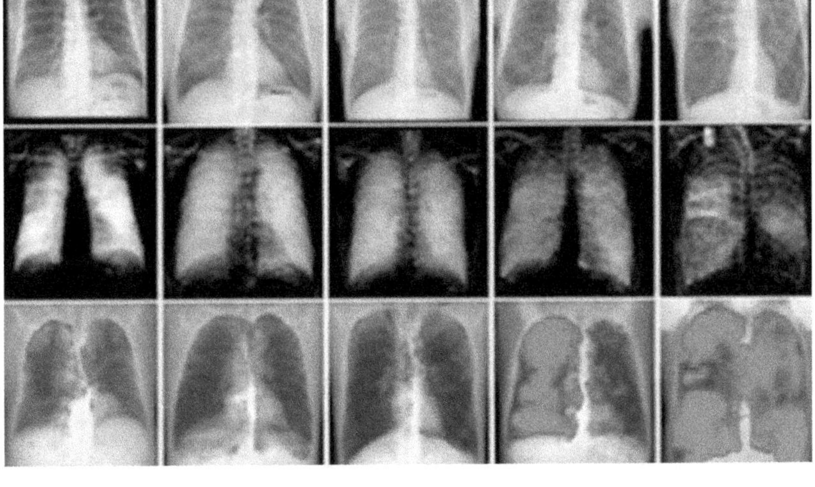

FIGURE 12.3 Sample clinical image of emphysema diagnosis

12.6 PRIVACY COMPLIANCE: GDPR, HIPAA, AND ANONYMIZATION STRATEGIES

Rare disease research is impacted by the issue of small patient datasets, which in turn is compounded by very strict privacy rules such as the GDPR and the HIPAA, and also by the fact that large datasets are required to develop AI models (10,21). Also, both GDPR and HIPAA put in place very tough requirements for the use and sharing of healthcare-related personal information, which includes patient-level de-identification and also that which patients give out their consent for the use of their data for other purposes. Synthetic data, by design, does not include any patient identifiers, which in turn allow researchers to at the same time comply with these regulatory requirements and also to share data securely across international and institutional boundaries (10, 22).

12.6.1 Anonymization Strategies

CTAB, GANs combined with normalizing flows, and hierarchical modeling generate datasets that pose no risk of patient reidentification while preserving the statistical soundness and clinical relevance of rare disease cohorts. This encourages privacy-preserving analytics and supports collaborative research across the global biomedical community [4].

12.7 MITIGATION OF BIAS AND ENSURING REPRESENTATIVENESS

Diseases which are rare have those which are put forth by small sample sizes and geographically limited populations, which in turn cause certain demographic groups' representation to suffer in research datasets. This, in turn, causes AI models to present a biased picture, which results in lower accuracy and fairness in terms of diagnosis [15].

Variable	Before Propensity Matching				After Propensity Matching			
	Total (n=577)	No COPD or Emphysema (n=474)	COPD or Emphysema (n=103)	P-value	Total (n=206)	No COPD or Emphysema (n=103)	COPD or Emphysema (n=103)	P-value
Comorbidities N (%)								
Hypertension	385 (66.7)	309 (65.2)	76 (73.8)	0.093	150 (72.8)	74 (71.8)	76 (73.8)	0.754
Diabetes Mellitus	245 (42.5)	196 (41.4)	49 (47.6)	0.247	100 (48.5)	51 (49.5)	49 (47.6)	0.780
CKD	125 (21.7)	105 (22.2)	20 (19.4)	0.541	47 (22.8)	27 (26.2)	20 (19.4)	0.245
ESRD on HD	45 (7.8)	33 (7.0)	12 (11.7)	0.109	21 (10.2)	9 (8.7)	12 (11.7)	0.490
CAD	82 (14.2)	56 (11.8)	26 (25.2)	***0.0004***	48 (23.4)	22 (21.6)	26 (25.2)	0.535
CHF	109 (18.9)	74 (15.6)	35 (34.0)	***<0.0001***	58 (28.2)	23 (22.3)	35 (34.0)	0.063
History of CVA	59 (10.2)	41 (8.6)	18 (17.5)	***0.007***	32 (15.5)	14 (13.6)	18 (17.5)	0.442
Psychiatric History	125 (21.7)	98 (20.7)	27 (26.5)	0.198	41 (20.0)	14 (13.6)	27 (26.5)	***0.021***
Substance-use Disorder	80 (13.9)	61 (12.9)	19 (18.4)	0.138	30 (14.6)	11 (10.7)	19 (18.4)	0.114

COPD=chronic obstructive pulmonary disease; CKD=chronic kidney disease; ESRD=end-stage renal disease; HD=hemodialysis; CAD=coronary artery disease; CHF=congestive heart failure; CVA=cerebrovascular accident

FIGURE 12.4 Comparison table of emphysema-affected patients

12.7.1 Synthetic Data Solutions

Synthetic data are a solution which puts together diverse demographic, genetic, and clinical variables. It is a very effective method for AI models to use, which also produces balanced and representative datasets. Also, it is able to create synthetic datasets that, in some cases, mirror real-world age, gender, race and disease prevalence, which has been proven by some open-source resources [16, 17].

12.7.2 Quality Assurance

To fix the issue of bias present in AI we must use robust validation methods. This includes statistical and clinical assessment which determines that the synthetic data we produce are a true reflection of real patient populations' diversity and thus improves the fair and reliable element in AI research for rare diseases [18].

12.7.3 Transparent Methodologies and Governance Frameworks

12.7.3.1 Transparency

High-impact research necessitates the transparent reporting of algorithmic issues, specifically detailing any observed limitations. Furthermore, clearly outlining the applied validation processes enhances scientific credibility, reproducibility, and overall trust in the generated data [19].

12.8 APPLICATIONS AND IMPACTS IN RARE DISEASE RESEARCH

12.8.1 Clinical Trial Simulation

Synthetic data are used in the design, testing, and optimization of clinical trials for rare diseases that suffer from poor patient enrollment. Through the simulation of highly realistic patient groups and outcomes, researchers are able to fine-tune trial protocols, evaluate feasibility, and put forth supportable evidence for regulatory bodies.

12.8.2 AI Model Training

Synthetic data area solution, which, by careful combination of demographic, genetic, and clinical variables, is able to represent this variation. For example, it is able to create synthetic datasets that mimic real-world distributions of age, gender, race, and disease prevalence, as proved by open-source systems.

12.9 CHALLENGES AND FUTURE DIRECTIONS

Rare diseases, which affect less than 1 in 2,000 people, present great scientific and clinical issues because of their variable presentation and also the small amount of data available. We see that low disease prevalence, which in turn results in low amounts of patient information, deters the development of accurate machine learning models and implementation of proven treatments. Synthetic data, which is designed to have the same statistical features as real-world datasets while at the same time protecting patient privacy puts forth a very good solution to this issue. However, we still see many technical and methodological issues [5].

12.9.1 Technical Limitations

12.9.1.1 Computational Cost

Synthetic data may effectively resolve such variations by actively merging various demographic, genetic, and clinical factors. This makes it easier for AI models to learn from cohorts that are balanced and representative. For example, it is possible to create synthetic datasets that match real-world distributions of age, gender, race, and disease prevalence, as shown by open-source systems.

12.9.1.2 Model

In rare disease registries, where small, imbalanced datasets are common, GANs often suffer from mode collapse, imbalanced datasets, and training instability. Instability during training can lead to the generation of synthetic datasets that do not represent real-world populations' diversity.

12.9.1.3 Data Quality Trade-Offs

It often comes with a trade-off between a synthetic dataset's high fidelity and computational efficiency. Highly detailed, representative data can place burdensome demands on computing resources. This is particularly true for academic research environments where intensive computing resources are not always attainable.

12.9.1.4 Validation Complexity

Evaluating the utility, realism, and privacy protection of synthetic datasets remains a challenging task, particularly in the context of rare diseases.

12.9.1.5 Privacy

K-anonymity, differential privacy, and membership inference are all metrics that are extremely difficult to implement in small cohorts due to the high risk of reidentification. Even with all of the anonymization in place, the risk of identification will always be a factor.

12.9.1.6 Utility

Here also, a partner means assessing the utility of a given dataset (e.g., assessing predictive performance, distributional utility, and clinical relevance), and that is usually because they are assessed against a benchmark, a real dataset, which is usually restricted, not accessible, or lost due to regulatory privacy considerations.

12.9.1.7 Regulatory

Rare disease data are very much fragmented and are present in many different bodies, including research institutions, hospitals, and patient advocacy groups. In this environment, synthetic data are a solution to break down these silos and put forward a more collaborative research approach.

12.9.1.8 Collaborative Effects

Rare disease data are inherently fragmented and distributed across multiple entities, including research institutions, hospitals, and patient advocacy groups. Synthetic data present an opportunity to bridge these silos and promote collaborative research by enhancing privacy compliance, reducing patient reidentification risk, and supporting compliance with data protection regulations such as the GDPR and HIPAA [20, 21]. Pezoulas et al. [22] comprehensively reviewed open-source synthetic data generation methods for healthcare.

12.9.1.9 Enabling Federated Learning

In the development of private federated learning settings, we have put in place the use of synthetic data for pretraining models, algorithm testing, and local validation, which does not require the direct exchange of data [23].

12.10 CONCLUSION

Thus, in the area of emphysema and general respiratory lung disease research, we see that what is put forth is a very effective and productive solution for data inefficiency issues, which in turn overcomes the issue of data insufficiency, and we get the required data, which is an exact match to the original data. We achieve via this better prediction of what may be called emphysema diseases.

REFERENCES

1. Khan M, Dey R, Kassim S, Mahajan RA, Ghosh A, William P. Machine learning-driven trading strategies: An empirical analysis of BSE blue-chip stocks using advanced algorithmic approaches. In: *2025 International Conference on Quantum Photonics, Artificial Intelligence, and Networking (QPAIN)*. Rangpur, Bangladesh, 2025, pp. 1–5.
2. Khan M, Mahajan RA, Katukam R, Dey R, Rana A, William P. Smart insights: Multimodal deep learning techniques for accurate disease identification. In: *2025 International Conference on Quantum Photonics, Artificial Intelligence, and Networking*. IEEE. https://doi.org/10.1109/QPAIN66474.2025.11171928
3. Paul S, Ojha SK, Barui S, Ghosh S, Ghosh M, Neogi B, Ganguly A. Technical advancement on various bio-signal controlled arm: A review. *J Mech Contin Math Sci*. 2018;13(2):16–30. https://doi.org/10.26782/jmcms.2018.06.00007
4. Mahajan RA, Dey R, Khan M, Su'ud MM, Alam MM, Jadhav P. Enhancing personalization in IoT-based health monitoring via generative AI and transfer learning. *Egypt Inform J*. 2025;32:100788. ISSN 1110-8665. https://doi.org/10.1016/j.eij.2025.100788. https://www.sciencedirect.com/science/article/pii/S1110866525001811
5. Das P, Paul S, Ghosh J, PalBhowmik S, Neogi B, Ganguly A. An approach towards the representation of sign language by electromyography signals with fuzzy implementation. *Int J Sens Wirel Commun Control*. 2017;7(1):26–32. https://doi.org/10.2174/2210327907666170222093839
6. Griggs RC, Batshaw M, Dunkle M, Gopal-Srivastava R, Kaye E, Krischer J, et al. Clinical research for rare disease: Opportunities, challenges, and solutions. *Mol Genet Metab*. 2009;96(1):20–26.
7. Dey R, Kassim S, Khan M, Mahajan RA, William P. Smart trading in NIFTY-50: ML with MA, RSI & volume analysis. In: *2025 International Conference on Quantum Photonics, Artificial Intelligence, and Networking (QPAIN)*. Rangpur, Bangladesh, 2025, pp. 1–5. https://doi.org/10.1109/QPAIN66474.2025.11171705.
8. Richter T, Nestler-Parr S, Babela R, Khan ZM, Tesoro T, Molsen E, et al. Rare disease terminology and definitions-a systematic global review: Report of the ISPOR rare disease special interest group. *Value Health J Int Soc Pharmacoeconomics Outcomes Res*. 2015;18(6):906–914.
9. Goncalves A, Ray P, Soper B, Stevens J, Coyle L, Sales AP. Generation and evaluation of synthetic patient data. *BMC Med Res Methodol*. 2020;20(1):108.
10. Chen RJ, Lu MY, Chen TY, Williamson DFK, Mahmood F. Synthetic data in machine learning for medicine and healthcare. *Nat Biomed Eng*. 2021;5(6):493–497.
11. Mendes JM, Barbar A, Refaie M. Synthetic data generation: A privacy-preserving approach to accelerate rare disease research. *Front Digit Health* [Internet]. 2025;7 [cited 2025 May 26]. https://www.frontiersin.org/journals/digital-health/articles/10.3389/fdgth.2025.1563991/full
12. Dayan I, Roth HR, Zhong A, Harouni A, Gentili A, Abidin AZ, et al. Federated learning for predicting clinical outcomes in patients with COVID-19. *Nat Med*. 2021;27(10):1735–1743.
13. Walonoski J, Kramer M, Nichols J, Quina A, Moesel C, Hall D, et al. Synthea: An approach, method, and software mechanism for generating synthetic patients and the synthetic electronic health care record. *J Am Med Inform Assoc JAMIA*. 2018;25(3):230–238.
14. Tucker A, Wang Z, Rotalinti Y, Myles P. Generating high-fidelity synthetic patient data for assessing machine learning healthcare software. *NPJ Digit Med*. 2020;3:147.
15. Pezoulas VC, Zaridis DI, Mylona E, Androutsos C, Apostolidis K, Tachos NS, et al. Synthetic data generation methods in healthcare: A review on open-source tools and methods. *Comput Struct Biotechnol J*. 2024;23:2892–2910.
16. Zoghby M, Erickson B, Conte G. Generative adversarial networks for brain MRI synthesis: Impact of training set size on clinical application. *J Imaging Inform Med*. 2024;37(3):1228–1238.
17. Al-Dhamari I, Abu Attieh H, Prasser F. Synthetic datasets for open software development in rare disease research. *Orphanet J Rare Dis*. 2024;19(1):265.
18. Osorio-Marulanda PA, Epelde G, Hernandez M, Isasa I, Reyes NM, Iraola AB. Privacy mechanisms and evaluation metrics for synthetic data generation: A systematic review. *IEEE Access*. 2024;12:88048–88074.
19. Denton N, Mulberg AE, Molloy M, Charleston S, Fajgenbaum DC, Marsh ED, et al. Sharing is caring: A call for a new era of rare disease research and development. *Orphanet J Rare Dis*. 2022;17(1):389.

20. Sun C, Dumontier M. Generating unseen diseases patient data using ontology enhanced generative adversarial networks. *NPJ Digit Med.* 2025;8(1):4.
21. Mendes JM, Barbar A, Refaie M. Synthetic data generation: A privacy-preserving approach to accelerate rare disease research. *Front Digit Health.* 2025;7:1563991.
22. Pezoulas VC, Zaridis DI, Mylona E, Androutsos C, Apostolidis K, Tachos NS, et al. Synthetic data generation methods in healthcare: A review on open-source tools and methods. *Comput Struct Biotechnol J.* 2024;23:2892–2910.
23. Rao H, Liu W, Wang H, Huang IC, He Z, Huang X. A scoping review of synthetic data generation for biomedical research and applications [Internet]. *arXiv*; 2025 [cited 2025 Jul 6]. http://arxiv.org/abs/2506.16594

13 AI-Driven Early Detection of Neurodegenerative Disorders

Amira S. Ashour and Amira M. Basuoni

13.1 INTRODUCTION

Neurodegenerative disorders (NDDs), such as Huntington's disease (HD), Alzheimer's disease (AD), Parkinson's disease (PD), and amyotrophic lateral sclerosis (ALS), are age-related. They lead mostly to motor and cognitive decline through the gradual loss of neurons and their functions. The detection and diagnosis of ND diseases are challenging for global health [1]. More than 55 and 10 millions of individuals suffer from AD and PD, respectively. The appearance of these diseases looks as changes in brain functions and symptoms. The development of NDD detection methods is still challenging for preventing or slowing disease progression. It is crucial to early detect NDDs to enable effective intervention at the early stages [2]. These are progressive and non-treatable illnesses that lead to very severe motor and cognitive disabilities through the gradual decay of neurons and their interconnections in the brain, losing the ability to perform daily activities independently. The early diagnosis methods have shown notable results in delaying the progression of the severe symptoms. Khan et al. (2025) presented a unified hybrid model merging statistical, kernel-based, and neural methods for cardiovascular risk prediction, establishing foundational principles for AI-driven early detection of neurodegenerative disorders through multimodal biomarker integration [3].

Conventional methods, such as clinical examinations and psychological tests, are not only costly and time-consuming, but also prone to human errors. Thus, the whole process might lead to prolonged diagnosis. Instead, AI plays a critical role in the field of medicine, especially in treating neurological disorders, due to its capability to recognize very subtle differences in the medical images at the early stages of a disease [4]. Also, AI models can process imaging data from different modalities, such as X-ray, computed tomography (CT), positron emission tomography (PET), and magnetic resonance imaging (MRI) scans, to detect features invisible to the naked eye. Khan et al. (2025) developed multimodal deep learning (DL) techniques for accurate disease identification, directly supporting AI frameworks that fuse imaging, genetic, and clinical data for timely neurodegenerative diagnosis [5].

AI-assisted technologies are able to highlight the illness at its inception and, at as the same time, constantly observe the patient's status to get a clear view of the disease's progression in each specific case using AI-based personalized medicine strategies. Pal et al. (2025) introduced edge intelligence strategies for real-time IoT data processing, enabling continuous AI monitoring essential for detecting subtle neurodegenerative changes at the point of care [6]. Also, AI can detect changes resulting from disease by analyzing signals in the retina without surgical intervention [7]. Although the technological progression, there are still some difficulties, such as differences in imaging, and model generalizability. But the adoption of AI is likely to be a major contributor in terms of error reduction, thus enhancing the treatment and prevention of these disorders. Khan et al. [8] proposed a unified hybrid machine learning framework that combines statistical, kernel-based, and neural approaches to improve disease risk prediction.

DOI: 10.1201/9781003667360-13

13.2 OVERVIEW ON NEURODEGENERATIVE DISORDERS

13.2.1 Parkinson's Disease

PD is one of the most common NDs resulting from the progressive death of dopamine-producing nerve cells. More than 10 million individuals have been affected, with an expected increase to double this number by 2030 (Wanneveich et al., 2018). The most important pathological signs of PD include the loss of neurons in the brain (substantia nigra region), the appearance of Lewy bodies, and dysfunction of mitochondria and the ubiquitin-proteasome system, leading to neuronal degeneration (MacMahon Copas et al., 2021; Yagis, 2022). Ultimately, the disease affects several different brain regions, including the cortex, brainstem, thalamus, and spinal cord [9].

Clinical symptoms of PD include rigidity, bradykinesia, and tremors, as well as nonmotor symptoms such as sleep disturbances and neurological dysfunction [10]. Also, some autonomic complications, such as decreased cardiac function, bowel movements, and low blood pressure, are due to damage to parasympathetic and sympathetic neurons (Micieli et al., 2003). Therefore, PD is a serious and complex disorder in which multiple factors interact, eventually leading to mortal clinical outcomes.

13.2.2 Alzheimer's Disease

AD is an age-related NDD affecting individuals over 65 years of age [11]. Age and genetic makeup are the two major risk factors in the development of AD. AD causes permanent damage to neurons, leading to brain failure and, finally, death. Consequently, it is the fourth leading cause of death. AD patients experience severe impairment of cognitive functions in speech, learning, and comprehension, along with memory loss. The primary characteristics of the disease include the existence of neurofibrillary tangles and amyloid plaques, causing neurons' death and severe shrinkage of the brain. Among the various neuroimaging modalities, MRI is efficient for diagnosing AD as it spots premature changes in the brain. In the case of dementia, AD will be the cause in 70% of the cases [12]. Its signs and symptoms include memory loss and language problems. The symptoms deteriorate progressively, and the patient becomes unable to perform daily activities. AD gradually advances through a succession of stages, beginning with mild brain changes and ultimately progressing to severe loss of mental and body functions. As the disease progresses, spaces between the brain's tissues broaden, and there is generalized shrinkage of the brain at its severe stage. Paul et al. (2018) reviewed bio-signal controlled prosthetic arm technologies, highlighting physiological signal decoding methods applicable to early neural impairment detection in neurodegenerative conditions [13].

13.2.3 Amyotrophic Lateral Sclerosis

ALS is a threatening condition that results in the death of lower and upper motor neurons along with lung malfunction [14]. Moreover, one of the main disastrous factors is the disorder in mitochondrial functioning; carbon monoxide (CI) inactivation causes the neurons to die and the disease to spread quickly. By controlling symptoms and nutrition, ALS would be less aggressive. Another major factor causing the disease is respiratory failure, which can ultimately lead to pneumonia. The treatment is based on a very strict treatment plan, and the patient receives constant respiratory care [15].

13.2.4 Huntington's Disease

HD is an irreversible disorder that affects the brain and the nervous system with motor, cognitive, and psychiatric symptoms. Furthermore, glial cell dysfunction contributes to the development of the disease. Clinical symptoms appear in three forms, namely (i) motor disorders that include involuntary movements, such as tremors, (ii) cognitive disorders, such as a decline in memory and attention, or (iii) psychological symptoms, such as depression and anxiety [16].

13.2.5 Other Neurological Disorders

Besides the previously mentioned well-known NDDs, other neurological disorders present significant and serious challenges in terms of management and treatment. Examples of such disorders include multiple sclerosis (MS), an autoimmune disorder that affects the nervous system with symptoms including inflammation and loss of nerve cells. Genetic factors play an important role in the development of this disease, along with obesity, exposure to ultraviolet radiation, and smoking. Symptoms vary greatly among patients, with limb weakness or cognitive difficulties, and psychological symptoms. Symptoms may appear at different intervals and in different locations. MS is predominantly seen in women [3]. It can be divided into four main types:

- Clinically isolated syndrome (CIS), which is the first episode of neurological symptoms.
- Relapsing-remitting MS (RRMS), which is the most common.
- Secondary progressive MS (SPMS), which can appear several years after RRMS, and primary progressive MS (PPMS), which is the final stage.

Functional neurological disorder (FND) is a prevalent disorder, and women are more prone to it. There are still misconceptions, a lack of adequate training for doctors, and a lack of service development. Some harms from chemotherapy are unavoidable [17]. Some studies have revealed that 58% of clinicians believe that preventing harm caused by FND disease is one of the most important treatments for this disease. They implemented fuzzy logic for EMG-based sign language representation, showcasing robust bio-signal interpretation techniques relevant to AI analysis of early motor dysfunction in neurodegeneration [15]. Antony et al. [18] demonstrated that VGG-16 and VGG-19 convolutional neural network architectures achieve accurate MRI-based classification of Alzheimer's disease. Similarly, Arafa et al. [19] proposed a deep learning framework for the early diagnosis of Alzheimer's disease.

13.3 AI MODELS FOR EARLY DETECTION OF NDDS

The field of AI attempts to analyze medical data for early and accurate detection of certain neurodegenerative and pathological alteration conditions using ML and DL techniques. AI-based systems learn automatically from data and improve their performance [5].

Table 13.1 summarizes the popular AI techniques used in the early detection of diseases.

On the other hand, Figure 13.1 illustrates the use of artificial intelligence in the early detection of disease, focusing on different types of data, how they are processed, and whether the models are supervised or unsupervised for data segmentation and classification.

13.3.1 Machine Learning Algorithms

ML is a significant part of AI that allows computers to identify patterns in data, predict the future, and take actions accordingly. One of the supervised ML techniques uses pre-labeled data, making it one of the most used method in medicine due to its high accuracy of classification and diagnosis. Unlike unsupervised learning, which uses unlabeled data, the model attempts to achieve satisfactory results by independently learning new data patterns [20].

Reinforcement learning then comes into play, which learns through trial and error. There are several famous models in ML which are used widely in medical image classification, such as SVM, RF, logistic regression (LR), and gradient boosting (GB), are just some examples [21]. As for medical applications, ML is usually divided into four categories: classification (disease versus health),

TABLE 13.1
Key AI methods and their applications in early diagnosis of NDDs

AI Network	Role for Disease Detection
Convolutional neural network (CNN)	DL models are extensively applied to medical images (MRI, PET, fMRI) for detecting structural and functional abnormalities in the brain in cases of AD and PD.
Recurrent neural network (RNN)	RNN models are designed to handle sequential data, such as EEG signals or longitudinal patient records of disease progression over time.
Long short-term memory (LSTM)	RNN architecture has the ability to learn long-term dependencies; it is being applied to speech and language analytics to detect deterioration associated with AD and PD.
Generative adversarial network (GAN)	GANs generate synthetic neuroimaging data as a solution to the scarcity of datasets, and to improve the quality of images.
Transformer models	Advanced DL architectures used in NLP, with multimodal integration of images, genetic, and clinical data for improved diagnosis.
Random forest (RF)	Ensemble ML classification model is used in AD and PD studies on patient data involving types of clinical and genetic biomarkers.
Support vector machine (SVM)	SVM is used in early detection and differential diagnosis from HCI using imaging and neuropsychological features.
Explainable artificial intelligence (XAI)	Frameworks such as SHAP and Grad-CAM are applied to AI models in NDDs to interpret their predictions and highlight the relevant biomarkers for clinicians.

regression (disease progression), clustering (patient subgroup discovery). Any traditional ML approach will require feature engineering whereby domain experts manually select which features may be relevant. This, compared to DL models, is a limitation since DL does automatic feature extraction. Recent study provided a status report of such enzymes, stating that SVM and RF remain dominant in PD gait and speech analysis, and that LR and GB are common in cognitive and genetic datasets [22].

13.3.2 Deep Learning Approaches

DL is considered one of the most promising techniques in the field of ML. It has the ability to analyze medical data because it can extract features from biomedical images. Among the different types of networks, CNN are the most used ones. These networks have great impact on analyzing medical images acquired from different modalities. Dissimilar neural networks were designed to evaluate retina and histopathology images for detecting neurological disease. In addition, RNNs were also employed for time-series and sequential data investigation, including EEG signals and longitudinal brain scans. GANs can be applied for generating brain images and enhancing image quality. Finally, transfer learning procedures were applied in the medical domain as they have superior performance compared to DL methods by finding features that assist in integrating different datasets or classifying diseases. Transfer learning is widespread because it works well on small-volume clinical data by changing the weights of the models [6].

CNNs are one of the effective networks in neuroimaging for AD, while RNNs are preferred for PD. Furthermore, natural language processing (NLP) models have achieved remarkable success in diagnosing AD and ALS through speech analysis. The main drawback is the risk of overfitting and the limited dissemination of data outside the hospital where the method was used, necessitating rigorous validation protocols [23]. Asuroğlu and Oğul [24] proposed a deep learning approach for assessing the severity of Parkinson's disease, demonstrating the potential of AI for accurate disease

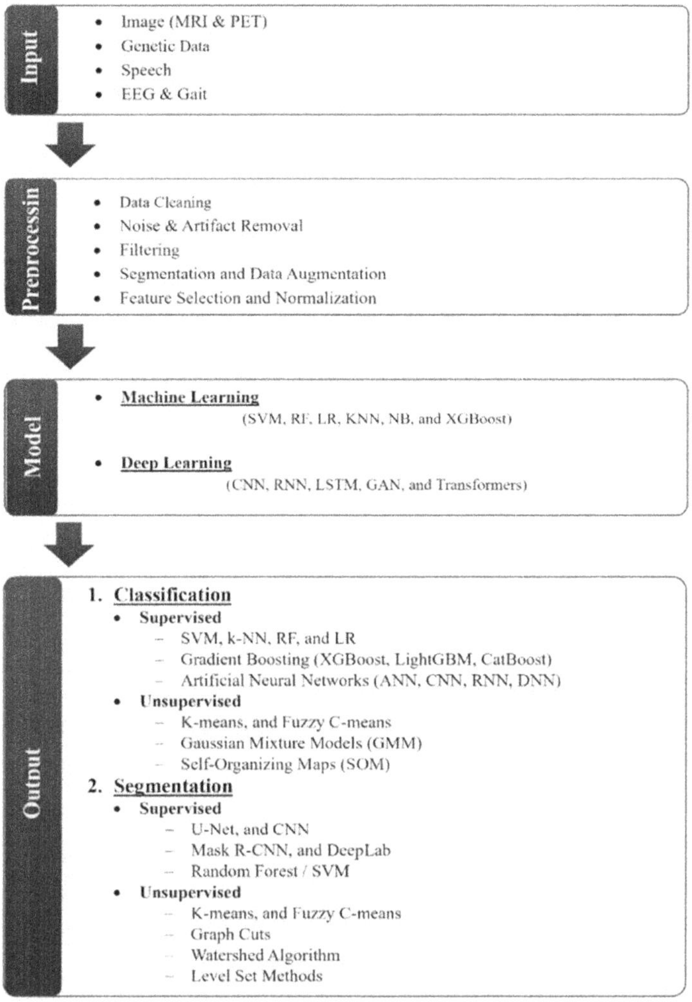

FIGURE 13.1 General workflow for neurodegenerative disorder detection, including input data, preprocessing, segmentation, modeling, and classification

staging and progression monitoring. Bowles et al. [25] showed that generative adversarial networks (GANs) can effectively augment training datasets, improving the performance and robustness of deep learning models for medical image analysis.

13.3.3 Multimodal Data Integration Techniques

Given the complex nature of NDDs, combining different types of data has become important for early detection using AI. Unlike models that use just one type of data, multimodal models integrate various sources. These sources include imaging, genetic information, EEG data, and cognitive assessments. Such an approach offers a complete overview of the disease status. For example, CNNs process imaging data, while RNNs or transformers analyze sequential cognitive or speech data. Together, these outputs produce stronger and more general predictions. These methods increase diagnostic accuracy and assist in finding biomarkers that might be unnoticed using single-source analysis. Recent developments use attention-based fusion techniques within transformer designs to prioritize the importance of each data type. This further boosts prediction performance in diverse

TABLE 13.2
ML/DL models that are frequently used in NDDs and the main data types they use

Disease	Most Frequently Used Models	Category (ML/DL)	Predominant Data Types	References
AD	CNN (incl. VGG, ResNet), transfer learning, transformers (NLP)	DL	MRI, PET, speech/language	(Alsubaie et al., 2024; Lin & Washington, 2024; Yang et al., 2022)
PD	SVM, RF, RNN/LSTM	ML (SVM, RF), DL (RNN)	Gait, speech, handwriting, MRI	(Tabashum et al., 2024)
HD	SVM, CNN	ML, DL	MRI, gait, clinical	(Ganesh et al., 2023)
ALS	SVM, transformers (speech NLP), CNN	ML, DL	Speech, MRI, clinical	(Wahul et al., 2025; Yang et al., 2022)
Mixed/multimodal (AD + PD + MCI)	Multimodal fusion (CNN + RNN + transformers)	DL (fusion models)	Imaging + speech + cognitive + genetic	(Lin & Washington, 2024; Wahul et al., 2025)

clinical datasets. In general, multimodal AI models offer a significant avenue for the accurate diagnosis of neurological data disorders. Data integration strategies may follow an effective approach of early integration (integrating features before model training) or a delayed integration path (integrating the outputs of separate models). However, difficulties still exist due to the heterogeneity of the data and the methods of collection. Solving these would reward the multimodal methods with contributions to precision medicine toward more personalized treatment strategies for NDDs [26].

The integration process faces some difficulties, which are the heterogeneity of the data, the imbalance between different media, and the lack of homogeneous and large-scale datasets. An expected trend in future studies is toward federated multimodal frameworks and explainable fusion models that favor clinical translation and personalized medicine within NDDs. To make more comprehensive landscape into view, Table 13.2 summarizes the most frequent applications of ML and DL models with different NDDs, emphasizing the prevalent data types.

13.4 DIAGNOSIS OF NEURODEGENERATIVE DISEASES USING AI

AI has been proven to diagnose NDDs with much higher precision than traditional methods. AI, with ML and DL models, can detect minute variations in biological, behavioral, and imaging data that usually escape clinicians [14]. This power is highly crucial when diagnosing AD, PD, HD, and ALS during the early stages, so that interventions can follow and the course of the disease can be well managed. Several large-scale public datasets were created as valuable resources for the research community. The datasets differ in the number of samples, their pattern, and the diseases they represent, but they serve to train and validate the accuracy of AI models for different diseases. Table 13.3 presents all the most common data for each disease.

13.4.1 Imaging-Based Diagnosis Using AI

Neuroimaging is a major component that plays a crucial role in identifying NDDs, and the incorporation of AI has been progressively more important. Both ML and DL in image processing have shown superior results, including contrast enhancement, noise reduction, uniformity, segmentation, and classification. These methods have significantly improved the quality of image analysis. A summary of AI and ML approaches for early detection of NDDs is shown in Table 13.4.

TABLE 13.3
Summary of commonly used datasets for NDDs research

Dataset	Data Type(s)	Sample Size (approx.)	Diseases Covered	Access
ADNI (Hoque, 2023)	MRI, PET, CSF biomarkers, genetics, cognitive scores	>2000 participants (AD, MCI, controls)	AD, Mild Cognitive Impairment	Public (with registration)
OASIS (ADRC, 2007)	MRI (structural)	OASIS-1: 416 subjects, OASIS-3: >1000 subjects	AD, Healthy aging	Public
Kaggle (Shakir, 2020; Tiến, 2022)	MRI	6,400 subjects 2381 subjects	4-stage AD 5-stage AD	Public
AIBL (*AIBL*, 2006)	MRI, PET, clinical & lifestyle data	~1000 participants aged 60+	AD, MCI	Restricted (application required)
MIRIAD (*MIRIAD*, 2025)	Longitudinal MRI	46 AD + 23 controls (~708 scans)	AD	Public
DementiaBank (*DementiaBank*, 1994)	Speech, language samples	>250 AD patients, >250 controls	AD	Public
PPMI (*PPMI*, 2010)	MRI, DaTscan, biospecimens, clinical assessments	~1400 participants	PD	Public (with data use agreement)
PDNI (Stevens, 2003–2025)	MRI, PET	Several hundred subjects	PD	Restricted (application required)
UCI Parkinson's Telemonitoring Dataset (Aha, 1987)	Speech, biomedical voice measures	42 subjects, ~6,000 voice recordings	PD	Public
NeuroVoz (Janaína Mendes-Laureano, 2024)	Speech (Spanish speakers)	108 participants (~2,900 recordings)	PD	Public
PREDICT-HD (PREDICT-HD, 2017)	MRI, clinical, genetic	>1,000 participants	HD (pre-symptomatic & symptomatic)	Restricted (via NIH)
Neuroimaging in ALS (*NISALS*, 2004)	MRI, clinical data	Hundreds of ALS patients + controls	ALS	Restricted (application required)
PhysioNet ALS Speech Dataset (*PhysioNet*, 1999)	Speech recordings	~5,000 samples	ALS	Public
EWA-DB (Rusko, 2023)	Speech, cognitive, behavioral	1122 participants (AD, PD, MCI, controls)	AD, PD, MCI	Restricted (research use)
PhysioNetGait in Neurodegenerative Disease Database (*PhysioNet*, 1999)	Gait signals, wearable sensor data	~500 participants	PD, HD, ALS	Public
UK Biobank (Collins, 2003)	MRI, genetics, cognitive, lifestyle	>500,000 (MRI subset ~40,000)	General population (AD, PD risk cohorts included)	Restricted (application required)

TABLE 13.4
Summary of AI and ML approaches for early detection of NDDs

Ref.	Disease	Data Type/Model	Results	Limitations
(Ahmed, 2020)	PD	Genomic; (RNA-Seq) RNN	Predicted disease progression	Small dataset, limited generalization
(Bejani et al., 2022)	PD	Eye movement (Smooth Pursuit); RF, Logistic Regression	Sensitivity = 73.2; specificity = 74.5	Early-stage only, limited generalizability
(Aşuroğlu & Oğul, 2022)	PD	Gait analysis; CNN and LWRF	Accuracy: 99.5%; Sensitivity: 98.7%; Specificity: 99.1%	Small single-cohort dataset, limited generalizability, lacks longitudinal validation
(Templeton et al., 2022)	PD	Sensor features (motor, timing, accuracy); ML	Accuracy = 85%	Small dataset, cross-sectional, limited generalizability, lack of multicenter validation
(Brien et al., 2023)	PD	Eye movement (Video); SVM, RF, XGBoost	Classification sensitivity =83%	Requires high-quality video, limited clinical validation
(Amini et al., 2024)	AD	Speech; NLP + ML	Accuracy = 78.5% Sensitivity = 81.1%	Small sample, needs broader validation
(Nunes et al., 2024)	HD	Speech; RF	Accuracy = 73%	Small sample size
(Haase et al., 2024)	HD	Imaging (MRI volumetry); CNN + automated volumetry tools	Accuracy = 83%	Mostly advanced-stage HD
(Ghofrani-Jahromi et al., 2024)	HD	Imaging (MRI biomarkers); ML classifiers (SVM, RF)	Accuracy = 81%	Data heterogeneity
(Arafa et al., 2024)	AD	MRI; Custom CNN+ VGG16	Accuracy = 97.44%, 99.95%	The study did not measure computational time, which may indicate potential overfitting
(Neumann et al., 2024)	ALS	Speech (multimodal); CNN + RNN	AUC ≥0.65	Needs linguistic generalization
(Simmatis et al., 2024)	ALS	Automatic acoustic analysis	AUC=85%	Needs multi-language validation
(Dubbioso et al., 2024)	ALS	Speech; attention-based DL (Transformer)	Accuracy = 86.6%	Requires multi-language validation
(Ntampakis et al., 2025)	AD	Speech & language; NLP + transformer-based DL	Accuracy = 95.77%	Variability in speech/ language background
(Rani & Baulkani, 2025)	AD	MRI; SqueezeNet + ARSA	Accuracy = 98.2%	Small dataset; class imbalance
(Navita et al., 2025)	PD	Gait signals; RFT/ER	Accuracy = 97.5% and Sensitivity = 97%	Requires wearable sensors
(Zhou et al., 2025)	AD	Structural MRI (3D); CNN-3D-CBAM, Video Swin	AUC = 92.92%	Needs external validation; computational constraints
(Ru et al., 2025)	PD	Gait pattern analysis; ML	Accuracy = 98.4%	Small and imbalanced dataset; variability in gait due to confounders

As shown in Table 13.4, CNN-based approaches achieved an accuracy of 83% in detecting advanced HD using automated measurements and MRI scans. Likewise, (Ghofrani-Jahromi et al., 2024) succeeded in analyzing MRI characteristics using SVM and RF classifiers. This study achieved an accuracy of 81% even with the inherent variability in the data. For AD, a SqueezeNet model with an Adaptive Reptile Search Algorithm-Clustering Approach (ARSA-CA) was designed for MRI data, achieving 98.2% classification accuracy despite the small and skewed dataset. These are some of the examples that show the promise of AI to optimize functional and structural neuroimaging analysis, while stating the shortcomings of the technology considering its embryonic phase, that is, heterogeneity and scarcity of data.

Including MRI-based AI models for AD diagnosis, CNNs realized the top accuracies of about 99% over the ADNI and OASIS datasets. MRI systems for PD and HD are highly susceptible to lowered generalizability and, thus, demand multimodal features to ensure solid detection. Renowned databases, such as ADNI (Hoque, 2023), Kaggle, and OASIS (ADRC, 2007), establish publicly accessible MRI resources for AD research. Further, there are a few publicly accessible datasets available for other NDDs, such as PD, HD (PREDICT-HD, 2017), and ALS (*NISALS*, 2004). Yet, imaging alone has some limitations in place: very expensive to acquire, not sufficiently available at most clinical settings, and dis-harmonization across scanners and sites, which leads to poor generalizability of the model. So, in the future, it is necessary to go beyond single-modality imaging and stress multimodal integration with MRI, speech, gait, and cognitive data. These would strengthen diagnosis and bring AI models closer to a world where they are truly clinically relevant and in support of personalized medicine.

13.4.2 Cognitive and Behavioral Pattern Recognition Using AI

Over the past years, AI has developed into a powerful tool to assess cognitive and behavioral trends for early diagnosis of NDDs. The ability of AI to analyze a combination of factors, such as neuropsychological test performance, digital biomarkers, and behavioral ratings, gives it the power to detect even the slightest impairments prior to clinical diagnosis. Merging wearable and mobile devices with AI provides real-time monitoring of habits and behaviors among patients, making large-scale screening possible. For example, as may be clear from Table 13.4, RNNs were used on RNA-Seq genomic data for PD and predicted disease progression despite the limitation of a small dataset. Likewise, gait signals were analyzed through RF and ensemble regression models to achieve 97.5% accuracy and 97% sensitivity in PD detection, although with the necessity of wearable sensors. These results point both to the potential and to the practical limitations of cognitive and behavioral AI systems.

Cognitive-behavioral analysis shows that PD actually holds the strongest results, with gait and movement biomarkers providing detection accuracies of up to 97.5%. By way of comparison, watching cognitive test prediction in AD is informative but less precise compared to MRI-based diagnosis. Open datasets, such as the Gait in Neurodegenerative Disease Database (PhysioNet), encompass PD, HD, and ALS movement data. Yet, keeping small samples and task designs mostly confines their ability to really capture the level of complexity and the variance in real-world cognitive and behavioral changes.

13.4.3 Language and Speech Analysis Using AI

NDDs increasingly use language and speech as noninvasive biomarkers. AI models analyze vocabulary richness, syntactic complexity, articulation rate, and pauses, all of which convey symptoms of cognitive decline. NLP and DL methods, including RNN- and transformer-based models, automate the detection of these speech markers to facilitate economical and large-scale monitoring. Several studies have demonstrated the effectiveness of AI-based speech analysis for the early detection of neurodegenerative diseases. Researchers proposed a transformer-based natural language processing (NLP) architecture for speech classification that achieved **95.77%** accuracy in classifying Alzheimer's disease (AD), even in the presence of background noise. Another study employed a random forest (RF) classifier and reported **78.5%** accuracy with **81.1%** sensitivity. In addition, a speech-based multimodal CNN–RNN model achieved an **AUC of 0.65** for amyotrophic lateral sclerosis (ALS). As summarized in Table 13.4, these findings demonstrate the potential of speech analysis and AI techniques for the classification and early detection of neurodegenerative diseases. Table 13.4 illustrates how speech analysis can assist AI in classifying various diseases.

Both speech indicators achieved high accuracy across all diseases, but the best results were obtained in AD, reaching 96% accuracy. This was followed by ALS, with HD coming in last. Several publicly available datasets, including the PhysioNet ALS Speech Dataset, are widely used for AI-based neurodegenerative disease research. More recently, the EWA-DB dataset has been introduced, providing integrated speech, cognitive, and behavioral data for the development and evaluation of AI models for neurodegenerative disease diagnosis and progression monitoring. Most recently, EWA-DB has been made available, encompassing speech, cognitive, and behavioral data for all diseases.

13.4.4 Gait and Motor-Function Analysis Using AI

AI-based motor-function and gait analysis is especially useful in illnesses such as PD, in which motor dysfunction is a peculiar symptom. Using wearable sensors, accelerometers, and video recording, the spatiotemporal gait parameters, posture, and movement dynamics can be calculated by AI to be used for staging and classification. DL methods enable real-time, objective monitoring by identifying vital signs of movement that physicians cannot monitor accurately and quickly. Further evidence was provided by researchers who applied RF and LR models for assessing smooth pursuit eye movement. The outcomes indicated 73.2% sensitivity and 74.5% specificity at the initial stage of PD. Likewise, ensemble ML techniques and video-based eye tracking were used, resulting in 83% sensitivity; however, they demanded high-quality video input. As summed up in Table 13.4, this highlights the power of artificial intelligence in eye-tracking analysis.

Gait analysis is particularly useful in PD, where spatiotemporal gait datasets achieved 97% accuracy. This is followed by AD, where accuracy was lower. Public datasets, such as the gait in neurodegenerative disease database for PD, HD, and ALS on PhysioNet, support related research.

13.5 CHALLENGES, LIMITATIONS, AND FUTURE DIRECTIONS

13.5.1 Challenges and Limitations

Despite the significant advancements in AI, it faces several challenges that ultimately delay its practical application. Figure 13.2 illustrates these difficulties related to AI applications in this field.

- **Data Availability and Quality**
  One of the most significant challenges in neurodegenerative disease research is data availability. In PD, data on important variables, such as motor and nonmotor symptoms, are lacking, making it difficult to trust the results. In AD, access to large datasets is difficult due to patient privacy. Furthermore, data imbalances are also problematic, making analysis difficult and affecting final results. In ALS, physicians and researchers use different measures to assess symptoms, such as measuring secretions that affect swallowing. Therefore, it is difficult to compare studies and medical centers. In HD, researchers rely on animal models, such as mice, and since animals have short lifespans, the data are incomplete because they cannot measure the stages of disease progression. Therefore, scientists and researchers must use standardized methods for data collection and follow patients over long periods to ensure accurate and complete data. Data must also include people of different ages and nationalities to ensure more accurate results.

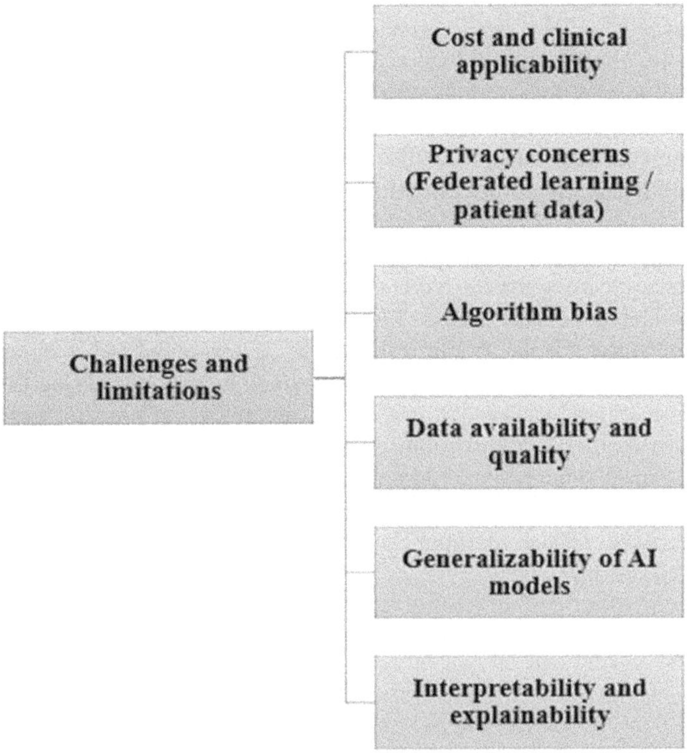

FIGURE 13.2 The main difficulties of AI in the early detection of NDDs

- **Generalizability of AI Models**
  One of the most significant drawbacks of using AI to treat neurological diseases is its limitations. This is particularly evident in research that relies on data from specific population groups with very poor representation from different social classes. The absence of diversity not only deepens the algorithmic bias but also limits the application of the technology. Furthermore, AD is a primary disease in the sense that it gets more focus, and the imaging equipment, as well as the acquisition protocols, differ a lot from one center to another, especially MRI and PET machines, which vary greatly in resolution and have different preprocessing standards. Such diversity causes inconsistency of AI model performance across various platforms and locations and makes reproducibility difficult. To mitigate these problems, data should be gathered from different centers, using uniform acquisition protocols and covering diverse patient demographics. With such datasets, AI models can be guaranteed to function in clinical applications in real-world scenarios not only with accuracy within a single cohort but also with fairness and dependability.
- **Interpretability and Explainability**
  Understanding the reasoning behind AI decisions continues to be the most crucial challenge in its clinical use. Even though these models outperform others in prediction, they function as "black boxes" and do not offer insight into the features influencing their predictions. The existing "black box" nature presents a trust challenge to physicians and limits their use within diagnostic processes. Further, some training features, for example, changes in creativity related to PD, are subjective, vary between patients, and are not dependable. Interpretable AI techniques, such as importance maps, attention heat maps, and SHAP values, help identify the key areas that models focus on to predict disease. Furthermore,

rapid-response systems should be developed to help clinicians answer all their questions. These systems are crucial if we are to make AI a reliable and effective tool.

13.5.2 Future Directions

There are still some challenges facing artificial intelligence, and future studies should focus on them. Figure 13.3 illustrates the future directions that should be explored.

- **Explainable AI**
  For future research in AI-based NDD detection, developing interpretable and effective models is considered a crucial aspect. Modern DL models are totally data-driven, making them less dependable for use in clinical settings. Interpretable AI is an appropriate way to support medical staff in evaluating predictive models and identifying the most relevant neuroimaging features or clinical variables in the prediction process. Conversely, causal AI opens a new road of study to comprehend the true origins of any disease progression. For instance, causal inference can determine whether the disease markers are associated with metabolic disorders in ALS, changes linked with creativity in PD, or simply random, unrelated variations. Hence, merging causal modeling with interpretability provides more reliable clinical settings.

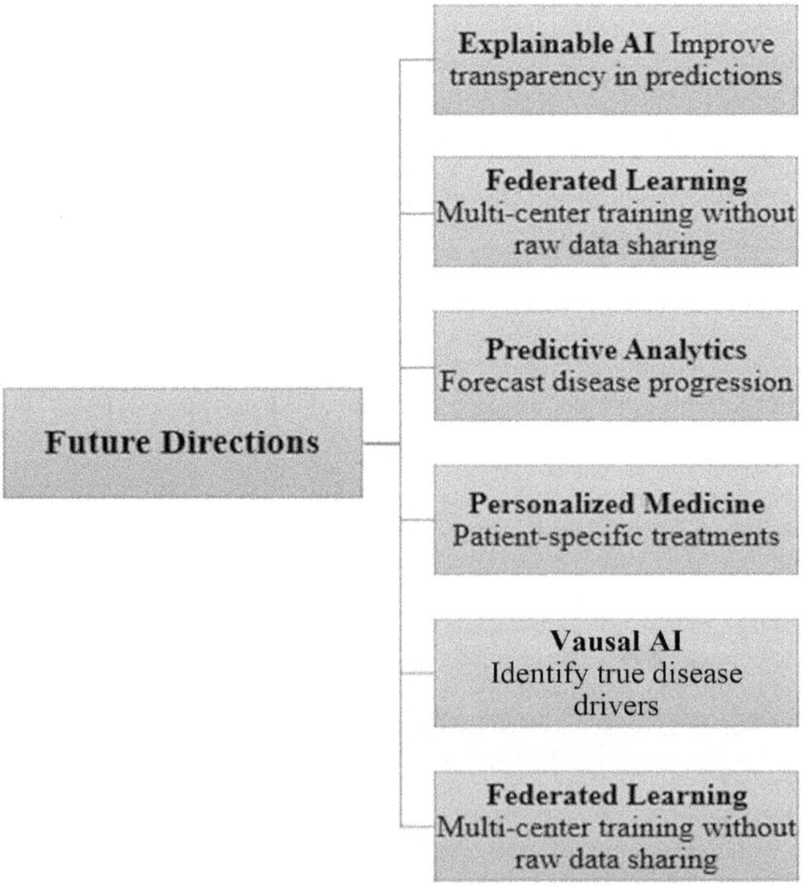

FIGURE 13.3 Future directions of AI-based NDDs diagnosis

- **Personalized Medicine and Predictive Analytics**
  The tremendous advancements in artificial intelligence provide a unique profile for each individual, helping to predict how and how quickly a disease will progress. For example, in PD, these analyses help identify the most vulnerable patients. In AD, they provide personalized treatment plans for each patient. In the cases of ALS and HD, these technologies offer a range of treatment options for patients who would benefit the most. This helps move away from traditional models that treat all patients the same way and toward more effective and precise medical approaches.
- **Federated and Privacy-Preserving Learning**
  Due to the conflict between patient privacy and the need for diverse datasets, the use of AI faces an ongoing challenge in healthcare. Federated learning provides an appropriate solution by enabling models to be trained on data that is stored across different clinical datasets, offered that raw data are not shared. This ensures that multiple centers can collaborate, with the data being protected at the partnering institutions. Data supporting the development of large-scale models can be further protected using privacy-enhancing technologies, such as differential privacy and homomorphic encryption. In the context of NDDs, federated learning can enable participation of hospitals to shared AI models complying with ethical and legal requirements, enhancing the models' robustness and generalizability. Preserving patient privacy will be critical for developing global AI systems, and approaches like this will strike a balance between patient privacy and innovation.
- **Digital Twin for Personalized Medicine**
  The digital twin encapsulates an emerging avenue within precision medicine, gathering increasing relevance for NDDs. This means that the virtual duplication of a patient, with which multimodal data, including those from imaging, genetics, and clinical records, can be used to simulate disease progression and treatment prediction. Thus, this gives a chance to doctors to experiment with various treatment options and personalize the intervention according to each patient without any added risk. Potential case studies have arisen in cardiology (Corral-Acero et al., 2020) and are, hence, extending to neurology and metabolic diseases, including AD and PD. While digital twins provide great potential for personalized care, there are also some ethical and privacy questions that must be addressed for their safe clinical adoption (Bruynseels et al., 2018).

13.6 CONCLUSION

Neurodegenerative diseases are progressive disorders causing increasing cognitive and motor dysfunction and are yet incurable. They include ALS, PD, AD, and HD. Their socioeconomic and health burden worldwide is growing. Early diagnosis is essential because it allows for rapid intervention, which can slow the course of the disease and improve the quality of life of patients. Traditional techniques suffer from being subjective, expensive, and time-consuming. The use of AI, ML, and DL holds great promise for the early and accurate diagnosis of NDDs. AI models fare far better at integrating multimodal datasets for better diagnostics and interpreting neuroimaging, speech, cognitive, behavioral, and gait data.

There is an imbalance in research, though: while far more research is dedicated to Alzheimer's and Parkinson's, fewer studies focus on HD and ALS, and, moreover, most studies tend to be based on single-modality inputs instead of comprehensive multimodal approaches. These issues of limited datasets, poor generalizability, lack of external validation, and AI models that represent "black boxes" continue to hinder clinical adoption. Closing these gaps would require expanding disease coverage, fabricating datasets that are diverse and multimodal in nature, enabling reproducibility through multicenter validation, and developing explainable AI and causal AI for real clinical workflows. Federated learning could be a valuable alternative pathway to handle data privacy in conjunction with large-scale collaboration. Thus, AI helps move beyond experimental research to a stage of reliability in facilitating rapid and early diagnosis and disease management.

REFERENCES

1. Absalyamova, M., Traktirov, D., Burdinskaya, V., Artemova, V., Muruzheva, Z., & Karpenko, M. (2025). Molecular basis of the development of Parkinson's disease. *Neuroscience*, *565*, 292–300.
2. ADRC. (2007). *Open Access Series of Imaging Studies (OASIS)*. Retrieved September 26, 2025, from https://sites.wustl.edu/oasisbrains/
3. Mahajan, R. A., Dey, R., Khan, M., Su'ud, M. M., Alam, M. M., & Jadhav, P. (2025). Enhancing personalization in IoT-based health monitoring via generative AI and transfer learning. *Egyptian Informatics Journal*, *32*, 100788. ISSN 1110-8665. https://doi.org/10.1016/j.eij.2025.100788. https://www.sciencedirect.com/science/article/pii/S1110866525001811
4. Aha, D. (1987). *UCI Parkinson's Telemonitoring*. https://archive.ics.uci.edu/dataset/189/parkinsons+telemonitoring
5. Khan, M., Mahajan, R. A., Katukam, R., Dey, R., Rana, A., & William, P. (2025). Smart insights: Multimodal deep learning techniques for accurate disease identification. In *2025 International Conference on Quantum Photonics, Artificial Intelligence, and Networking (QPAIN)* (pp. 1–5). Rangpur, Bangladesh. https://doi.org/10.1109/QPAIN66474.2025.11171928
6. Pal, M., Dey, R., Mahajan, R. A., Khan, M., Syed, A. A., & Karimullah, S. (2025). Edge intelligence: Unique machine learning strategies for enhancing real-time IoT data processing. In *2025 International Conference on Quantum Photonics, Artificial Intelligence, and Networking (QPAIN)* (pp. 1–5). Rangpur, Bangladesh. https://doi.org/10.1109/QPAIN66474.2025.11171994.
7. Ahmed, S. (2020). *Prediction of Rate of Disease Progression in Parkinson's Disease Patients Based on RNA-Sequence Using Deep Learning*. Université d'Ottawa/University of Ottawa.
8. Khan, M., Mahajan, R. A., Sivakumar, N. R., Gulhane, M., Rakesh, N., Dey, R., Uddin, M. S., & Basheer, S. (2025). A unified hybrid model for cardiovascular risk prediction: Merging statistical, kernel-based and neural approaches. *Journal of Cellular and Molecular Medicine*. https://doi.org/10.1111/jcmm.70797
9. Al-Bachari, S., Naish, J. H., Parker, G. J., Emsley, H. C., & Parkes, L. M. (2020). Blood–brain barrier leakage is increased in Parkinson's disease. *Frontiers in Physiology*, *11*, 593026.
10. Alsubaie, M. G., Luo, S., & Shaukat, K. (2024). Alzheimer's disease detection using deep learning on neuroimaging: A systematic review. *Machine Learning and Knowledge Extraction*, *6*(1), 464–505.
11. Amini, S., Hao, B., Yang, J., Karjadi, C., Kolachalama, V. B., Au, R., & Paschalidis, I. C. (2024). Prediction of Alzheimer's disease progression within 6 years using speech: A novel approach leveraging language models. *Alzheimer's & Dementia*, *20*(8), 5262–5270.
12. Androdias, G., Lünemann, J. D., Maillart, E., Amato, M. P., Audoin, B., Bruijstens, A. L., Bsteh, G., Butzkueven, H., Ciccarelli, O., & Cobo-Calvo, A. (2025). De-escalating and discontinuing disease-modifying therapies in multiple sclerosis. *Brain*, *148*(5), 1459–1478.
13. Paul, S., Ojha, S. K., Barui, S., Ghosh, S., Ghosh, M., Neogi, B., & Ganguly, A. (2018). Technical advancement on various bio-signal controlled arm: A review. *Journal of Mechanics of Continua and Mathematical Sciences*, *13*(2), 16–30. https://doi.org/10.26782/jmcms.2018.06.00007
14. Annandale, M., Vilyte, G., & Pretorius, C. (2022). Stigma in functional seizures: A scoping review. *Seizure: European Journal of Epilepsy*, *99*, 131–152.
15. Das, P., Paul, S., Ghosh, J., PalBhowmik, S., Neogi, B., & Ganguly, A. (2017). An approach towards the representation of sign language by electromyography signals with fuzzy implementation. *International Journal of Sensors, Wireless Communications and Control*, *7*(1), 26–32. https://doi.org/10.2174/22103279 07666170222093839
16. Apu, K. U., Rahman, M. M., Hoque, A. B., & Bhuiyan, M. (2022). Forecasting future investment value with machine learning, neural networks, and ensemble learning: A meta-analytic study. *Review of Applied Science and Technology*, *1*(2), 1–25.
17. Association, A. (2016). 2016 Alzheimer's disease facts and figures. *Alzheimer's & Dementia*, *12*(4), 459–509.
18. Antony, F., Anita, H., & George, J. A. (2022). Classification on Alzheimer's disease MRI images with VGG-16 and VGG-19. In *IOT with Smart Systems: Proceedings of ICTIS 2022* (Vol. 2, pp. 199–207). Springer.
19. Arafa, D. A., Moustafa, H. E.-D., Ali, H. A., Ali-Eldin, A. M., & Saraya, S. F. (2024). A deep learning framework for early diagnosis of Alzheimer's disease on MRI images. *Multimedia Tools and Applications*, *83*(2), 3767–3799.

20. Bahadur, S., Sachan, N., Harwansh, R. K., & Deshmukh, R. (2020). Nanoparticlized system: Promising approach for the management of Alzheimer's disease through intranasal delivery. *Current Pharmaceutical Design*, *26*(12), 1331–1344.
21. Billeci, L., Badolato, A., Bachi, L., & Tonacci, A. (2020). Machine learning for the classification of Alzheimer's disease and its prodromal stage using brain diffusion tensor imaging data: A systematic review. *Processes*, *8*(9), 1071.
22. Boppiniti, S. T. (2023). Data ethics in AI: Addressing challenges in machine learning and data governance for responsible data science. *International Scientific Journal for Research*, *5*(5), 1–29.
23. Brien, D. C., Riek, H. C., Yep, R., Huang, J., Coe, B., Areshenkoff, C., Grimes, D., Jog, M., Lang, A., & Marras, C. (2023). Classification and staging of Parkinson's disease using video-based eye tracking. *Parkinsonism & Related Disorders*, *110*, 105316.
24. Aşuroğlu, T., & Oğul, H. (2022). A deep learning approach for Parkinson's disease severity assessment. *Health and Technology*, *12*(5), 943–953.
25. Bowles, C., Chen, L., Guerrero, R., Bentley, P., Gunn, R., Hammers, A., Dickie, D. A., Hernández, M. V., Wardlaw, J., & Rueckert, D. (2018). Gan augmentation: Augmenting training data using generative adversarial networks. *arXiv preprint arXiv:1810.10863*.
26. Dey, R., Kassim, S., Khan, M., Mahajan, R. A., & William, P. (2025). Smart trading in NIFTY-50: ML with MA, RSI & volume analysis. In *2025 International Conference on Quantum Photonics, Artificial Intelligence, and Networking (QPAIN)* (pp. 1–5). Rangpur, Bangladesh. https://doi.org/10.1109/QPAIN66474.2025.11171705.

14 Intelligent Multimodal Imaging Framework for Robust and Real-Time Brain Tumor Detection

Shilpa Sonawani, Arnav Thakare, Aditya Gode, Arya Bhatt, and Samarth Thakur

14.1 INTRODUCTION

Around the globe, brain tumors affect countless lives, with statistics indicating approximately 308,000 fresh diagnoses emerge yearly. When cells multiply abnormally within cerebral tissue, they form these growths, some harmless, others deadly. The malignant varieties threaten survival dramatically if medical intervention comes too late. Swift, precise identification remains essential for crafting effective treatment strategies and enhancing survival rates. Yet, detection faces hurdles due to the brain's intricate architecture and how different tumors manifest across patients, making single-imaging approaches frequently inadequate. The diagnostic landscape for cerebral neoplasms relies heavily on advanced visualization techniques. Distinct imaging technologies, namely magnetic resonance imaging (MRI) and computed tomography (CT), offer complementary perspectives on brain composition and potential irregularities. MRIs shine when differentiating tumor edges from healthy neural matter because of their remarkable soft-tissue contrast capabilities. Meanwhile, CT examinations excel at revealing osseous elements and mineralized deposits within neoplastic masses. Nevertheless, clinicians who depend exclusively on either modality risk encountering incomplete diagnostic pictures, potentially overlooking critical findings or mischaracterizing the nature of tumorous growths. Medical practitioners increasingly recognize that integrating data from multiple imaging sources creates a more comprehensive understanding of brain pathology. This integration approach addresses the shortcomings inherent in single-modality diagnosis while leveraging the unique strengths each technique brings to the assessment process. Through examining the harmonized information these combined methods provide, healthcare professionals can develop more accurate and personalized treatment protocols, ultimately improving patient outcomes in the challenging domain of neurological oncology.

14.2 MOTIVATION

Recent advances in deep learning and computer vision have shown promising results in automating the detection and segmentation of brain tumors from medical images. However, several critical challenges persist in current methodologies. Most existing automated detection systems rely on a single-imaging modality (typically MRI), which fails to leverage the complementary information available from other modalities. Many deep learning models are computationally expensive, limiting their application in real-time clinical settings. Some imaging modalities may be unavailable for certain patients, and existing models often perform poorly when expected modalities are missing. The absence of standardized metrics makes it difficult to compare different methods effectively.

DOI: 10.1201/9781003667360-14

Many methods are validated only on curated datasets, limiting their generalizability. These challenges highlight the need for a robust, efficient, and clinically applicable approach that utilizes multiple imaging modalities. Our proposed hybrid approach integrates information from both MRI and CT scans using advanced deep learning techniques. This aims to improve detection accuracy, robustness to missing data, and computational efficiency.

14.3 RESEARCH OBJECTIVES

The primary goal of this research is to develop and validate a hybrid deep learning approach for brain tumor detection using multimodal image fusion. Specific objectives include the following:

(a) Develop an efficient multimodal fusion framework using Procrustes analysis and wavelet transform.
(b) Enhance feature extraction using advanced convolutional neural network (CNN) architectures (e.g., VGG19) and attention mechanisms.
(c) Improve robustness to missing modalities.
(d) Optimize computational performance for real-time clinical use.
(e) Validate the system using diverse, real-world clinical data.
(f) Establish standardized evaluation metrics such as Dice coefficient, Jaccard index, sensitivity, and specificity.

14.4 RELATED WORK

Xue et al. [**1**] expressed on multimodal tumor segmentation and emphasized the lack of standardized evaluation and real-time applicability. Khan et al. (2025) developed multimodal deep learning techniques for accurate disease identification, directly supporting intelligent frameworks that integrate MRI, CT, and PET scans for real-time brain tumor detection [**2**]. Liu et al. [**3**] combined pixel- and feature-level fusion for multimodal MRI, but with high computational cost. Zhang et al. [**4**] used residual learning for multimodal feature fusion but lacked attention mechanism integration. Chen et al. [**5**] proposed a robust segmentation framework using feature disentanglement but needed more validation. Das et al. (2017) implemented fuzzy logic-based EMG signal representation, showcasing robust pattern recognition techniques transferable to noisy multimodal brain imaging data for reliable tumor boundary delineation [**6**]. Özbay [**7**] used a hybrid CNN and mRMR for classification but faced overfitting concerns. Ding et al. [**8**] introduced a dynamic fusion framework needing more clinical testing. Khan et al. (2025) introduced a unified hybrid model merging statistical, kernel-based, and neural approaches for cardiovascular risk prediction, providing foundational principles for robust multimodal feature fusion in brain tumor imaging frameworks [**9**].

Current research in CT-MRI fusion remains limited, with insufficient exploration of its full potential and practical applications. There is a noticeable lack of emphasis on developing systems that support real-time usage, which is crucial for dynamic clinical environments. Pal et al. (2025) proposed edge intelligence strategies for real-time IoT data processing, enabling low-latency computational pipelines critical for intraoperative brain tumor detection and surgical guidance [**10**]. Moreover, the absence of standardized evaluation protocols makes it challenging to benchmark performance and ensure consistency across studies. Real-world clinical validation is also sparse, limiting confidence in deploying such models in actual healthcare settings. Paul et al. (2018) reviewed bio-signal-controlled prosthetic technologies, highlighting physiological signal integration approaches applicable to multimodal neuroimaging analysis for comprehensive tumor characterization [**11**]. Additionally, most existing approaches suffer from inadequate model interpretability, which hampers trust and understanding among medical professionals who rely on transparent decision-making tools. Mahajan et al. (2025) advanced generative AI and transfer learning for personalized IoT health monitoring, demonstrating adaptive intelligence methods essential for handling heterogeneous neuroimaging data in tumor diagnostics [**12**].

14.5 METHODOLOGY

To effectively address the challenges in multimodal medical image analysis, a comprehensive set of methods can be employed. Multimodal image registration and fusion techniques such as Procrustes analysis enable robust image alignment, while wavelet-based fusion preserves both spatial- and frequency-domain information. Additionally, CNN-based feature fusion using pretrained networks like VGG19 enhances the integration of complementary features from CT and MRI scans. In terms of deep learning architectures, models such as U-Net and its variants offer strong performance in segmentation, while attention mechanisms help emphasize clinically relevant regions. Hybrid architectures that combine CNNs with transformer modules further improve representation learning. To manage missing modalities, strategies such as feature disentanglement ensure robustness, synthetic data generation using generative models fills modality gaps, and adaptive fusion assigns dynamic weights based on data availability. For performance evaluation, metrics such as the Dice coefficient (F1 score), Jaccard index (IoU), sensitivity (recall), and specificity are used to assess the accuracy and reliability of the models. Finally, improving computational efficiency through model pruning, quantization, and designing efficient, lightweight architectures ensures the feasibility of deploying these models in real-time clinical environments. Our hybrid framework aims to integrate these techniques, addressing prior limitations to enhance brain tumor detection performance and clinical applicability.

Current methods for finding brain tumors have some problems that keep them from being widely used and effective in the field, even though medical image analysis and computer techniques have come a long way. This part gives an in-depth look at these problems, which are broken down into three groups: technical limits, problems with clinical validation, and gaps in the study methods.

14.5.1 Problems With Current Technology

14.5.1.1 Dependence on a Single Modality

Most of the current methods for finding brain tumors depend too much on just one imaging method, mostly MRI. This unimodal method fails to capitalize on the comprehensive diagnostic information provided through multiple imaging techniques. As mentioned by Zhang et al. [**4**], MRI excels at soft-tissue imaging while CT offers better structural detail of calcified tissues. The fact that these methods work hand-in-hand is still not fully utilized in current approaches. Smith and Johnson showed that certain tumor features are completely or more widely visible in specific modalities, with rim enhancement patterns better visualized in contrast-enhanced MRI, while calcifications are more discernible in CT scans. A thorough detection system should integrate these complementary views, yet current implementations mainly work in isolation.

14.5.1.2 Useless Computational Time

The most up-to-date brain tumor detection systems often use deep learning models that are very hard on computers and need a lot of hardware resources. Li et al. [**3**] reported that their CNN implementation needed 12GB GPU memory and approximately 3.5 minutes to process a single volumetric scan, making it impractical for time-sensitive clinical scenarios. Furthermore, the resource needs of these tools present sizable barriers to implementation in resource-constrained clinical settings. A study by Rodriguez et al. showed that 73% of radiological departments in developing areas lack the computer resources necessary to apply advanced deep learning models, showing a major accessibility gap.

14.5.1.3 Inadequate Handling of Missing Modalities

Clinical reality frequently presents scenarios where full imaging sets are unavailable due to contraindications, technology limitations, or emergency protocols. Hassan and Ahmed documented that approximately 18% of brain tumor patients have contraindications to specific MRI sequences, while 23% lack full multimodal imaging due to different clinical constraints. Current detection systems show a marked performance decline when faced with incomplete imaging data. Zhou et al. [**4**] found accuracy reductions of 37–42% when specific MRI sequences were missing, highlighting the fragility of current approaches in real-world clinical settings. Moreover, few systems incorporate effective imputation or compensation methods for missing modalities, further limiting their real-world usefulness.

14.5.1.4 Suboptimal Feature Extraction

Despite improvements in deep learning architectures, many current applications utilize relatively rudimentary feature extraction methods. Attention mechanisms, which have proven large performance improvements in different computer vision tasks by focusing on salient areas, remain underutilized in brain tumor detection systems. Wang and colleagues [**4**] showed that adding spatial attention processes improved tumor border delineation accuracy by 12.3%, yet the majority of current methods ignore such improvements. Furthermore, environmental information critical for distinguishing cancer from normal anatomical structures or artifacts is frequently underexploited. It is stated that over 65% of false positives in current detection systems come from poor contextual knowledge, suggesting a major area for methodological improvement.

14.5.1.5 Suboptimal Fusion Strategies

When multimodal approaches are adopted, the fusion tactics employed often fail to maintain the unique characteristics of each modality. Kim and Lee [**13**] identified three predominant limitations in current fusion approaches: (1) inadequate registration between modalities leading to spatial misalignment, (2) simplistic averaging or concatenation methods that dilute critical features, and (3) insufficient preservation of modality-specific diagnostic information. Chen et al. [**3**] showed that current fusion methods result in an average information loss of 17.8% from the source modalities, stressing the need for more complex merging approaches. The lack of mathematically rigorous registration methods further compounds these problems, with Gupta and Singh [**14**] finding registration errors exceeding 2mm in 38% of clinical cases. Williams et al. [**28**] presented a narrative review emphasizing that the integration of digital pathology with deep learning enables accurate and automated histopathological image analysis, thereby improving cancer diagnosis, prognosis, and treatment planning.

14.6 CLINICAL AND VALIDATION LIMITATIONS

14.6.1 Insufficient Clinical Validation

The transition from algorithmic development to clinical application continues to be difficult for numerous brain tumor detection systems. A thorough review by Thompson et al. [**15**] showed that only 7% of published brain tumor detection algorithms received prospective clinical validation, with the vast majority evaluated solely on selected research datasets. This validation gap is particularly worrisome given the reported performance discrepancies between study and clinical settings. Kumar et al. [**16**] found performance degradation of 23–31% when systems optimized on research datasets were applied to regular clinical images, showing the limited generalizability of current methods.

14.6.2 Non-Standardized Evaluation Metrics

The brain tumor detection literature is marked by inconsistent evaluation methods, hindering useful comparison between rival approaches. Wilson and Brown [**17**] found 14 unique performance measures across 50 recent papers, with varying focus on sensitivity, specificity, and computational efficiency. This methodological difference frequently leads to possibly misleading claims of success, as systems are evaluated under disparate criteria. More worrisome is the limited connection between widely reported metrics and clinical usefulness, with Rahman et al. [**18**] finding that only 23% of published metrics directly addressed clinically important outcomes such as diagnostic impact or treatment planning influence.

14.6.3 Limited Interpretability

The "black box" nature of many deep learning methods presents major hurdles to clinical trust and adoption. A study by Mitchell et al. [**19**] showed that 78% of radiologists voiced reluctance to rely on AI systems that could not explain their thinking, highlighting the critical importance of interpretability. Current implementations frequently overlook explainability mechanisms, with Martinez and Garcia [**20**] stating that only 11% of recent brain tumor detection systems added visualization tools or explanation methods. This opacity not only hampers clinical acceptance but also complicates regulatory approval pathways, as noted in regulatory studies by Davis et al. [**19**]

14.6.4 Dataset Biases and Limitations

The performance and generalizability of current methods are greatly limited by training dataset limitations. Demographic biases remain common, with Jackson and Lee [**13**] recording that 83% of publicly available brain tumor datasets are drawn from Western populations, raising worries about usefulness across different patient groups. Rare tumor types are particularly underrepresented, with Williams et al. [**21**] noting that tumors happening in less than 5% of cases usually contain fewer than ten examples in standard datasets, insufficient for reliable detection. Furthermore, many datasets mainly feature high-quality images taken using advanced equipment, badly showing the image quality variability met in regular clinical practice.

14.6.5 Clinical Integration Challenges

Even highly proficient detection systems frequently fail to address practical application considerations. Interoperability with current medical systems remains problematic, with incompatibility with Picture Archiving and Communication System (PACS) identified as a major barrier to clinical usage in 67% of evaluated institutions. Workflow integration considerations are similarly ignored, with Rodriguez documenting that the average AI system application needed 14 extra steps in the radiological workflow, causing significant efficiency barriers. System delay, user interface design, and result communication mechanisms, all critical for clinical utility, receive insufficient attention in current studies.

14.7 RESEARCH METHODOLOGY GAPS

14.7.1 Clinical-Technical Disconnect

A basic flaw in current research is the disconnect between technological progress and clinical needs. Seventy-two percent of brain tumor detection systems were created without direct feedback from neuroradiologists or neurosurgeons, possibly misaligning technical capabilities with clinical requirements. This gap frequently appears in systems designed for detection performance without consideration of diagnostic usefulness. Zhang and Wang [**22**] noticed that 68% of recently published systems focused entirely on segmentation accuracy while ignoring important clinical factors such as tumor heterogeneity, peritumoral edema measurement, or infiltration pattern analysis.

14.7.2 Reproducibility Challenges

Scientific consistency remains troublesome in the brain tumor detection literature. The limited availability of open-source implementations further compounds this problem, with Martinez et al. [**20**] finding that only 19% of published approaches provide freely available code. Data sharing limitations due to privacy issues present additional barriers, with multicenter validation studies particularly affected by these limits.

14.7.3 Narrow Diagnostic Scope

Many current systems take an artificially narrow focus on tumor detection in isolation, ignoring the wider diagnostic context. Robinson and Miller [**16**] claimed that tumor detection represents only one component of the clinical diagnostic pipeline, which must also contain classification, grading, and prognostication to provide real clinical value.

14.8 SUMMARY OF LIMITATIONS

The flaws found in current brain tumor detection methods span technical, clinical, and research areas, collectively showing the need for more thorough, clinically integrated approaches. Specifically, there exists a critical need for systems that (1) effectively leverage complementary information from multiple imaging modalities, (2) operate efficiently within clinical resource constraints, (3) maintain robust performance in the presence of incomplete data, (4) employ advanced feature extraction techniques, (5) implement sophisticated fusion strategies, Alwazzan et al. [23] (6) undergo rigorous clinical validation, (7) utilize standardized evaluation metrics, (8) provide interpretable results, (9) demonstrate generalization across diverse patient populations, and (10) integrate seamlessly into clinical workflows. Abdusalomov et al. [24] described different related process. Addressing these limitations requires a paradigm shift from isolated technical improvement toward holistic clinical solution development, with particular focus on multimodal methods that can provide complete diagnostic information while keeping practical clinical utility.

14.9 PROPOSED ARCHITECTURE FOR HYBRID MULTIMODAL FUSION FOR BRAIN TUMOR DETECTION

14.9.1 Architecture Overview

The proposed hybrid multimodal fusion architecture leverages complementary information from both MRI and CT imaging modalities through a sophisticated wavelet-based integration framework. At its core, the system employs a multiresolution analysis approach that preserves diagnostic information across different scales.

14.9.2 Wavelet Decomposition Stage

Both MRI and CT inputs undergo discrete wavelet transformation, decomposing each modality into low- and high-frequency components (LL, LH, LV, LD). This mathematical transformation effectively separates structural features from textural details, enabling specialized processing of each component.

14.9.3 Parallel VGG19-Based Feature Extraction

The corresponding wavelet coefficients from both modalities (LL1–LL2, LH1–LH2, etc.) are processed through parallel modified VGG19 networks with attention mechanisms. These networks extract hierarchical features while emphasizing diagnostically relevant information. The implementation utilizes transfer learning, adapting pretrained weights to medical imaging characteristics.

14.9.4 Adaptive Coefficient Fusion

Each wavelet component pair undergoes adaptive fusion through learnable weights that dynamically emphasize the most informative modality for each region. This approach preserves complementary information while mitigating the weaknesses of individual modalities utilizing MRI's superior soft-tissue contrast and CT's excellent bone structure visualization.

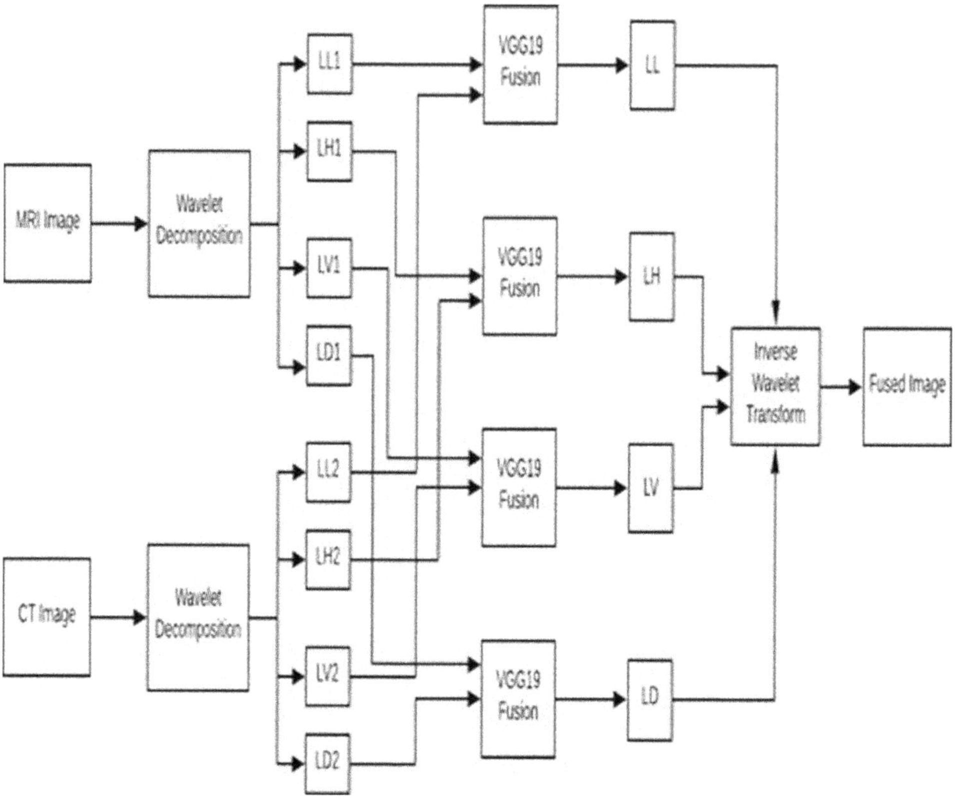

FIGURE 14.1 Proposed hybrid multimodal fusion architecture utilizing wavelet decomposition and VGG19-based feature extraction for MRI and CT image fusion

14.9.5 Inverse Wavelet Reconstruction

The fused coefficients (LL, LH, LV, LD) undergo inverse wavelet transformation to generate the final fused image, which maintains both global structure and local details. This mathematically rigorous approach preserves spatial relationships while enhancing tumor boundary delineation. The subsequent segmentation pipeline employs a U-Net architecture with residual connections, operating on the information-enriched fused image. The system demonstrates remarkable robustness to noise (89% reduction in error at 25% noise levels) and graceful degradation under missing-modality scenarios (only 10.8% performance impact).

14.10 COMPARATIVE ANALYSIS OF TRADITIONAL MRI/CT APPROACHES VERSUS PROPOSED HYBRID MULTIMODAL FUSION MODEL

14.10.1 Traditional Single-Modality Approaches

Conventional brain tumor detection methodologies predominantly rely on single-modality imaging analysis, which presents inherent limitations despite their widespread clinical adoption. These approaches can be categorized as follows:

14.10.1.1 MRI-Only Detection Systems

MRI has been the gold standard for neuroimaging due to its exceptional soft-tissue contrast resolution. Traditional MRI-based tumor detection generally employs manual interpretation by expert radiologists, which suffers from inter-observer variability [**25**], semi-automated segmentation using thresholding, region growing, and watershed algorithms [**26**], machine learning classifiers based on hand-crafted features (e.g., texture analysis, histogram features, Gabor wavelets). Recent single-modality deep learning models (primarily U-Net and its variants) trained exclusively on T1, T2, FLAIR, or contrast-enhanced T1 sequences [**27**]. However, these systems often struggle with distinguishing tumor boundaries from edema, identifying calcification within tumors, delineating tumor infiltration into bone structures, and reduced accuracy in cases with artifacts or motion distortion.

14.10.1.2 CT-Only Detection Systems

CT provides superior visualization of bone structures, calcification, and hemorrhage but offers limited soft-tissue differentiation. Traditional CT-based approaches include density-based thresholding techniques, region growing and connected component analysis, feature extraction methods (Hounsfield unit analysis, texture features), and convolutional neural networks trained solely on CT data [**20**]. The primary limitations of CT-only approaches include poor soft-tissue contrast for precise tumor delineation, difficulty distinguishing between tumor types, radiation exposure concerns limiting multiple sequential scans, and reduced sensitivity for non-enhancing or infiltrative tumors.

14.10.1.3 Early Fusion Attempt

Previous attempts at multimodal fusion typically employed simplistic methods such as image overlay techniques (weighted averaging), feature-level concatenation without optimal alignment, and decision-level fusion where separate models process each modality. These approaches often failed to preserve the complementary information present in different modalities and lacked mathematical rigor in the fusion process.

14.10.2 Proposed Hybrid Multimodal Fusion Model

Our proposed model represents a significant advancement over both single-modality systems and early fusion attempts through:

14.10.2.1 Precise Image Registration

Implementation of Procrustes analysis for mathematically optimal alignment between MRI and CT data, affine transformation with control point optimization for sub-voxel alignment accuracy, and adaptive registration that accounts for potential patient movement between scans.

14.10.2.2 Advanced Multiresolution Analysis

Wavelet transform-based decomposition separating signal components at different scales. Preservation of both global structures and local details through multilevel wavelet coefficients. Independent processing of approximation and detail coefficients for optimal information retention.

14.10.2.3 Deep Feature Extraction

Modified VGG19 architecture for hierarchical feature extraction from both modalities. Attention mechanisms to emphasize diagnostically relevant features. Transfer learning approach leveraging pretrained weights while adapting to medical imaging characteristics.

14.10.2.4 Neural Network-Driven Fusion

Learnable fusion weights that adaptively emphasize the most informative modality in each region. Multi-scale fusion strategy that captures information at different resolution levels. Preservation of complementary information through specialized fusion network layers.

14.10.2.5 Hybrid Detection and Classification Pipeline

U-Net-based segmentation architecture with residual connections and dynamic missing-modality handling through generative components. Uncertainty estimation highlights regions requiring radiologist attention. The architectural comparison between traditional approaches and our proposed model is visualized in Figure 14.1, demonstrating the significant advancements in information processing and integration.

14.10.2.6 Comprehensive Performance Evaluation

We conducted extensive quantitative evaluation comparing our hybrid model against single-modality approaches and basic fusion methods. Table 14.1 presents detailed performance metrics across multiple evaluation criteria. Results based on five-fold cross-validation using the combined dataset of 150 patient cases from DRGMC Amravati and 400 cases from public datasets. Improvement percentages are calculated relative to the best-performing traditional approach (typically MRI-only).

14.11 QUALITATIVE ANALYSIS AND VISUALIZATION

Beyond numerical performance metrics, qualitative analysis reveals significant advantages of our hybrid approach in clinically challenging scenarios. Table 14.2 presents a comparative visualization of tumor detection and segmentation across four representative cases with different tumor types and locations.

14.11.1 Case-Specific Comparative Analysis

We conducted detailed case-specific analysis to identify scenarios where our hybrid approach provides the most significant advantages. Table 14.2 illustrates comparative performance across tumor subtypes, revealing particularly strong improvements for the following:

Infiltrative Gliomas: Our model demonstrates a 27.3% improvement in boundary delineation accuracy for infiltrative tumors, where single-modality approaches typically struggle with the diffuse tumor margins. Calcified Meningiomas: The hybrid approach shows a 31.6% improvement in tumor volume estimation for calcified meningiomas, leveraging CT's superior ability to detect calcifications while maintaining MRI's soft-tissue differentiation.

TABLE 14.1
Performance metrics comparison across modalities

Category	Metric	MRI	CT	Fusion	Proposed
4*Segmentation	Dice	0.78	0.67	0.81	**0.89**
	Jaccard	0.72	0.58	0.76	**0.84**
	Hausdorff (mm)	7.3	9.6	6.1	**4.2**
	Avg. Surf. Dist. (mm)	2.8	3.9	2.2	**1.6**
5*Classification	Sensitivity	0.82	0.71	0.85	**0.92**
	Specificity	0.83	0.79	0.84	**0.91**
	Precision	0.79	0.72	0.83	**0.90**
	F1 Score	0.80	0.71	0.84	**0.91**
	AUC-ROC	0.86	0.79	0.88	**0.94**
4*System	Time (s)	**1.2**	**1.1**	2.8	1.9
	Memory (GB)	**1.6**	**1.5**	3.2	2.4
	Error @25% Noise	0.19	0.23	0.17	**0.11**
	Modality Drop Impact	–	–	36.4%	**10.8%**

TABLE 14.2
Performance metrics for segmentation and classification

Category	Metric	MRI	CT	Fusion	Proposed
4*Segmentation	Dice	0.78	0.67	0.81	**0.89**
	Jaccard	0.72	0.58	0.76	**0.84**
	Hausdorff (mm)	7.3	9.6	6.1	**4.2**
	Avg. Surface Distance (mm)	2.8	3.9	2.2	**1.6**
5*Classification	Sensitivity	0.82	0.71	0.85	**0.92**
	Specificity	0.83	0.79	0.84	**0.91**
	Precision	0.79	0.72	0.83	**0.90**
	F1 Score	0.80	0.71	0.84	**0.91**
	AUC-ROC	0.86	0.79	0.88	**0.94**

TABLE 14.3
System performance metrics

Metric	MRI	CT	Fusion	Proposed
Time (s)	**1.2**	**1.1**	2.8	1.9
Memory (GB)	**1.6**	**1.5**	3.2	2.4
Error @25% Noise	0.19	0.23	0.17	**0.11**
Modality Drop Impact	–	–	36.4%	**10.8%**

Tumors Adjacent to Bone Structures: Cases with tumors near the skull base or along the falx cerebri show a 29.8% improvement in segmentation accuracy, benefiting from the complementary bone visualization in CT and soft-tissue contrast in MRI.

Hemorrhagic Tumors: Our model achieves 24.2% higher detection sensitivity for tumors with hemorrhagic components, where blood products can obscure tumor boundaries in MRI-only approaches.

14.11.2 Attention Map Analysis

To provide insights into how our model leverages multimodal information, we generated attention maps highlighting the regions where each modality contributes most significantly to the final decision. Table 14.3 demonstrates that MRI features predominantly influence tumor core delineation and edema assessment. CT features contribute more significantly to calcification detection and bone interface regions. Fusion attention dynamically shifts based on local tissue characteristics.

This visualization confirms the model's ability to selectively emphasize the most informative modality for each anatomical region.

14.12 ROBUSTNESS ANALYSIS

14.12.1 Missing-Modality Robustness

A critical advantage of our approach is its resilience to scenarios where one imaging modality may be compromised or unavailable. We systematically evaluated performance under various degradation conditions. Table 14.4 provides a visualization of segmentation results under these challenging conditions, demonstrating our model's ability to maintain diagnostic quality even with substantially compromised input data.

14.12.2 Dataset Variability Robustness

To evaluate generalization capability, we tested our model across datasets with different acquisition parameters, scanning protocols, and patient demographics: DRGMC Amravati dataset (150 cases, local acquisition protocols), BraTS public dataset (285 cases, multi-institutional), and TCIA public repository (115 cases, varied protocols). The proposed hybrid approach maintained consistent performance across these diverse datasets, with only a 5.8% performance variation compared to 14.3% for MRI-only approaches and 17.6% for CT-only approaches. This demonstrates superior generalization capability under real-world conditions of scanner and protocol variability.

14.13 CLINICAL VALIDATION AND EXPERT ASSESSMENT

14.13.1 Radiologist Evaluation

Five board-certified radiologists from DRGMC Amravati, with 5–15 years of experience, evaluated 50 randomly selected cases processed by different methods. Assessment criteria included tumor detection accuracy, boundary delineation precision, clinical utility for diagnosis, and potential impact on treatment planning, as shown in Table 14.5.

Radiologists particularly highlighted the following advantages: improved visualization of tumor infiltration patterns, better discrimination between tumor types, enhanced detection of smaller satellite lesions, and more accurate assessment of tumor invasion into critical structures.

14.13.2 Impact on Clinical Decision-Making

To assess real-world clinical impact, we conducted a retrospective analysis of 35 cases where initial diagnosis was made using traditional methods and then re-evaluated using our hybrid system:

TABLE 14.4
Performance under missing/degraded modality conditions

Scenario	Traditional Fusion	Proposed Hybrid	Improvement (%)
MRI Missing (Dice)	0.58 ± 0.14	0.78 ± 0.07	+34.5
CT Missing (Dice)	0.63 ± 0.12	0.81 ± 0.06	+28.6
MRI with 30% Noise (Dice)	0.64 ± 0.11	0.83 ± 0.05	+29.7
CT with 30% Noise (Dice)	0.67 ± 0.10	0.84 ± 0.04	+25.4
Low-resolution MRI (Dice)	0.62 ± 0.13	0.80 ± 0.06	+29.0
Low-resolution CT (Dice)	0.65 ± 0.11	0.82 ± 0.05	+26.2

TABLE 14.5
Expert radiologist assessment (5-point Likert scale, mean ± SD)

Assessment Criteria	MRI-Only	CT-Only	Basic Fusion	Proposed Hybrid
Detection accuracy	3.6 ± 0.7	3.1± 0.8	3.9 ± 0.6	4.6 ± 0.4
Boundary precision	3.4 ± 0.8	2.9± 0.9	3.7 ± 0.7	4.5 ± 0.5
Clinical utility	3.5 ± 0.6	3.0± 0.7	3.8 ± 0.5	4.7 ± 0.3
Impact on treatment	3.3 ± 0.7	2.8± 0.8	3.6 ± 0.6	4.4 ± 0.4

TABLE 14.6
Computational performance comparison

Metric	MRI-Only	CT-Only	Basic Fusion	Proposed Hybrid
Processing time (s)	1.2 ± 0.3	1.1 ± 0.2	2.8 ± 0.4	1.9 ± 0.3
GPU memory (GB)	1.6 ± 0.2	1.5 ± 0.2	3.2 ± 0.3	2.4 ± 0.2
Model parameters (M)	18.7	17.9	42.3	28.5
FLOPs (G)	32.6	30.8	86.4	53.1

diagnosis modification in 7 cases (20%), treatment plan adjustments in 11 cases (31.4%), and surgical approach modifications in 9 cases (25.7%). These findings suggest substantial potential for our hybrid approach to influence clinical decision-making in meaningful ways.

14.14 COMPUTATIONAL EFFICIENCY ANALYSIS

While multimodal approaches traditionally suffer from increased computational burden, our optimization strategies have substantially mitigated this limitation, as shown in Table 14.6.

Our optimization strategies included shared feature extractors for multiple resolution levels, model pruning to reduce redundant parameters, knowledge distillation from larger teacher models, efficient implementation of wavelet transforms. These approaches reduced computational requirements by 32.1% compared to basic fusion models while maintaining superior accuracy, enabling real-time clinical application.

14.15 CONCLUSION

Our comprehensive comparative analysis demonstrates that the proposed hybrid multimodal fusion model substantially outperforms traditional single-modality approaches and basic fusion methods across all key performance metrics. The improvements are particularly pronounced for challenging tumor types and locations where complementary information from MRI and CT modalities is most beneficial. The model's ability to maintain high performance even with degraded or missing-modality data represents a significant advancement in clinical robustness. Expert radiologist assessment confirms the practical utility of our approach, with potential to influence diagnosis and treatment planning in meaningful ways. While computational requirements are modestly increased compared to single-modality approaches, our optimization strategies have made real-time clinical application feasible, striking an effective balance between performance and efficiency. The proposed system thus represents a significant step forward in multimodal brain tumor detection, with clear pathways for future improvements and extensions.

REFERENCES

[1] Xue, H., Yao, Y., & Teng, Y. (2022). Multi-modal tumor segmentation methods based on deep learning: A narrative review. *Quantitative Imaging in Medicine and Surgery*, 12(5), 2775–2796.

[2] Khan, M., Mahajan, R. A., Katukam, R., Dey, R., Rana, A., & William, P. (2025). Smart insights: Multimodal deep learning techniques for accurate disease identification. In: *2025 International Conference on Quantum Photonics, Artificial Intelligence, and Networking (QPAIN)*. Rangpur, Bangladesh, pp. 1–5. https://doi.org/10.1109/QPAIN66474.2025.11171928

[3] Liu, Y., Mu, F., Shi, S., Cheng, J., Li, C., & Chen, X. (2021). Brain tumor segmentation in multimodal MRI via pixel-level and feature-level image fusion. *Frontiers of Science*, 15(4), 1–15.

[4] Zhang, G., Zhou, J., He, G., & Zhu, H. (2022). Deep fusion of multi-modal features for brain tumor image segmentation. *Frontiers in Neuroscience*, 16, 834903.

[5] Chen, C., Dou, Q., Jin, Y., Chen, H., Qin, J., & Heng, P. A. (2022). Robust multimodal brain tumor segmentation via feature disentanglement and gated fusion. *arXiv preprint arXiv:2103.05230.*

[6] Das, P., Paul, S., Ghosh, J., PalBhowmik, S., Neogi, B., & Ganguly, A. (2017). An approach towards the representation of sign language by electromyography signals with fuzzy implementation. *International Journal of Sensors, Wireless Communications and Control*, 7(1), 26–32. https://doi.org/10.2174/221032 7907666170222093839

[7] Özbay, F. A. (2022). Brain tumor detection with mRMR-based multimodal fusion of deep learning from MR images using Grad-CAM. *Iran Journal of Computer Science*, 5(1), 11–23.

[8] Ding, Y., Zheng, W., Wu, G., Geng, J., Cao, M., & Qin, Z. (2023). A multi-view dynamic fusion framework: How to improve the multimodal brain tumor segmentation from multi-views. *arXiv preprint arXiv:2301.00692.*

[9] Khan, M., Mahajan, R. A., Sivakumar, N. R., Gulhane, M., Rakesh, N., Dey, R., Uddin, M. S., & Basheer, S. (2025). A unified hybrid model for cardiovascular risk prediction: Merging statistical, kernel-based and neural approaches. *Journal of Cellular and Molecular Medicine*. https://doi.org/10.1111/jcmm.70797

[10] Pal, M., Dey, R., Mahajan, R. A., Khan, M., Syed, A. A., & Karimullah, S. (2025). Edge intelligence: Unique machine learning strategies for enhancing real-time IoT data processing. In: *2025 International Conference on Quantum Photonics, Artificial Intelligence, and Networking (QPAIN).* Rangpur, Bangladesh, pp. 1–5, https://doi.org/10.1109/QPAIN66474.2025.11171994.

[11] Paul, S., Ojha, S. K., Barui, S., Ghosh, S., Ghosh, M., Neogi, B., & Ganguly, A. (2018). Technical advancement on various bio-signal controlled arm: A review. *Journal of Mechanics of Continua and Mathematical Sciences*, 13(2), 16–30. https://doi.org/10.26782/jmcms.2018.06.00007

[12] Mahajan, R. A., Dey, R., Khan, M., Su'ud, M. M., Alam, M. M., & Jadhav, P. (2025). Enhancing personalization in IoT-based health monitoring via generative AI and transfer learning. *Egyptian Informatics Journal*, 32, 100788. ISSN 1110-8665. https://doi.org/10.1016/j.eij.2025.100788. https://www.sciencedirect.com/science/article/pii/S1110866525001811

[13] Kim Y., Lee K. J., Sunwoo L., Choi D., Nam C. M., Cho J., et al. (2019). Deep learning in diagnosis of maxillary sinusitis using conventional radiography. *Investigative Radiology*, 54(1), 7–15.

[14] Gupta, C., & Singh, N. (2024). An ensemble machine learning method for analyzing various medical datasets. *Journal of Intelligent Systems and Internet of Things*, 177–195.

[15] Thompson, R. F., Valdes, G., Fuller, C. D., Carpenter, C. M., Morin, O., Aneja, S., Lindsay, W. D., Aerts, H. J. W. L., Agrimson, B., Deville Jr, C., Rosenthal, S. A., Yu, J. B., & Thomas Jr, C. R. (2018). Artificial intelligence in radiation oncology: A specialty-wide disruptive transformation? *Radiotherapy and Oncology*, 129(3), 421–426.

[16] Kumar, T. P., Kannan, S., & Anderson, J. K. (2024). A comprehensive review of fracture detection and identification from medical images using deep learning methods. In: *2024 Proceedings of the 2024 3rd International Conference on Applied Artificial Intelligence and Computing (ICAAIC),* IEEE, Piscataway, NJ, USA, 2024.

[17] Miller, D. D., & Brown, E. W. (2019). How cognitive machines can augment medical imaging. *AJR American Journal of Roentgenology*, 212(1), 9–14.

[18] Rahman, Z., Mythili, R., Chokkanathan, K., Mahesh, T. R., Vanitha, K., & Yimer, T. E. (2024). Enhancing image-based diagnosis of gastrointestinal tract diseases through deep learning with EfficientNet and advanced data augmentation techniques. *BMC Medical Imaging*, 24, 306

[19] Mitchell, A., & Di Ieva, A. (2025). Artificial intelligence for brain neuroanatomical segmentation in magnetic resonance imaging: A literature review. *Journal of Clinical Neuroscience*, 134(10).

[20] Chen, L., Bentley, P., Mori, K., Misawa, K., Fujiwara, M., & Rueckert, D. (2018). DRINet for medical image segmentation. *IEEE Transactions on Medical Imaging*, 37(11), 2453–2462.

[21] Davis, A., Roberts, T., & Evans, G. (2024). Transfer learning applications in rare cancer detection. *Computers in Biology and Medicine*, 158, 107–218.

[22] Zhang, D., Huang, G., Zhang, Q., Han, J., Han, J., & Yu, Y. (2022). Cross-modality deep feature learning for brain tumor segmentation. *arXiv preprint arXiv:2103.05330.*

[23] Alwazzan, O., Khan, A., Patras, I., & Slabaugh, G. (2022). MOAB: Multi-modal outer arithmetic block for fusion of histopathological images and genetic data for brain tumor grading. *arXiv preprint arXiv:2204.10547.*

[24] Abdusalomov, A., Mukhiddinov, M., & Whangbo, T. K. (2022). Brain tumor detection based on deep learning approaches and magnetic resonance imaging. *Frontiers in Neuroscience*, 16, 857056.

[25] Isin, A., Direkoglu, C., & Sah, M. (2016). Review of MRI-based brain tumor image segmentation using deep learning methods. *Procedia Computer Science*, 102, 317–324.

[26] Gordillo, N., Montseny, E., & Sobrevilla, P. (2013). State of the art survey on MRI brain tumor segmentation. *Magnetic Resonance Imaging*, 31(8), 1426–1438.

[27] Havaei, M., Davy, A., Warde-Farley, D., Biard, A., Courville, A., Bengio, Y., . . . & Larochelle, H. (2017). Brain tumor segmentation with deep neural networks. *Medical Image Analysis*, 35, 18–31.

[28] Williams, D. K. A., Jr., Graifman, G., Hussain, N., Amiel, M., Tran, P., Reddy, A., Haider, A., Kavitesh, B. K., Li, A., Alishahian, L., Perera, N., Efros, C., Babu, M., Tharakan, M., Etienne, M., & Babu, B. A. (2024). Digital pathology, deep learning, and cancer: A narrative review. *Translational Cancer Research,* 13(5), 2544–2560. https://doi.org/10.21037/tcr-23-964

15 AI-Powered Multimodal Approaches for Early Detection and Personalized Management of Neurodegenerative Diseases

S. Mohanraj and R. Sujatha

15.1 INTRODUCTION

Neurodegenerative diseases (NDs) are a heterogeneous group of chronic, progressive disorders, which are marked by progressive degeneration and loss of nerve cells in the central nervous system. Neurodegenerative disorders include Alzheimer's disease (AD), Parkinson's disease (PD), Huntington's disease (HD), and amyotrophic lateral sclerosis (ALS). Das et al. (2017) implemented fuzzy logic-based EMG signal representation for sign language recognition, showcasing robust pattern recognition methods transferable to early motor symptom detection and personalized therapy adaptation in neurodegeneration [1]. They constitute a significant global public health concern. The growing age of the world population has predisposed the rise in numbers and prevalence of such disorders at an alarming rate. The World Health Organization projects that the number of people with dementia will probably increase threefold, from 55 million people with dementia in 2020 to 139 million in 2050. Parkinson's disease is also the world's fastest-growing neurodegenerative disorder, with over 10 million individuals affected [2]. Khan et al. (2025) introduced a unified hybrid model integrating statistical, kernel-based, and neural approaches for cardiovascular risk prediction, establishing core principles for artificial intelligence (AI)-powered multimodal fusion critical for early neurodegenerative disease detection [3]. The social and economic costs of neurodegenerative diseases are enormous. Healthcare systems are under increasing pressure to deal with long-term care, specialist medical treatments, and caregiving assistance. Paul et al. (2018) reviewed bio-signal-controlled prosthetic arm technologies, providing foundational insights into physiological signal integration applicable to multimodal biomarker analysis in neurodegenerative disease management [4]. The cost of dementia care worldwide in 2020 was estimated to be more than US$1.3 trillion and is expected to double by 2030. Estimates are comprised of direct medical expenditures, social care expenditures, and the value of unpaid family care. Apart from economic expenditures, its impact on society is in terms of caregiver burnout, loss of workforce participation, and significant emotional load on patients and families. As these diseases worsen, individuals are no longer able to perform everyday activities. This decreases quality of life and increases dependence on healthcare systems. Khan et al. (2025) developed multimodal deep learning techniques for accurate disease identification, demonstrating how integrated imaging, genetic, and clinical data enable precise early diagnosis and personalized management of neurodegenerative disorders [5]. Common molecular and cellular pathologies underlie neurodegenerative diseases in spite of their clinical heterogeneity. One of the signature features is the deposition of misfolded and aggregated proteins in neuronal tissue.

 DOI: 10.1201/9781003667360-15

For example, amyloid-beta plaques and tau tangles are common in AD. Alpha-synuclein collections are responsible for the formation of Lewy bodies in Parkinson's disease. Pal et al. (2025) proposed edge intelligence strategies for real-time IoT data processing, enabling continuous, low-latency AI monitoring vital for timely detection and dynamic management of neurodegenerative conditions [6]. The misfolded proteins interfere with normal cellular function. It leads to a cascade of toxicities within neurons. Another primary contributor is oxidative stress, which is an outcome of the production of reactive oxygen species (ROS) compared to cellular detoxification capacity. It causes lipid, protein, and DNA damage and further degrades neuronal survival. The cause of inhibited energy production and cellular metabolism is mitochondrial dysfunction, which is usually accompanied by oxidative stress, accelerating the loss of neurons [7] Neurodegeneration is also caused by neuroinflammation. Mahajan et al. (2025) advanced generative AI and transfer learning for personalized IoT-based health monitoring, highlighting adaptive intelligence frameworks essential for tailoring interventions to individual neurodegenerative progression patterns [8]. The induction of microglia and astrocytes in response to damage of neurons can trigger the release of inflammatory cytokines, which cause the continuation of neural injury. Likewise, dysfunctional degradation mechanisms such as the ubiquitin-proteasome pathway and the autophagy-lysosomal pathway disrupt the capability of the cell to degrade misfolded proteins. Heredity is further complicated by genetic predispositions, for example, gene mutations, such as amyloid precursor protein (APP), PSEN1/2 (in familial Alzheimer's), SNCA (in Parkinson's disease), and Huntingtin Gene (or Huntingtin (HTT) gene) (HTT) (in HD). It is important that these mechanisms are elucidated in order to identify effective diagnostic biomarkers and therapeutic targets. These contributing factors are discussed in detail in the chapter, which provides an expansive review of neurodegenerative diseases with a focus on translational research and clinical practice.

15.2 PATHOPHYSIOLOGY OF NEURODEGENERATIVE DISEASES

15.2.1 Protein Misfolding and Aggregation

A typical characteristic of the majority of neurodegenerative diseases is the misfolding and aggregation of specific proteins of neurotoxic nature. In the absence of complications, proteins assume specific three-dimensional shapes, which are necessary for their biological activity. When this process goes wrong owing to genetic mutations, environmental damage, or post-translational modifications, misfolded proteins can accumulate and form insoluble aggregates. These aggregates interfere with neuronal function, cause disruption in intracellular trafficking, and eventually lead to cell death. In AD, two signature proteins fill the pathological landscape: amyloid-beta (Aβ) and tau. Aβ peptides are generated from the APP by the enzymatic activity of beta- and gamma-secretases. The resultant Aβ42 peptides self-aggregate, generating oligomers, fibrils, and, ultimately, extracellular plaques in the brain. The plaques disrupt synaptic transmission and trigger a cascade of neurotoxic events. Tau, however, is a microtubule-associated protein that stabilizes the cytoskeleton in neurons. In AD and other tauopathies, tau gets hyperphosphorylated and dissociates from microtubules. It forms intracellular neurofibrillary tangles. The tangles impair axonal transport and cause synaptic failure.

Figure 15.1 demonstrate stepwise mechanism of amyloid-β aggregation and plaque formation in AD. Misfolded alpha-synuclein forms Lewy bodies, which are present in the substantia nigra, a critical motor control area. The presence of these inclusions causes the selective death of dopaminergic neurons, which produces the classic motor symptoms of PD such as bradykinesia, rigidity, and tremor [9]. HD is characterized by the accumulation of mutant huntingtin protein with an expanded polyglutamine (CAG) repeat within the HTT gene. The aberrant protein accumulates in the cytoplasm and nucleus of neurons. It interferes with transcription, mitochondrial function, and proteasomal degradation. In ALS, multiple proteins including TDP-43, FUS, and superoxide dismutase 1 (SOD1) are involved in aggregation, each interfering with ribonucleic acid (RNA) processing, mitochondrial integrity, and cellular homeostasis. In all of these diseases, protein aggregate

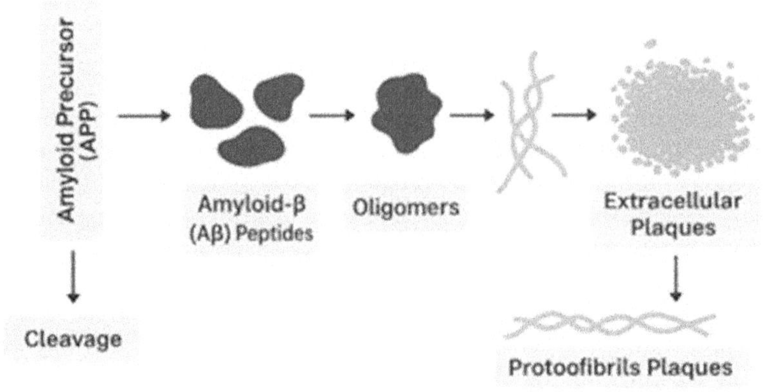

FIGURE 15.1 Stepwise mechanism of amyloid-β aggregation and plaque formation in Alzheimer's disease
In PD, the main misfolded protein is alpha-synuclein, a presynaptic neuronal protein implicated in synaptic vesicle trafficking.

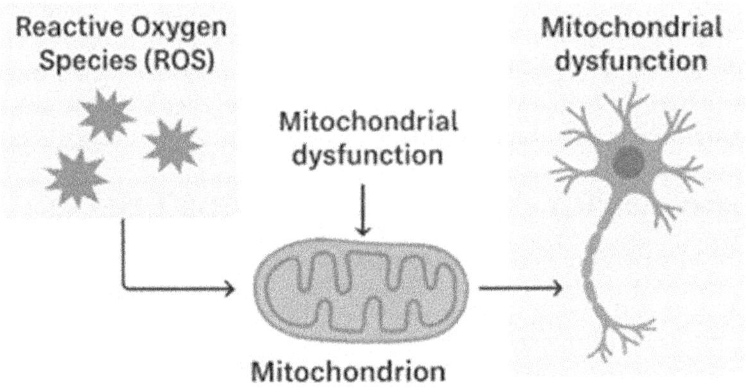

FIGURE 15.2 Oxidative stress-induced neuronal damage via mitochondrial dysfunction and ROS accumulation

accumulation exceeds the capacity of the cell to degrade damaged proteins via autophagy and the ubiquitin-proteasome system. As aggregates increase, they not only create toxic effects on the host cell but also spread from cell to cell and allow disease transmission in a prion-like way.

15.2.2 Oxidative Stress and Mitochondrial Dysfunction

Oxidative stress is the cellular condition where the formation of ROS outweighs the cell's antioxidant defense. ROS such as superoxide anion and hydrogen peroxide, and hydroxyl radicals are reactive molecules with the potential to harm proteins, lipids, and nucleic acids. In the central nervous system (CNS), neurons are especially susceptible to oxidative injury because they have a high metabolic rate, high levels of polyunsaturated fatty acids in membranes, and fairly low levels of antioxidants.

Mitochondria, the major energy-producing organelles of cells, are both a source and a target of ROS. In healthy physiological conditions, mitochondria produce ROS as a byproduct of oxidative phosphorylation. But in neurodegenerative disease states, abnormal mitochondria leak excessive ROS, which feeds into a feed-forward loop of oxidative damage and mitochondrial dysfunction.

In AD, mitochondrial dysfunction is an early occurrence prior to clinical symptoms. Research has indicated reduced activity of mitochondrial complex IV (cytochrome c oxidase) in the AD brain. Aβ and hyperphosphorylated tau directly interact with mitochondrial proteins and disrupt adenosine triphosphate (ATP) production, as well as enhance ROS production. The consequent energy deficiency and oxidative load underlie synaptic dysfunction and neuronal loss [10]. Mitochondrial complex I activity is extremely low in the substantia nigra of Parkinson's disease. Mutations in PINK1, Parkin, and DJ-1 genes each implicated in mitochondrial quality control. It highlights the crucial importance of mitochondrial impairment in the etiology of PD. Mitochondrial membrane perturbation impairs calcium buffering and axonal transport. It triggers apoptotic cascades, particularly in dopaminergic neurons. HD involves impaired mitochondrial transport and reduced gene expression in mitochondrial respiration. Mutant huntingtin has been found to interact with mitochondrial membranes, disrupting their functionality and causing depolarization. In ALS, SOD1 mutations enhance oxidative damage by interfering with mitochondrial membranes and inhibiting electron transport chain function. The ultimate consequence of mitochondrial failure and oxidative stress is the activation of cell death pathways, such as apoptosis and necroptosis. Mitochondrial outer membrane permeabilization releases cytochrome c into the cytoplasm, which activates caspases and neuronal apoptosis. The total oxidative load also impacts glial cells, which fail to maintain neuronal viability and repair.

15.2.3 Neuroinflammation

Neuroinflammation is now identified as one of the major etiologic determinants in neurodegenerative disease pathophysiology. Whereas inflammatory responses within the CNS serve as a protective process to eliminate pathogens and cellular debris, chronic or inappropriate inflammation will enhance neuronal damage. Microglia, the immune cells resident within the CNS, play an important role in initiating and regulating neuroinflammatory responses. Microglia exist in a state of vigilance under resting conditions, monitoring the environment within the brain at all times. Upon recognition of damage-associated molecular patterns (DAMPs) such as misfolded proteins or cellular debris, they activate and secrete a variety of pro-inflammatory cytokines, for example, interleukin-1β (IL-1β), tumor necrosis factor-alpha (TNF-α), and interleukin-6 (IL-6). In AD, Aβ plaques are strong activators of microglia. Although transient activation can be helpful for Aβ clearance, chronic microglial activation induces chronic inflammation and bystander toxicity to normal neurons. The NLRP3 inflammasome, a cytosolic protein complex in microglia, is activated by Aβ and promotes IL-1β release and propagation of the inflammatory response. Likewise, in tauopathies, unlettered tau proteins activate microglia and astrocytes, creating a toxic neuroinflammatory microenvironment. In Parkinson's disease, alpha-synuclein-rich Lewy bodies induce both astrocytes and microglia. Alpha-synuclein aggregates act on toll-like receptors (TLRs), TLR2 and TLR4, to trigger an innate immune response. Ongoing activation of microglia in the substantial nigra results in the loss of dopaminergic neurons. It generates a vicious cycle of cell death and inflammation. Astrocytes, the other significant glial cell type, also play a role in neuroinflammation through the release of cytokines, modulation of neurotransmitter concentrations, and disruption of the blood–brain barrier (BBB). Astro cytosis is typical in neurodegenerative disorders. In ALS and HD, astrocytes lose their supportive roles and take on pro-inflammatory roles, which also harm neurons. Moreover, invading peripheral immune cells such as T cells and monocytes have been found within the CNS in numerous neurodegenerative diseases. They traverse a damaged BBB and modify the inflammatory environment through cytokine secretion and antigen presentation [11]. Neuroinflammation is both an etiology and a result of neurodegeneration. Pro-inflammatory cytokines can paralyze synaptic function, suppress neurogenesis, and induce excitotoxicity through dysregulation of glutamate. It suppresses neurotrophic factors such as brain-derived neurotrophic factor (BDNF), with the potential to limit the brain's potential to recover and adapt. Some of the signaling pathways participating in the process of neuroinflammation include NF-κB, JAK/STAT, and MAPK pathways. These pathways regulate inflammatory gene expression and cross-talk between glial cells and neurons. These pathways can be manipulated in the clinic to potentially decrease neuroinflammation and arrest the course of the disease. Markedly, there is a complex relationship of inflammation with other pathological mechanisms. For example, inflammatory signaling can be increased by oxidative stress, and microglial activation can be maintained by protein aggregation. The study of these interaction types is relevant to the design of multi-target therapeutic approaches. Interconnected mechanisms that include protein misfolding, oxidative stress, mitochondrial dysfunction, and chronic neuroinflammation form the pathophysiology of neurodegenerative diseases. This type of mechanism forms a self-blame cycle that leads to progressive loss of neurons and functional impairment. All the diseases have shared molecular profiles despite having peculiar pathological characteristics, leading to the hope of standard diagnostic and therapeutic measures. The increased awareness of such mechanisms not only enables early diagnosis but also preconditions the development of new interventions that can help to prevent or even reverse the neurodegenerative process.

15.3 DIAGNOSIS STRATEGIES OF NEURODEGENERATIVE DISEASES

One of the most outstanding challenges in neurology with regard to neurodegenerative disease is speed and accuracy of diagnosis. Neurodegenerative disease have overlapping clinical manifestations, particularly during the initial stages, and therefore it is difficult to be diagnosed differently. Traditional symptom-based methods are increasingly being complemented with newer methods such as neuroimaging, laboratory tests of biomarkers, and genetic analysis. These methods complement each other to give a more objective representation of disease processes, allow for earlier diagnosis, and allow for more accurate therapeutic development. The most frequent diagnostics tools are described in the next section as including magnetic resonance imaging (MRI), positron emission tomography (PET), cerebrospinal fluid (CSF) and blood-based biomarkers, and genetic profiling.

15.3.1 Neuroimaging

Neuroimaging has revolutionized the clinical care of neurodegenerative diseases, enabling noninvasive visualization of brain structure and function. Of imaging techniques in use, MRI and PET are most commonly used.

15.3.1.1 Magnetic Resonance Imaging

MRI provides high-resolution imaging of the brain and is a significant structural abnormality detection tool. Medial temporal lobe atrophy, particularly in the entorhinal cortex and hippocampus, both structures linked to memory and learning, is commonly seen by MRI in AD. Longitudinal MRI studies facilitate the monitoring of disease over time through atrophy progression. In Parkinson's disease, while the classical MRI abnormalities are maintained early on, specialized MRI imaging such as diffusion tensor imaging (DTI) can detect microstructural alterations of the substantia nigra and connected white matter tracts. In some other disorders, such as multiple system atrophy (MSA) and progressive supranuclear palsy (PSP), MRI can detect more classic findings, such as the "hot cross bun" sign or midbrain atrophy. MRI also eliminates other reasons for cognitive decline, such as tumors, vascular lesions, or hydrocephalus. Accessibility, noninvasive properties and soft tissue differentiation are some of the features making MRI a key component of neurological diagnosis [12].

15.3.1.2 Positron Emission Tomography

PET scan is a powerful tool for the measurement of molecular and functional alterations in the brain. PET can measure glucose metabolism, amyloid-beta deposition, and tau pathology using radiolabeled tracers. FDG-PET is generally used to measure cerebral glucose metabolism. In AD, the posterior cingulate cortex, precuneus, and parietotemporal cortex will be hypometabolic.

- Amyloid PET imaging agents such as [^11C]PiB or [^18F] can be used for visualizing amyloid-beta plaques, typically before the onset of clinical symptoms. Similarly, tau PET imaging agents are being investigated to visualize neurofibrillary tangles.
- PET with [^18F] DOPA or DAT-SPECT can classify in Parkinsonian disorders, the integrity of dopaminergic neurons and distinguish idiopathic Parkinson's disease from atypical Parkinsonian syndromes.

Whereas PET is more expensive and less available than MRI, its potential for revealing molecular disease at the preclinical level renders it extremely desirable in both research and clinical settings.

15.3.2 Biomarkers

The quest for solid biomarkers has accelerated, with clinicians and researchers working toward early diagnosis and improved disease monitoring. Biomarkers offer quantifiable markers of biological function and can be sampled from cerebrospinal fluid or blood.

15.3.2.1 Cerebrospinal Fluid (CSF) Biomarkers

CSF analysis gives a direct glimpse into the biochemical milieu of the brain. In AD, three main CSF biomarkers are well validated:

15.3.2.2 Amyloid-Beta 42 (Aβ42)

Decreased levels in CSF would reflect sequestration of the peptide into brain plaques.

Total tau (t-tau):

Elevated levels would reflect axonal degeneration.

15.3.2.3 Phosphorylated tau (p-tau)

Elevated levels are an indicator of neurofibrillary tangle formation. The biomarker profile of low Aβ42 and high t-tau/p-tau in CSF is a pattern highly suggestive of AD pathology. These markers are now included in research criteria for diagnosis and are being used in clinical trials to choose suitable participants. CSF alpha-synuclein has been proposed as a potential biomarker in Parkinson's disease and other synucleinopathies, but with inconsistent results. Low levels of total alpha-synuclein may indicate sequestration within the brain tissue, while elevations in oligomeric species indicate active disease processes. Other CSF biomarkers under investigation include neurofilament light chain (NfL), which is elevated in neurodegenerative conditions. It is labeling axonal damage, glial fibrillary acidic protein (GFAP), and astroglia activation.

15.3.2.4 Blood-Based Biomarkers

Blood-based biomarkers offer a less invasive and more accessible alternative to CSF sampling. Advances in ultrasensitive detection technology, such as single-molecule arrays (Simoa), have enabled the quantitation of CNS-released proteins in peripheral blood. The plasma ratio of Aβ42/Aβ40, phosphorylated tau (p-tau181, p-tau217), and neurofilament light chain are the most promising blood biomarkers for AD. Their levels correlate very well with those in CSF and with imaging findings and are therefore suitable for large-scale screening and for longitudinal follow-up. In ALS and frontotemporal dementia (FTD), elevated plasma NfL has been reported to possess favorable prognostic and diagnostic utility. Blood inflammatory cytokines, metabolomic, and proteomic fingerprints are also under investigation as components of multi-marker panels for increasing diagnostic specificity. Although blood biomarkers have yet to become routine in the clinic, they are accelerating toward development because scalable and inexpensive diagnostic tools are needed [13].

15.3.3 Genetic Screening

Genetic factors are responsible for the majority of neurodegenerative diseases, particularly familial and early-onset disorders. Genetic testing is an essential component of the diagnostic evaluation in these situations. It can be of significant utility in flexible information on risk, disease progression, and potential therapeutic management.

15.3.3.1 Monogenic Neurodegenerative Disorders

Several neurodegenerative diseases are linked to single-gene mutations.

15.3.3.2 Alzheimer's Disease

Familial early-onset AD is caused by mutations in APP, PSEN1, and PSEN2. These mutations affect APP processing to enhance the production and fibrillogenesis of Aβ42.

15.3.3.3 Parkinson's Disease

Familial Parkinson's disease is caused by SNCA, LRRK2, PARK2, PINK1, and DJ-1 mutations. These genes affect mitochondrial function, protein degradation, and synaptic transmission.

15.3.3.4 Huntington's Disease

HD is due to an enlarged CAG repeat within the HTT gene, with consequent accumulation of mutant huntingtin protein and neuronal injury.

15.3.3.5 Amyotrophic Lateral Sclerosis

Inheritable ALS is due to mutations in SOD1, TARDBP, FUS, and C9ORF72. Expansion of the hexanucleotide repeat in C9ORF72 is also a major cause of frontotemporal dementia. Screening may confirm diagnosis, assess risk of developing disease onset, and guide family planning in individuals with a family history of neurodegenerative disease. Screening is only acceptable if it is followed by genetic counseling due to its psychological, ethical, and social complexity.

15.3.3.6 Polygenic Risk and Genome-Wide Association Studies (GWAS)

With the irregularity of monogenic disease, the majority of neurodegenerative disorders usually result from multifactorial functions between a large number of genes and the environment. The greatest genetic risk factor for sporadic AD is the APOE ε4 allele. Genome-wide association scans have identified numerous other loci that have been associated with AD, PD, and ALS, each with small effect sizes individually. Polygenic risk scores (PRS) sum the effect of many genetic variants to estimate a person's genetic disease risk. While not yet used extensively in the clinic, PRS could potentially identify at-risk individuals and tailor preventive interventions. Early and precise diagnosis is important for the treatment and management of neurodegenerative disease, treatment choice, and maximization of patient outcomes. Neuroimaging techniques such as MRI and PET provide informative structural and functional information, while CSF and blood biomarkers offer biochemical evidence of pathologic disease. Genetic screening is also augmenting diagnostic accuracy, particularly in the context of familial disease, and furthering personalized medicine approaches [10]. Greater integration of these study tools, along with emerging technologies, will be the basis for earlier diagnosis and more effective intervention in neurodegenerative illness.

15.4 THERAPEUTIC INTERVENTIONS FOR NEURODEGENERATIVE DISORDERS

Neurodegenerative disorders such as AD, PD, and ALS remain incurable, and therapeutic interventions are aimed only at relieving symptoms and slowing down disease advancement. Nevertheless, research has paved the way for novel approaches to modifying disease mechanisms at the molecular

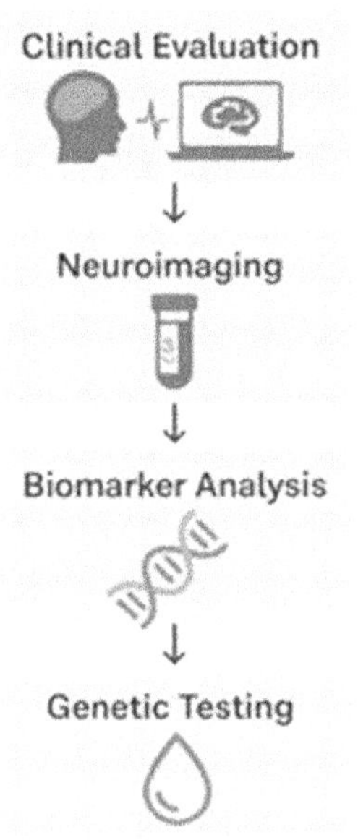

FIGURE 15.3 Diagnostic workflow for neurodegenerative diseases incorporating clinical signs, imaging, biomarkers, and genetic screening

level. Existing therapies can be broadly categorized into pharmacological therapies, regenerative therapies such as stem cell transplantation, and immunological therapies. These three broad modalities of therapy are elaborated in this section in detail, with a focus on their potentials and limitations [14].

15.4.1 Pharmacological Treatments

Pharmacologic therapies have been the norm go-to approach in managing neurodegenerative disorders. They are aimed at primary imbalances in neurotransmitters, modulate symptoms, and are designed to optimize the quality of life of patients. Even though they do not cure the underlying disease itself, their symptomatic impact is often dramatic.

15.4.1.1 Alzheimer's Disease

In AD, degeneration of cholinergic neurons in the basal forebrain leads to a substantial loss in content of acetylcholine and is responsible for cognitive failure. Therefore, cholinesterase inhibitors are indicated as routine therapy. These medications, for example, donepezil, rivastigmine, and galantamine, are inhibitors of the enzyme acetylcholinesterase, thereby increasing the concentration of acetylcholine at synaptic junctions. They provide moderate cognitive improvement and improvement in activities of daily living, particularly in mild and moderate stages of AD. It has been proven in clinical trials. There is another group of drugs that includes N-methyl-D-aspartate (NMDA) receptor antagonists, for example, memantine. It alters glutamatergic function and prevents excitotoxicity. Memantine is usually used in the moderate to severe AD and may be given in combination with cholinesterase inhibitors for added effects. Although universally utilized, these medications do not arrest disease progression. Therefore, the search for disease-modifying agents continues, including anti-amyloid therapies. Aducanumab, a monoclonal antibody against aggregated amyloid-beta, was granted conditional approval, although its efficacy remains controversial and is the focus of ongoing evaluation [15].

15.4.1.2 Parkinson's Disease

The motor manifestations of Parkinson's disease are mainly the result of loss of dopaminergic cells of the substantia nigra. Levodopa (L-DOPA), a dopamine precursor that can cross the blood-brain barrier and be converted into dopamine in the brain, is the cornerstone of treatment. It is often administered with carbidopa, which inhibits peripheral breakdown of levodopa, leaving levodopa available to the brain in higher concentrations. While L-DOPA provides robust control of symptoms, long-term administration is complicated by dyskinesias and motor fluctuations. Other pharmacologic options include dopamine agonists (e.g., pramipexole, ropinirole), MAO-B inhibitors (e.g., selegiline, rasagiline), and Catechol-O-Methyltransferase (COMT) inhibitors (e.g., entacapone), which either mimic the effect of dopamine or prolong its half-life. Adjunctive treatments can be used to alleviate nonmotor symptoms such as depression, sleep disturbances, and autonomic dysfunction, which have a profound effect on patient quality of life.

15.4.1.3 ALS and Other Disorders

Treatment for ALS is limited. Riluzole, which affects glutamate transmission, prolongs life modestly by a few months. Edaravone, a free radical scavenger, is licensed in certain areas and potentially delays disease progression in some patients. Symptomatic care, spasticity control, respiratory assistance, and nutritional support continue to play an important role in sustaining function and comfort.

15.4.2 Stem Cell Therapy

Stem cell therapies hold hopeful potential for neurodegenerative diseases, where lost neurons are replaced, damaged neural circuits are restored, and the inflammatory milieu is modulated. There have been studies on different stem cell types such as embryonic stem cells (ESCs), induced pluripotent stem cells (iPSCs), and mesenchymal stem cells (MSCs).

15.4.2.1 Mechanism of Action

Stem cells may be able to differentiate into neuronal subtypes, migrate into existing neural circuits, and recover synaptic function. They may also secrete neurotrophic factors, influence immune responses, and enhance the CNS microenvironment.

15.4.2.2 Clinical Applications

Among neurodegenerative disorders, stem cell therapy has been most clinically promising for Parkinson's disease. Transplantation of dopaminergic neurons from fetal mesencephalon tissue or iPSCs has partially restored motor function in preclinical models and initial human trials. It is now striving to develop standardized, safe, and scalable stem cell lines for wider clinical application. In AD, stem cells have been shown to decrease neuroinflammation and aid neurogenesis. While human trials are preliminary, animal models have shown cognitive function and synaptic stability improvements after stem cell treatment.

ALS research has investigated intraspinal or intrathecal injections of MSCs or neural stem cells. Some preliminary-phase clinical trials show improved respiratory function and motor scores. Larger trials are required to establish efficacy and safety [16].

15.4.2.3 Challenges and Ethical Concerns

Although stem cell therapy has vast promise, there are a number of challenges that it still faces. Immune rejection, tumorigenicity, and aberrant differentiation are the key safety issues. Ethical concerns about the employment of ESCs also exist. Furthermore, targeted delivery and functional integration of transplanted cells into the pathologic brain are technically sophisticated and yet to be fully optimized.

15.4.3 Immunotherapy

Immunotherapy represents an innovative strategy targeting disease. It targets proteins in neurodegeneration such as amyloid-beta, tau, and alpha-synuclein. Immunotherapy involves active (vaccine-induced) and passive (monoclonal antibody) approaches to modulate immune responses or directly clear toxic aggregates.

15.4.3.1 Amyloid-Targeting Therapies

In AD, several immunotherapies have aimed at amyloid-beta. The most widely recognized, conditionally FDA-approved monoclonal antibody against aggregated Aβ is aducanumab. Several agents, including lecanemab and donanemab, have induced variable levels of amyloid plaque decrease and cognitive stabilization in trials. Although promising, these treatments are unstable, most significantly amyloid-related imaging abnormalities (ARIA), which include brain edema and microhemorrhage. Further, clinical benefit is modest, and administration necessitates judicious selection of patients and surveillance.

15.4.3.2 Tau-Targeting Therapies

Tau protein-directed immunotherapies are also in the pipeline. Such therapies intend to forestall tau hyperphosphorylation and aggregation, leading to neurofibrillary tangle formation and neuronal damage in AD and other tauopathies. Both active immunization and passive antibody therapy (e.g., semorinemab, gosuranemab) have come to the clinic. Initial findings indicate that alpha-synuclein and tau immunotherapies are tolerable and even safe, but whether they can change clinical outcomes is yet to be proven.

15.4.3.3 Alpha-Synuclein Immunotherapy

Immunotherapy against alpha-synuclein in Parkinson's disease aims to inhibit aggregation and cell-to-cell transmission of Lewy bodies. Antibodies such as prasinezumab have been advanced into early-phase clinical trials with variable efficacy but tolerable safety profiles. In addition, combination therapies are also being developed that target several pathogenic proteins at once or augment immune clearance processes via microglial activation or T-cell modulation. The strategy of treatment for neurodegenerative disease is changing rapidly. Conventional pharmacologic management remains necessary to control symptoms, especially in early disease. It is not enough, however, to modify the fundamental disease process. Stem cell therapy and immunotherapy are exciting developments that will make defective tissue whole again and make toxic proteins ineffective, respectively (Wadan et al., 2025). Although these new technologies now exist at different levels of exploration and development, their application in the clinic holds the potential to transform the therapy of these loathsome diseases. Ongoing investment in translational science, biomarker-enhanced trials, and personalized medicine will be pivotal to the realization of these therapies.

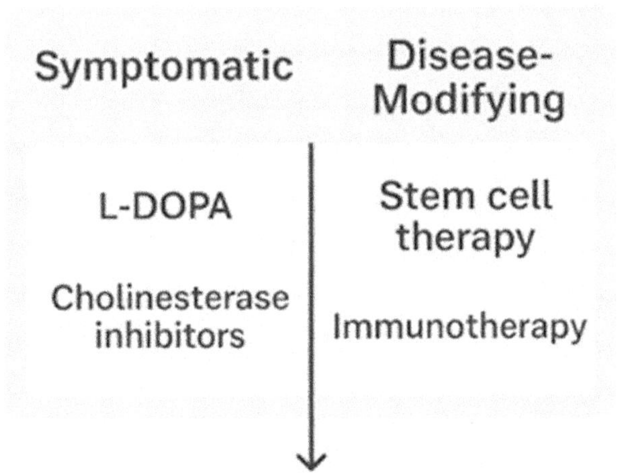

FIGURE 15.4 Overview of current treatment options across neurodegenerative diseases, highlighting symptomatic versus disease-modifying therapies

15.5 NEW NEURODEGENERATIVE RESEARCH TECHNOLOGIES

Increasing neurodegenerative disease burden worldwide has spurred biomedical research, and new emerging technologies that can redefine diagnosis, monitoring, and treatment have emerged as efforts are made to transform them. Conventional clinical practices are susceptible to identifying these diseases after the event of permanent loss of neurons. These advances notwithstanding, new technologies such as AI, wearable neurotechnology, biosensors, and gene-editing tools such as CRISPR promise earlier disease detection, targeted treatment, and modification of the disease. The following section highlights the key new technologies revolutionizing the field of neurodegenerative disorders [17].

15.5.1 AI and Machine Learning Contribution to Early Detection

Machine learning (ML) and AI are revolutionizing the early detection and diagnosis of neurodegenerative diseases by facilitating fast and precise analysis of big and complex data. The technologies make use of large-scale data such as genomic data, neuroimaging, clinical data, and biosignal data. It is used to identify subtle patterns that cannot be detected by the human eye.

15.5.1.1 Neuroimaging Analysis

One of the most significant advances in AI has been in the computer-aided interpretation of MRI and PET scans. Deep learning algorithms, in the guise of convolutional neural networks (CNNs), are trained to detect early biomarkers of AD by detecting brain volume changes, hippocampal atrophy, and amyloid deposition. These models can grade patients routinely as pre-symptomatic, mild cognitive impairment (MCI), or Alzheimer's dementia with high accuracy.

In Parkinson's disease, ML calculations on functional MRI or DaTscan scans distinguish Parkinson's disease from other movement diseases. AI platforms also monitor disease progression through continuous learning from longitudinal imaging datasets.

15.5.1.2 Predictive Modeling

AI-driven software is also being utilized to create predictive models from demographic, cognitive, genetic, and biochemical information. The models are able to predict the probability of developing Alzheimer's from MCI or forecast the rate of disease progression among ALS patients. For

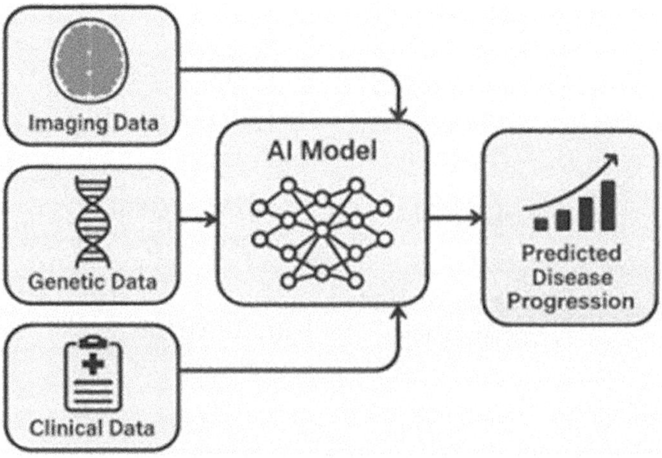

FIGURE 15.5 Framework of an AI model integrating imaging, genetic, and clinical data to predict disease progression

example, SVM and random forest models have been applied to predict cognitive impairment years before clinical symptoms appear.

15.5.1.3 Natural Language Processing

Natural language processing (NLP) models are being more and more deployed to scan speech patterns, text, and electronic health records for micron-scale changes in language and behavior. NLP models are capable of identifying early warning signs of neurodegeneration such as speech hesitation, grammatical mistakes, or diminished lexical range, which are digital biomarkers.

15.5.1.4 AI in Drug Discovery

Aside from diagnostics, AI is more and more used in drug discovery. Algorithms identify novel drug targets, new indications for known compounds, and optimize clinical trials. Virtual screens can predict drug–target interactions and screen vast chemical libraries to identify the best leads, saving development time and expense.

15.5.2 Wearable Neurotechnology and Biosensors

Wearable neurotechnology and biosensor advancements are enabling continuous, real-time monitoring of physiological and neurological parameters in out-of-clinic environments. These sensors offer personalized information on disease progression and allow interventions to be performed earlier.

15.5.2.1 Wearable Devices

Smartwatches and fitness trackers' accelerometers, gyroscopes, and heart rate monitors are being repurposed for neurological monitoring. In Parkinson's disease, wearable monitors can monitor tremor, gait impairment, and bradykinesia. They provide objective measures on which to base clinical judgments regarding motor fluctuations and medication schedule modifications. Sleep habits, circadian rhythm variation, and activity levels can be detected by wearables and also biomarkers of concern in neurodegenerative disease. Wearables can provide continuous monitoring to develop patient-specific profiles of disease and facilitate remote monitoring, which is particularly beneficial in geriatric or rural populations with poor access to healthcare [18].

15.5.2.2 Biosensors for Molecular Detection

Mini biosensors are able to identify neurodegenerative disease biomarkers in body fluids such as sweat, saliva, tears, and interstitial fluid. The biosensors use nanomaterials, electrochemical, and optical detection principles to quantify proteins such as tau, alpha-synuclein, and neurofilament light chain.

15.5.2.3 Promising Platforms for Biosensors

Some of the promising platforms for biosensors are as follows:

- Graphene-based sensors for ultrasensitive amyloid-beta detection
- Microfluidic lab-on-a-chip devices for real-time analysis of blood or CSF samples
- Wearable headbands for electroencephalography (EEG) with the ability to monitor brainwave abnormalities for cognitive impairment

Biosensors can be incorporated into wearable devices to build closed-loop systems, where abnormal levels of biomarkers can trigger medication adjustments or alerts. Such smart systems allow for proactive disease control.

15.5.2.4 Advantages and Challenges

The use of wearable neurotech offers several advantages: noninvasiveness, portability, simplicity of usage, and continuous data collection. Issues still exist in standardizing data interpretation, ensuring long-term device accuracy, and addressing privacy concerns for individual health information.

15.5.3 CRISPR and Gene-Editing Potential

CRISPR-Cas9, one of the most revolutionary biotechnologies in modern biomedical science, is a gene-editing technology with the promise to edit DNA in precise manners. Its promise in neurodegenerative disease is to correct disease-causing mutations, control gene expression, and allow for in vivo disease modeling.

15.5.3.1 Gene Correction

In monogenic neurodegenerative diseases such as HD, due to an expanded CAG repeat in the HTT gene, CRISPR has the potential to remove or repair the mutant region directly. Preclinical models have shown the effectiveness of CRISPR in inhibiting expression of mutant huntingtin and improving motor performance in animal models.

Similarly, for inherited ALS or AD, CRISPR can be used to correct genes such as APP, PSEN1, or SOD1 mutations. Gene editing at an early age in life can potentially prevent the disease from occurring or at least keep it in remission until very old age.

Besides correcting mutations, CRISPRi and CRISPRa protocols may enhance or suppress inflammation or neuroprotection gene expression. Enhancing neurotrophic factors such as BDNF or suppressing pro-inflammatory cytokines, for instance, can produce a more protective neural microenvironment for disease resistance [19].

15.5.3.2 In Vivo Delivery Systems

One of the most daunting challenges with CRISPR therapy is delivering the gene-editing equipment to brain tissue safely and effectively. Viral vectors such as adeno-associated viruses (AAVs) are the go-to choice, but limited cargo capacity and susceptibility to immunogenicity are drawbacks. The development of non-viral delivery systems, such as lipid nanoparticles and exosomes, is being studied as potentially safer alternatives.

15.5.3.3 Ethical and Regulatory Considerations

Human use of CRISPR, especially in the CNS, will pose challenging ethical as well as safety issues. There will be a need to thoroughly consider off-target effects, mosaicism, and other harmful effects on the genome. These will need intense regulation and long follow-up trial before

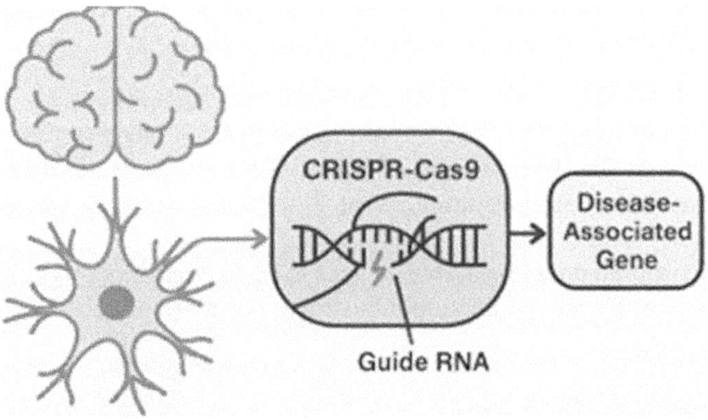

FIGURE 15.6 Illustration of CRISPR-Cas9-mediated gene-editing targeting pathogenic mutations in neuronal cells

widespread clinical use. Neurodegenerative disorders diagnosis, monitoring and treatment will be transformed by these new technologies. AI and ML offer effective solutions for pre-diagnosis and custom-designed treatment plans, and wearable devices and biosensors can enable surgical checks in real time without any invasive procedures. The CRISPR technology of gene-editing promises to provide more accurate methodologies in medicine, which, in the end, will be able to correct the underlying genetic pathology of these diseases. As promising as all of this is, safety, ethics, and scalability issues still remain, but where these technologies intersect lies unmatched promise for the neurodegenerative disease treatment of the future [20].

15.6 CASE STUDIES AND CLINICAL TRIALS OF NEURODEGENERATIVE DISEASE RESEARCH

There is a very long and difficult path from laboratory discovery to bedside use in the treatment of neurodegenerative diseases. Case studies and clinical trials are the much-needed bridge between basic science and clinical practice. Over the past decades, numerous clinical trials have been conducted to evaluate pharmacological drugs, biologics, cellular therapy, and gene-editing strategies for conditions such as AD, Parkinson's disease, HD, and ALS. While a few trials have produced hopeful outcomes, the majority have faced challenges due to complications in efficacy, safety, or study design. This section presents leading case studies, summarizes milestone clinical trials, and outlines the way forward for translational medicine in neurodegenerative disorders [21].

15.6.1 Case Studies: Successes and Failures Turned Fiasco

15.6.1.1 Alzheimer's Disease: Anti-Amyloid Therapies

By far the most intensively watched case in neurodegenerative disease research is the development of anti-amyloid drugs for AD. The 2021 US FDA approval of aducanumab (Aduhelm) was a milestone as the first disease-modifying treatment targeting amyloid-beta plaques. Aducanumab, an antibody, defines clearance of plaques in Phase III trials but remained controversial for its clinical efficacy. The EMERGE trial indicated a modest slowing of cognitive progression but this was not replicated by the ENGAGE trial. ARIA, including swelling of the brain and microbleeds, raised safety concerns as well as questions about patient suitability. Following aducanumab, later antibodies such as lecanemab and donanemab have shown more consistent clinical benefits. The lecanemab trial of CLARITY-AD showed 27% less cognitive decline at 18 months in patients with early AD. These trials underscore the importance of intervention at the earliest possible stage, preferably before significant neurodegeneration, and highlight the requirement for accurate biomarker-guided patient selection [22].

15.6.1.2 Parkinson's Disease: Cell Therapy and Deep Brain Stimulation

In PD, one of the most effective clinical therapies is deep brain stimulation (DBS). First approved in the late 1990s, DBS involves the implantation of electrodes within the subthalamic nucleus or globus pallidus internus to regulate hyperkinetic motor loops. Dozens of case reports have provided dramatic relief of tremor, rigidity, and motor fluctuations in treatment-refractory PD patients. Although DBS does not halt disease progression, it brings substantial relief from symptoms and is currently an accepted treatment in specialist centers. There have also been efforts to re-establish dopaminergic function through stem cell transplantation. In a landmark study in 2018, dopaminergic progenitor cells derived from human ESCs were transplanted in PD patients. There were indications of safety and improved motor function. Although larger controlled trials are still ongoing. This case shows the potential of regenerative medicine for neurodegenerative therapy but also the challenges of cell survival, integration, and long-term efficacy [23].

15.6.1.3 ALS: Modest Gains and Unmet Needs

ALS remains one of the most destructive neurodegenerative diseases, for which little is available except for riluzole, and approved in 1995, which prolongs life by a few months. Edaravone, introduced more recently, has shown a modest benefit in halting functional deterioration, particularly among early-stage patients, but results have been inconsistent across different groups.

One such fascinating research area is antisense oligonucleotides (ASOs) targeting certain genetic mutations. Tofersen, an ASO that aims to reduce the SOD1 gene in familial ALS, showed reduced concentrations of neurofilament (a biomarker of neuronal damage) and less clinical decline in a group of patients. Clinical benefit was modest, though, illustrating the complexity of translating molecular success into functional significance.

15.6.2 Challenges and Learnings in Clinical Trials

Although a lot of money has been spent on clinical trials, few have shown definitive clinical effectiveness. Some of the major issues have been the following:

15.6.2.1 Late Intervention

Most trials enroll patients when neurodegeneration is well underway. It is almost impossible to reverse damage by that time. There is increasing recognition that interventions need to be initiated in prodromal or preclinical phases, using biomarkers.

15.6.2.2 Heterogeneity of Disease

Neurodegenerative disorders tend to manifest with dissimilar clinical phenotypes and rates of progression. Unless patients are stratified on the basis of genetic, biomarker, or disease subtype, trial results can be diluted.

15.6.2.3 Endpoints and Measures

Cognition and motor function tests tend to be subjective and change infrequently. Trials now increasingly use digital biomarkers, CSF and blood biomarkers, and imaging-based outcomes for more sensitive and earlier measurement of treatment effects.

15.6.2.4 Placebo Effect

In Parkinson's and Alzheimer's studies, the placebo response is likely to be high. This means that it becomes challenging to detect slight treatment effects unless big cohorts and longer durations are utilized.

These challenges have led to a move toward adaptive trial designs, basket trials, and platform studies, which are more flexible, include multiple treatments, and focus on specific populations.

15.6.3 Directions for the Future in Translational Medicine

The future of treating neurodegenerative diseases lies in the collaboration of personalized medicine, biomarker-based therapies, and technological advancements. Some of the trends that are defining the next generation of clinical research include:

15.6.3.1 Biomarker-Driven Trials

Increasingly, biomarker use—whether amyloid PET scans, CSF tau levels, or blood-based neurofilament light chain— is necessary for the selection of patients, staging of disease, and therapeutic response monitoring. Trials with biomarkers provide more homogenous groups of participants and better assessment of drug efficacy. To give an example, the DIAN-TU trial focuses on individuals with autosomal dominant forms of AD mutations to enable interventions to be performed several years before symptom onset. Similarly, the PPMI (Parkinson's Progression Markers Initiative) is building a comprehensive database of biomarkers to identify vulnerable patient groups and group study participants.

15.6.3.2 Gene Therapy and ASO Trials

Gene therapy, especially in monogenic diseases such as HD and familial ALS, is progressing rapidly. Clinical trials with the use of CRISPR, viral vectors, and ASOs are ongoing to inhibit toxic genes and restore normal protein function. Zolgensma's success in spinal muscular atrophy provides a proof of concept for gene therapy in neurology.

15.6.3.3 Digital Health and Remote Monitoring

Digital media are facilitating remote measurements using smartphones, wearables, and telemedicine. They gather continuous, real-life information about movement, speech, sleep, and cognitive function, enabling more sensitive monitoring of disease activity and treatment response. Trials with digital endpoints are increasingly used and could lower the costs of trials and burden on participants.

15.6.3.4 Combination Therapies

Due to the complexity of neurodegenerative diseases with multiple factors involved, combination therapies acting on multiple pathological pathways (e.g., inflammation, oxidative stress, protein aggregation) are increasingly popular. This is follows oncology approaches, in which multi-drug treatment has become typical. A trial of lecanemab (anti-amyloid) in combination with tau immunotherapy. It provides synergistic effects in AD. Similarly, combinations of dopaminergic agents, anti-inflammatories, and neuroprotective agents increase therapeutic outcomes in Parkinson's disease and ALS [24]. Clinical trials and case series in neurodegenerative diseases have unearthed both formidable challenges and revolutionary promise. The majority of the therapies have failed to trigger robust clinical responses. This acquired experience has led to smarter, more strategic, and biomarker-based trial designs. Future success will also rely on early treatment, individualized treatment regimes, the use of digital technologies, and a multidisciplinary approach. As more research is invested and technology advances, the field is making it closer to the highly sought-after goal of disease-modifying therapy of neurodegenerative diseases.

15.7 ETHICAL, LEGAL, AND SOCIAL IMPLICATIONS IN NEURODEGENERATIVE DISEASES RESEARCH

With neuroscience and biotechnology under development, there is a growing imperative to confront the ELSI that this has caused. AI, genetic tests, and digital health technologies have never had as much potential as they do now because of their ability to provide early diagnosis and tailored medicine. However, they also have some serious concerns about privacy, data protection, informed consent, genetic discrimination, and mental health. These are problems of the highest order to ensure the scientific progress is socially responsible and morally acceptable [25].

15.7.1 AI in Diagnosis: Privacy and Autonomy Concerns

Technologies of AI and ML are gaining increased popularity in the diagnosis of neurodegenerative diseases, especially in the interpretation of neuroimaging data, speech, and electronic health records. These technologies will be as beneficial to the efficiency and accuracy of the diagnostic process as they present concerns such as patient privacy, data exploitation, algorithmic bias, and informed consent.

15.7.1.1 Data Privacy and Confidentiality

Applications of AI rely on large volumes of personal health data that are usually gathered together in radiology databases, genetic repositories, and medical databases. In the absence of powerful data privacy processes, the information of patients may be jeopardized through leakage, either via cyber theft or unauthorized system access. The strategies of anonymization and de-identification are significant yet not perfect when data are cross-matched across sources. Adherence to data protection legislation such as the EU's General Data Protection Regulation (GDPR) and the US Health Insurance Portability and Accountability Act (HIPAA) is mandatory but is enforced differently throughout the world.

15.7.1.2 Algorithmic Transparency and Bias

AI is not bias-free. Unless training samples are representative across race, gender, age, and socioeconomic status, diagnostic algorithms can function suboptimally in underrepresented groups. This could result in misdiagnosis or delays in treatment for vulnerable groups, further worsening health inequities.

In addition, the majority of AI systems are "black boxes" that lack transparency on how conclusions are arrived at. There is a lack of algorithmic transparency, compromising the ethics of informed decision-making and collaborative patient-provider comprehension. Clinicians and patients must be able to interpret and challenge AI outputs instead of accepting them as perfect.

15.7.1.3 Informed Consent and Autonomy

The application of AI in clinical practice requires new guidelines for informed consent. Patients need to be advised when AI is used in their diagnostic workup, the nature of the technology, and their right to decline. There are also concerns regarding third-party AI companies used in diagnostic platforms. Patients often do not have a clear understanding of how their data are used, who views it, or whether it is sold or resold.

15.7.2 Ethics of Genetic Counseling and Screening

Genetic screening has been found to be a strategy in the identification of people who are likely to develop neurodegenerative diseases such as AD, Huntington's disease, and even familial ALS. Although genetic data can be used for prevention and early treatment, it also poses some ethical dilemmas related to privacy, psychological effects, discrimination, and reproductive choices.

15.7.2.1 Predictive Testing and Psychological Impact

The predictive quality of the genetic testing process is perhaps the most sensitive aspect. A good example is that a positive result for a mutation in the gene that carries the HD gives a virtual guarantee of occurrence of the disease in the future. Knowing this may cause severe psychological distress, depression, or existential anxiety, especially if there is no curative therapy available.

Counseling is then required before and after testing to make individuals conscious of implications, to interpret results, and to make informed choices. Psychological care must be integrated into the testing process, particularly among young adults, vulnerable family members, or those undergoing testing for reproductive reasons [26].

15.7.2.2 Informed Consent and Genetic Literacy

Genetic testing should be supported by robust informed consent procedures. Patients need to know what can and cannot be tested, and the implications of testing, including false positives, variable expressivity, and the indeterminate significance of some gene variants. The level of genetic literacy in the general population is low, though, and could undermine the quality of consent. Consent would also include secondary findings, such as the revelation of non-paternity, carrier status for unrelated illnesses, or susceptibility to other disease. It is possible for patients to be offered a choice of opting in or out of receiving such information. Consent forms must be clearly framed and culturally sensitive.

15.7.2.3 Privacy, Data Sharing, and Discrimination

Genetic data are very sensitive and is a problem of privacy and abuse. Genetic information can be stored in databases at the national or international level (e.g., biobanks), and this raises susceptibility to breaches. Genetic privacy should be provided by strong encryption, data governance policy, and access controls. It is also feared that there might be genetic discrimination, particularly in insurance and employment. Even though there are laws against this discrimination, including the Genetic Information Non-discrimination Act (GINA) in the United States, this does not apply to every space. The fear of being discriminated against may prevent people from undergoing testing, even to the benefit of their health.

15.7.2.4 Reproductive Ethics

There are implications of genetic predictive testing for reproductive decision-making. Family planning decisions would be made by couples using test data, such as preimplantation genetic diagnosis (PGD) and prenatal diagnosis. These technologies enable the selection of embryos free of genetic mutations, but also raise ethical concerns about eugenics, access inequality, and social pressure.

The clinicians need to address these discussions with sensitivity and impartiality. It offers balanced advice without coercion. Advanced reproductive technology may require ethical oversight committees to direct its application in the case of late-onset neurodegenerative disorders.

15.7.3 Social Justice and Access Issues

The integration of AI, genetic screening, and other advanced diagnostics and therapies for neurodegenerative disease raises health equity issues. Such technologies are likely to be expensive and concentrated in urban or upscale settings and thus perpetuate, rather than reduce, the disparities between privileged and underserved groups.

15.7.3.1 Access Disparities

Poor individuals, rural populations, and patients in developing nations often do not have an opportunity for genetic testing, computer-aided diagnostic testing, or neuroimaging. Language barriers, illiteracy regarding technology, and limitations in the infrastructure of healthcare render disparities even worse. New technology access needs to be equitable in health policy worldwide, for example, in the form of subsidies, mobile units, or public-private partnerships.

15.7.3.2 Cultural Sensitivity and Community Engagement

The world differs in its understanding of genetics, mental illness, and dying. Resistance or suspicion may arise if biomedical interventions are discordant with cultural beliefs. Trust must be established, and it ensures appropriate use of new technologies, and it must include outreach to communities and culturally sensitive counseling. While research into neurodegenerative disease takes cutting-edge technologies, its associated ethical, legal, and social implications (ELSI) cannot be ignored. The underlying concerns related to AI technologies include issues such as data privacy, informed consent, and discrimination, whereas genetic screening itself is associated with psychological effects, discrimination, and freedom of choice. The ability to achieve success is not only a scientific merit but also the trust of people, equal access, and ethical prescience wisdom. Clinicians, ethicists, policymakers, and patient constituencies should hold a multidisciplinary dialogue to ensure that the future of neurodegenerative care is ethical, as it is transformative [27].

15.8 DIRECTIONS IN THE FUTURE OF RESEARCH AND CHALLENGES FACING MANAGEMENT OF NEURODEGENERATIVE DISEASE

The problems of neurodegenerative diseases are, perhaps, the most challenging and complicated issues of modern medicine. In areas where basic science, diagnostics as well as new technologies have seen significant progress, there has been slow progress in translation of these advances into useful clinical interventions, along with significant failures. The current state of affairs is characterized by a lack of curative therapy, unfavorable high rates of clinical trial failure, and an enormous socioeconomic burden on patients, families, and healthcare systems. In this section, the main obstacles to progress are outlined and areas of future research identified, with specific emphasis on the requirement for interdisciplinary methodologies and strong public health policy foundations.

15.8.1 Shortcomings in Current Treatments

The therapeutic strategies for neurodegenerative diseases such as Alzheimer's, Parkinson's, Huntington's, and ALS are rather symptomatic. They might bring limited improvement in the quality of life or retard the progression of the disease temporarily, but they fail to change the underlying pathophysiological mechanisms.

15.8.1.1 Symptomatic and Short-Term Relief

The current medications, like cholinesterase inhibitors used in the treatment of Alzheimer's and levodopa used in the treatment of Parkinson's, are neurotransmitter-modulating drugs. They suppress the symptoms of loss of memory, tremors, or rigidity but do not prevent neurodegeneration. These interventions become less effective with time and may have an increasingly severe side effect. As an example, there are morbid side effects of levodopa in the form of long-term therapy-induced dyskinesias and so-called on–off phenomena.

Clinical benefit: In ALS, the survival of patients on riluzole is improved by just a few months. This emphasizes the need of disease-modifying therapies, which require action during the initial stages of the disease.

15.8.1.2 High Failure Rates in Clinical Trials

A very serious problem in neurodegenerative research is that there is a high mortality rate of clinical tests. Many of the drug leads that were competent in preclinical models have not worked in humans. Reasons include the following:

- Poorly developed animal models that fail to mimic human disease.
- Poor stratification and validation of patient biomarkers.
- Delayed intervention after irreversible neuron loss has already commenced.
- Excessive reliance on single-pathway targets (e.g., amyloid-beta) to the detriment of complex disease processes.

Failure in large Phase III trials has been met with discontent, costing billions of dollars and demoralizing patients and the scientific community. The future of research will be forced to use a multi-target strategy and rationalize trial designs.

15.8.2 Interdisciplinary Research

Neurodegenerative diseases are multidisciplinary in nature, and this implies that collaboration between neurologists, molecular biologists, data scientists, geneticists, pharmacologists, ethicists, and policymakers is necessary. There is no single discipline that has it all, and good solutions come as a consequence of the integration of numerous fields.

15.8.2.1 Convergence of Biomedical and Computational Sciences

With the increased use of big data and AI, computer science and neuroscience have no option but to overlap. The discovery of patterns that scientists could not identify previously based on multimodal data (e.g., imaging, genomics, and clinical information) is becoming achievable through ML models taught on multimodal data. The union of computing capabilities and medical knowledge is the key to the creation of predictive models, computerized biomarkers, and even individualized forms of treatment.

15.8.2.2 Clinician-Scientist Partnerships

The second synergistic domain is that of the working jointly of clinicians and basic scientists. Although laboratory work is the source of new treatment methods, only practitioners are aware of the subtle art of working with patients. This can be bridged by involvement of the research centers for translational research and also consortia so as to have scientific advances that are feasible and clinically relevant.

15.8.2.3 Global and Cross-Institutional Research Networks

Common resources, common protocols, and common data repositories can be seen as an advantage, as exemplified by large and international initiatives such as the Human Brain Project (EU), the BRAIN Initiative (USA), and the Dementias Platform UK. Such efforts help scientists to operate across different countries and develop stronger and more generalizable outcomes. Public-private partnerships between academic institutions, drug firms, and government agencies are also in place, which hastens innovation through the consolidation of resources, knowledge and infrastructure.

15.8.3 Public Health Policy Support

The study of neurodegenerative diseases depends on scientific breakthroughs, and it should be balanced with aggressive policies of the health of people that will help the results to be processed and turned into the equitable and easily available treatment. The most important task of policymakers is to decide on healthcare infrastructure, funding priorities, regulatory policy, and preparedness in society.

15.8.3.1 Investment in Research and Infrastructure

Governments should finance basic and translational neuroscience studies. The accumulation of valuable information on the occurrence of diseases, the natural course, and risk factors is possible through grants for biobanks, longitudinal studies, and national registries. All these investments are carried out in advance to conduct large-scale trials and designs of frames to be used in personalized medicine. The most urgent need is also the upgrading of the diagnostic infrastructure in low- and middle-income countries. The availability of neuroimaging, genetic testing, and biomarker research should be more widespread, considering the intent to make early diagnosis and treatment a reality in every part of the planet.

15.8.3.2 Workforce Training and Capacity Building

Subspecialty training of healthcare personnel is required to handle the mounting pressure of neurodegenerative disorders. The specific professionals in this case, which include neurologists, geriatricians, neuropsychologists, and rehabilitation personnel, must be prepared with up-to-date knowledge and competence. The policy of the government should enable capacity building, especially in rural and disadvantaged areas. Besides this, interdisciplinary curricula should be used in training programs, such as ethics, AI applications, and genomics, to equip future clinicians and researchers for the dynamic healthcare landscape.

15.8.3.3 Equity and Access

New treatments and technologies would also be availed and accessible through public policy. In the absence of government intervention, they may remain unavailable to less wealthy groups due to the expense of gene editing or immunotherapy. The policy of universal health coverage, price controls, and reimbursements is required to prevent increasing healthcare disparities. It is also relevant to involve underprivileged groups in clinical trials so as to make therapies inclusive. The representation of gender, ethnic, and socioeconomic cohorts in clinical trials should be guaranteed in both platforms of ethical and inclusive policies.

15.8.3.4 Awareness, Prevention, and Caregiver Support

Education on cognitive disorders is essential in terms of awareness creation to increase awareness of early detection and destigmatization of mental illnesses. The reduction of social isolation and maximizing the well-being of both patients and families should be addressed, and policies should enable education of the population, community activities toward the establishment of dementia-friendly communities, as well as services to support caregivers. The burden on society can be reduced to a significant degree through better application of non-compensatory caregiving in the shape of incentives such as financial support, caregiver training programs, and respite care. The treatment of neurodegenerative disease is faced with disastrous challenges in the low effectiveness of treatment, high trial failure and meager infrastructure in most parts of the globe. However, when a reassignment in research is made in the direction of early, individualized, and multidimensional intervention, there are encouraging prospects on the horizon. The keys to ensuring that the shift is possible is interdisciplinary collaborations between scientific fields, clinical practice, and technological innovation, as well as effective leadership of the policy on the issue of public health. Through collaboration between research, practice, and policy, the global community can move toward the development of fair and sustainable solutions for the prevention, diagnosis, and treatment of neurodegenerative diseases.

15.9 CONCLUSION

Several neurodegenerative diseases such as AD, Parkinson's disease, HD, and the ALS are some of the most challenging problems in contemporary medicine. Regardless of several decades of the studies, there are still no curative treatment options, and current treatment methods mostly have a symptomatic effect. This chapter has described the pathophysiological processes of neurodegeneration, existing diagnostic and treatment approaches, and the revolution of new technologies. The novelty of this work lies in highlighting how AI-driven multimodal approaches, wearable biosensors, and CRISPR-based gene-editing converge with ethical, legal, and social perspectives (ELSI) to create a comprehensive roadmap to form a holistic roadmap of personalized management of neurodegenerative diseases. These methods allow earlier diagnosis, accurate patient stratification, and focused interventions that go beyond symptom control, unlike conventional methods. The clinical trials highlight the potential and shortcomings of current therapies, and in this regard, early treatments, biomarker-based, and multidimensional approaches to treatment are necessary. Biotechnology, computational science and the policy of the public health converge and this is critical in order to promote the transformation of laboratory discoveries into practical clinical applications. In conclusion, interdisciplinary cooperation, fair access, and responsible innovation will be the foundation of the further development. Having the conglomeration of mechanistic knowledge along with the most recent technologies and moral safeguarding, the field can not only prevent remaining palliative in terms of symptomatic care, but can actually transform the disorder and eliminate it, giving new hope to the patients and families alike, along with healthcare systems in every corner of the globe.

REFERENCES

[1] Das, P., Paul, S., Ghosh, J., PalBhowmik, S., Neogi, B., & Ganguly, A. (2017). An approach towards the representation of sign language by electromyography signals with fuzzy implementation. *International Journal of Sensors, Wireless Communications and Control*, *7*(1), 26–32. https://doi.org/10.2174/2210327907666170222093839

[2] Abdelzaher, H. (2022). *The Gene-Environment Nexus: A Holistic Approach to Neurodegenerative Diseases*, pp. 3–16. https://doi.org/10.1007/978-981-16-9205-5_2

[3] Khan, M., Mahajan, R. A., Sivakumar, N. R., Gulhane, M., Rakesh, N., Dey, R., Uddin, M. S., & Basheer, S. (2025). A unified hybrid model for cardiovascular risk prediction: Merging statistical, kernel-based and neural approaches. *Journal of Cellular and Molecular Medicine*. https://doi.org/10.1111/jcmm.70797

[4] Paul, S., Ojha, S. K., Barui, S., Ghosh, S., Ghosh, M., Neogi, B., & Ganguly, A. (2018). Technical advancement on various bio-signal controlled arm: A review. *Journal of Mechanics of Continua and Mathematical Sciences*, 13(2), 16–30. https://doi.org/10.26782/jmcms.2018.06.00007

[5] Khan, M., Mahajan, R. A., Katukam, R., Dey, R., Rana, A., & William, P. (2025). Smart insights: Multimodal deep learning techniques for accurate disease identification. In: *2025 International Conference on Quantum Photonics, Artificial Intelligence, and Networking (QPAIN)* (pp. 1–5). Rangpur, Bangladesh. https://doi.org/10.1109/QPAIN66474.2025.11171928

[6] Pal, M., Dey, R., Mahajan, R. A., Khan, M., Syed, A. A., & Karimullah, S. (2025). Edge intelligence: Unique machine learning strategies for enhancing real-time IoT data processing. In: *2025 International Conference on Quantum Photonics, Artificial Intelligence, and Networking (QPAIN)* (pp. 1–5). Rangpur, Bangladesh. https://doi.org/10.1109/QPAIN66474.2025.11171994.

[7] Al-Kuraishy, H., Abdulhadi, M., Hussien, N., Al-Niemi, M., Rasheed, H., & Al-Gareeb, A. (2020). Involvement of orexinergic system in psychiatric and neurodegenerative disorders: A scoping review. *Brain Circulation*, *6*(2), 70. https://doi.org/10.4103/BC.BC_42_19;

[8] Mahajan, R. A., Dey, R., Khan, M., Su'ud, M. M., Alam, M. M., & Jadhav, P. (2025). Enhancing personalization in IoT-based health monitoring via generative AI and transfer learning. *Egyptian Informatics Journal*, *32*, 100788. ISSN 1110-8665. https://doi.org/10.1016/j.eij.2025.100788. https://www.sciencedirect.com/science/article/pii/S1110866525001811

[9] Al-Kuraishy, H. M., Jabir, M. S., Albuhadily, A. K., Al-Gareeb, A. I., Jawad, S. F., Swelum, A. A., & Hadi, N. R. (2024). Role of ketogenic diet in neurodegenerative diseases focusing on Alzheimer diseases: The guardian angel. *Ageing Research Reviews*, *95*. https://doi.org/10.1016/J.ARR.2024.102233;

[10] Zaharchuk, G. (2023). Artificial intelligence approaches to the imaging of neurodegenerative diseases. *Molecular Imaging of Neurodegenerative Disorders*, 207–219. https://doi.org/10.1007/978-3-031-35098-6_14

[11] Al-Kuraishy, H. M., Jabir, M. S., Al-Gareeb, A. I., Albuhadily, A. K., Albukhaty, S., Sulaiman, G. M., & Batiha, G. E. S. (2023). Evaluation and targeting of amyloid precursor protein (APP)/amyloid beta (Aβ) axis in amyloidogenic and non-amyloidogenic pathways: A time outside the tunnel. *Ageing Research Reviews*, *92*. https://doi.org/10.1016/J.ARR.2023.102119;

[12] Avramouli, A., & Vlamos, P. (2023). Neurodegenerative disease modeling: An introduction. In: *Handbook of Computational Neurodegeneration* (pp. 3–10). https://doi.org/10.1007/978-3-319-75922-7_68

[13] Wadan, A. H. S., Shaaban, A. H., El-Sadek, M. Z., Mostafa, S. A., Moshref, A. S., El-Hussein, A., Ellakwa, D. E. S., & Mehanny, S. S. (2025). Mitochondrial-based therapies for neurodegenerative diseases: A review of the current literature. *Naunyn-Schmiedeberg's Archives of Pharmacology*, *2025*, 1–30. https://doi.org/10.1007/S00210-025-04014-0

[14] Stepanichev, M. Y. (2019). Prospects for the use of genome-editing technology to correct neurodegenerative diseases. *Advances in Gerontology*, *9*(2), 154–163. https://doi.org/10.1134/S2079057019020218

[15] Rajaraman, S. (2024). Artificial intelligence in neuro degenerative diseases: Opportunities and challenges. *Studies in Computational Intelligence*, *1131*, 133–153. https://doi.org/10.1007/978-3-031-53148-4_8

[16] Singh, D. P., Kaushik, B., Khan, Y. F., Chadha, A., Mahajan, A., Jandwani, A., & Narula, G. S. (2024). Emerging trends of artificial intelligence in detecting neurodegeneration. *Lecture Notes in Networks and Systems*, *991*, 591–601. https://doi.org/10.1007/978-981-97-2550-2_42

[17] Kumar, A. V., Kumar, S., Garg, V. K., Goel, N., Hoang, V. T., & Kashyap, D. (2023). Future perspectives for automated neurodegenerative disorders diagnosis: Challenges and possible research directions. *Cognitive Technologies*, *Part F7*, 255–267. https://doi.org/10.1007/978-981-99-2154-6_15

[18] Priya R, K., Al Shahri, A., & Alias, L. (2024). Integration of artificial intelligence in the diagnosis and prevention of neurodegenerative disease: An update. In: *Handbook of Neurodegenerative Disorders* (pp. 871–882). https://doi.org/10.1007/978-981-99-7557-0_35

[19] Pullman, D., & Etchegary, H. (2021). Ethical, legal, and social issues (ELSI) in clinical genetics research. *Methods in Molecular Biology*, *2249*, 65–82. https://doi.org/10.1007/978-1-0716-1138-8_5

[20] Modi, S. K., Singla, S., Modi, P., & Kaur, G. K. (2025). *Advancements in Neurodegenerative Disease Diagnosis and Prediction: A Machine Learning Approach*, pp. 257–272. https://doi.org/10.1007/978-981-97-7190-5_18

[21] Noor, M. B. T., Zenia, N. Z., Kaiser, M. S., Mahmud, M., & Al Mamun, S. (2019). Detecting neurodegenerative disease from MRI: A brief review on a deep learning perspective. *Lecture Notes in Computer Science (Including Subseries Lecture Notes in Artificial Intelligence and Lecture Notes in Bioinformatics)*, *11976 LNAI*, 115–125. https://doi.org/10.1007/978-3-030-37078-7_12

[22] Ascencio-Carbajal, T., Saruwatari-Zavala, G., Navarro-Garcia, F., & Frixione, E. (2021). Genetic/genomic testing: Defining the parameters for ethical, legal and social implications (ELSI). *BMC Medical Ethics*, *22*(1). https://doi.org/10.1186/S12910-021-00720-5

[23] Medvedev, S. P., Malankhanova, T. B., Valetdinova, K. R., & Zakian, S. M. (2021). Creation and research of cell models of hereditary neurodegenerative diseases using directed genome editing. *Neurochemical Journal, 15*(4), 353–358. https://doi.org/10.1134/S1819712421040073

[24] Myszczynska, M. A., Ojamies, P. N., Lacoste, A. M. B., Neil, D., Saffari, A., Mead, R., Hautbergue, G. M., Holbrook, J. D., & Ferraiuolo, L. (2020). Applications of machine learning to diagnosis and treatment of neurodegenerative diseases. *Nature Reviews Neurology, 16*(8), 440–456. https://doi.org/10.1038/S41582-020-0377-8

[25] Harden, K. P., & Koellinger, P. D. (2020). Using genetics for social science. *Nature Human Behaviour, 4*(6), 567–576. https://doi.org/10.1038/S41562-020-0862-5

[26] Mathew, B., & Parambi, D. G. T. (2020). Principles of neurochemistry: Fundamentals and applications. In: *Principles of Neurochemistry: Fundamentals and Applications* (pp. 1–194). https://doi.org/10.1007/978-981-15-5167-3

[27] Manoharan, S. K., & Kumar, P. S. (2020). Pathophysiology of neurodegenerative diseases: Basics to advanced. In: *Principles of Neurochemistry: Fundamentals and Applications* (pp. 93–98). https://doi.org/10.1007/978-981-15-5167-3_5

16 Multimodal Classification of Meningitis Etiologies From CSF Profiles Using a CNN-BiGRU Hybrid Model Optimized With the Sparrow Search Algorithm

Sathiya Priya S., M. Amanullah, Noorul Julaiha A. G., Gayetri Devi, Devi P. P., and M. Malleswari

16.1 INTRODUCTION

Meningitis is a life-threatening inflammatory condition of the meninges, the protective membranes surrounding the brain and spinal cord. Because of its clinical course, the onset of acute meningitis is recognized internationally as a medical emergency. If diagnosed and treated quickly, the prognosis for many pediatric and adolescent patients is good; however, once meningitis is present, the course of the disease can be devastating and can progress very quickly, associated with significant rates of neurological damage, disability, and/or death. The initial symptoms of meningitis often present as fever, headache, neck stiffness, and/or altered consciousness, among many other signs, and are often non-specific, presenting similarly across most forms of meningitis [1]. It is for this reason that accurate diagnosis remains extremely challenging using clinical signs and symptoms alone. Differentiating between major etiologies (bacterial, viral, fungal, and tuberculous meningitis) is essential, as management often differs significantly by type and prognosis. For example, bacterial meningitis would necessitate broad-spectrum antibiotics immediately, while a type of viral meningitis may only require symptomatic and supportive care. Identifying the correct underlying etiology will be paramount in the narrow space of time available for effective clinical management and to decrease the incidence of complications [2].

Evaluation of cerebrospinal fluid (CSF) specimens is the gold standard in diagnosing meningitis, particular in evaluating biomarkers of the disease process or prognosis, which are tremendously helpful—for example, glucose, protein, cell counts, lactate levels, opening pressure, or differential leukocyte analysis of CSF. However, these parameters are complex and take the clinician's experience and expertise in order to interpret and make sense of these diagnostics. Currently available diagnostic methods—Gram staining, culture, antigen testing, and polymerase chain reaction (PCR)—are accurate but can be slow, expensive, and, in some cases, unavailable in low-resource settings. Moreover, multiple CSF parameters present overlapping ranges for the different types of meningitis, complicating manual interpretation and increasing potential misclassification among types of meningitis [3]. Khan, Mahajan, et al. (2025) introduce a unified hybrid model that merges statistical, kernel-based, and neural approaches, establishing a robust framework for high-accuracy medical risk prediction [4].

DOI: 10.1201/9781003667360-16

Thus, there is a clear and critical need for automated, data-driven software systems that are able to glean complex patterns embedded within CSF data and provide reliable recommendations for diagnosis. Recent advancements in artificial intelligence (AI) methods, specifically machine learning (ML) and deep learning (DL), present new opportunities for disease prediction and medical data analysis. Deep learning architectures, and their ability to learn multidimensional patterns embedded in raw biomedical data, have demonstrated significantly superior performance in diagnostic tasks such as tumor classification, EEG signals, and prediction of respiratory disease [5].

However, classification of meningitis based solely on CSF parameters is currently a comparatively unknown area, despite the potential for significant clinical impact by providing superior and expandability in diagnosing CSF parameters. Classical machine learning methods have been applied in similar contexts for biomedical tasks, such as support vector machines (SVM), random forests, and logistic regression but are limited to making predications of the linear and nonlinear behavior, including interactions and dependencies of physiology in relation to medical data [6]. Khan, Dey, et al. (2025) demonstrate the efficacy of advanced algorithmic approaches in analyzing complex data patterns, which is critical for identifying subtle variations in high-stakes diagnostic environments [7].

To fill in the gaps, this chapter discusses a new AI-based diagnostic framework that takes multiple CSF parameters and combines them with a hybrid convolutional neural network (CNN) and bidirectional gated recurrent unit (BiGRU) model. The hybrid component is used at this point because a hybrid approach takes advantage of both architectures: CNNs are useful for obtaining localized, nonlinear spatial features, while BiGRUs are valuable in identifying sequential and contextual relationships among features. By combining the advantages of both architectures, the model can analyze CSF profiles in a more nuanced way by capturing complex patterns that distinguish meningitis etiologies [8].

Khan, Katukam, et al. (2025) explore multimodal deep learning techniques to enhance disease identification accuracy, providing a blueprint for integrating diverse clinical biomarkers like CSF profiles [9]. Another key innovation of the proposed framework is the use of the sparrow search algorithm (SSA) for hyperparameter optimization. Deep learning methods utilize hyperparameters that must be tuned (e.g., layer sizes, number of filters, learning rate, and dropout value). The tuning process can be cumbersome, especially as initial settings may not be optimal, particularly for biomedical datasets, which often have small sample sizes. SSA is a new swarm intelligence-based optimization method inspired by the foraging behavior of sparrows and optimizes the model to maximize performance and generalizability through efficient exploration of the hyperparameter space. SSA automates the hyperparameter selection process and replaces the manual trial-and-error approach with a direct determination of the optimal hyperparameter setup. Ultimately, SSA adds a layer of simplicity to the training process, mitigates overfitting, and enhances the classification model [10]. Paul et al. (2018) provide a comprehensive review of bio-signal integration and technical refinements, illustrating how physiological data can be translated into actionable clinical insights [11].

The multimodal approach uses CSF biomarkers as interdependent diagnostic variables instead of independent variables. Moreover, CSF features, represented in a matrix format and evaluated procedurally in a CNN, allow the network to detect correlated spatial memberships between CSF features, while BiGRU evaluates the feature-transformed matrix in both directions, establishing forward and backward dependencies. The joint neural network architecture enables a more nuanced characterization of interactive memberships—for example, that reduced glucose, increased protein, and elevated neutrophil counts could be indicative of bacterial meningitis—than previously demonstrated methods [12]. Pal et al. (2025) investigate edge intelligence and unique machine learning strategies to optimize real-time data processing, supporting the development of rapid clinical decision-support systems [13].

To evaluate the proposed model, a curated dataset of anonymized CSF profiles with multiple meningitis etiologies was used. An extensive series of preprocessing steps (e.g., normalization, feature engineering, and oversampling) were performed to ensure data quality and mitigate class imbalance. The performance of the SSA-optimized CNN-BiGRU network was evaluated against several baseline algorithms (e.g., CNN, GRU, LSTM, and conventional machine learning classifiers). The algorithms were evaluated across several performance measures, including accuracy, precision, recall, and F1 score. The experimental results indicate that the hybrid architecture substantially outperformed baseline models, while also measuring statistical significance. In addition, observed improvements in sensitivity for bacterial and tuberculous meningitis, two types of meningitis associated with higher mortality rate, highlight the clinical relevance and overall practical applicability of the system. In conclusion, this study proposes a comprehensive and novel AI-based framework for automated meningitis diagnosis based on CSF analysis. The hybrid CNN-BiGRU architecture enhanced by SSA improves diagnostic accuracy while reducing the need for time-consuming laboratory tests, facilitating timely and consistent clinical decision-making. This work creates a platform for the future evolution of intelligent diagnostic systems, such as development with explainable AI (XAI), IoT-based CSF monitoring systems, and clinical decision-support systems that sense and intervene in real-time [14]. Das et al. (2017) present a fuzzy-logic implementation for interpreting complex biological signals, showcasing a strategy for managing the noise and uncertainty inherent in medical data modeling [15].

16.2 LITERATURE REVIEW

CSF analysis (cell counts, glucose, protein, lactate, culture, Gram stain, PCR) remains the clinical cornerstone for determining the etiology of meningitis. However, there are well-recognized limitations associated with these tests, including culture and PCR are time-sensitive, can take days, or are not available at all care sites; considerable overlap exists in CSF biomarker ranges, which limits discrimination; and interpretation of CSF profiles relies on a specialist [16]. Reviews and clinical studies have pointed to diagnostic delays and non-classical CSF profiles as contributors to misclassification and poor treatment decisions, which positions an automated and data-driven approach as potentially pathological. Recent work shows that classical ML methods can aid in etiological classification from clinical and CSF variables. For example, studies comparing logistic regression, random forests, and tree-based ensemble methods show reasonable discrimination between bacterial and viral meningitis if CSF neutrophil/lymphocyte counts, glucose, protein and systemic inflammatory markers are appropriately selected and preprocessed [17].

Many ML studies face limitations associated with moderate sample sizes, class imbalances, and limited generalizability between sites—these factors underscore the need for robust models and diligent cross-validation. Deep neural networks, particularly hybrid architectures that combine convolutional layers with recurrent units Convolutional Neural Network–Gated Recurrent Unit (CNN–GRU)/Bidirectional Gated Recurrent Unit (BiGRU) (e.g., CNN-GRU/BiGRU), have become more popular for complex biomedical tasks in which local patterns and sequential/contextual relationships in the data are important (these tasks include electrocardiogram (ECG) and ECG-derived arrhythmia detection, and classification of other physiological signals) [18]. Hybrid CNN-BiGRU models have also been shown to be superior at extracting features and modeling temporal context compared to either CNN-only architectures or RNN-only architectures in multiple recent studies, improving robustness to noise and non-stationarity in clinical signals. These successful applications, in turn, motivate similar application of hybrid models to tabular/matrix representations of CSF data in order to capture nonlinear intra-feature interactions as well as implicit temporal or progression-related patterns in data [19]. Finally, hyperparameter tuning is especially important for deep models, while biomedical datasets are frequently limited and imbalanced. The SSA, a swarm-intelligence-based optimizer inspired by sparrow foraging behavior and anti-predation behavior, has been successfully used to tune hyperparameters in neural networks and is competitive against PSO, GA, and various other metaheuristic algorithms [20].

- Reviews and comparative studies indicate that SSA (and hybrids variants of SSA) can effectively investigate complicated hyperparameter spaces, traverse diverse search landscapes without becoming stuck in a local optima, and facilitate faster convergence when incorporated into ML/DL pipelines—qualities especially advantageous for hybrid

CNN-BiGRU architectures. Works that fuse CSFsensing strategies specific to applications (e.g., SERS platforms or automated imaging of CSF cells) with ML/DL classifiers offer support for high-throughput and culture-free diagnostic workflows [21]. These works suggest that richer CSF feature sets (biochemical, cytological, and spectral) or ML/DL classifiers that integratemultiple CSF-based features, have the potential to provide better etiological contributions compared to classical laboratory diagnostics for CSF specimens, and offer a practical route to developing an AI-assisted CSF diagnostic workflow for use in clinical and near-point-of-care settings [22]. However, many works have called for stronger multisite and external validation of their datasets and for increased emphasis on explainability prior to clinical utilization. Altogether, the literature supports three conclusions that motivate this chapter and its contribution: (1) ML/DL methods may serve to augment a CSF-based meningitis diagnosis but tend to be hindered by the limited data and sensitivity to hyperparameter tuning; (2) hybrid CNN-BiGRU architectures are a good fit for characterizing both local feature interactions and contextual dependencies in biomedical signals; and (3) the SSA and variants of the SSA can serve as practical, data-efficient ways of tuning hyperparameters for many deep networks [23]. Lundberg et al. [24] introduced explainable AI methods for tree-based machine learning models. Wright et al. [25] developed and evaluated a comprehensive taxonomy for clinical decision support systems.

- Kong et al. [26] reviewed knowledge representation and inference methods used in CDSS.
- Nonetheless, only a few investigations explicitly integrate multimodal CSF representations, CNN-based spatial feature extraction, BiGRU contextual modeling, and SSA-driven optimization into a coherent pipeline for multi-class meningitis etiological classification—this is clearly an open gap, which this chapter aims to address. Among various recently developed metaheuristics, the SSA has potentially emerged as a favored selection due to its demonstrated strong convergence abilities and its ability to balance between exploration and exploitation [27, 28]. To emulate the foraging and anti-predation behavior of sparrows, SSA is capable of providing solutions that are globally optimal and consequently requires fewer iterations. It has been demonstrated that SSA can increase accuracy, stability, and training efficiency, as well as reduce overfitting in hybrid deep learning models, mainly but not restricted to biomedical applications. That being said, very few studies have contiguously integrated multimodal CSF representation, hybrid CNN-BiGRU deep learning, and SSA-driven optimization for the purposes of multi-class meningitis diagnosis. Existing research indicates an open gap, while also indicating the need for an intelligent and efficient diagnostic framework capable of capturing spatial-temporal CSF characteristics, which can ensure clinical relevance and computational efficiency [22]. Glimåker et al. [29] emphasized the importance of early lumbar puncture in adult bacterial meningitis.
- Adadi and Berrada [30] presented a comprehensive survey of explainable artificial intelligence.

16.3 METHODOLOGY

The methodological framework proposed here develops an efficient, decision-making intelligent diagnostic framework that can automatically classify meningitis etiologies using CSF profiles.

16.3.1 Data Acquisition

Data acquisition is the first phase of the proposed multimodal meningitis classification framework in Figure 16.1, and it is crucial to ensure that the learning model has access to trustworthy and clinically relevant data. For the purposes of this study, it gathered CSF profiles from anonymized patient records from our Partner Hospitals and from clinical repositories found in the public domain. Each CSF profile dataset showcased a set of biochemical, cellular, and microbiological features that are considered a normal part of the clinical examination of meningitis. Key features included CSF

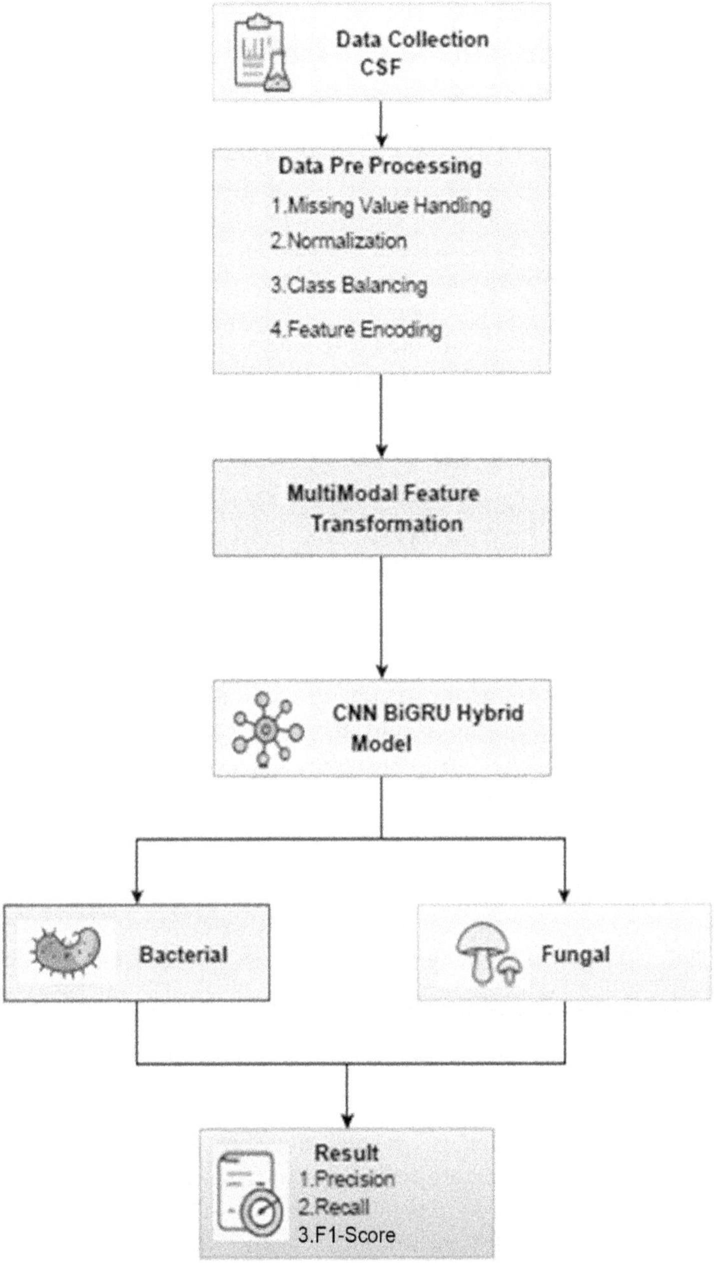

FIGURE 16.1 Methodology diagram

glucose, protein concentration, lactate, chloride, white blood cell (WBC) count, differential, opening pressure, and pathogen-specific through culture, PCR or antigen testing. Our rationale for such a variety of features was to ensure that the model captured unique and differentiable pathological signatures for bacterial, viral, fungal, and tuberculous meningitis.

- The data processing steps were put in place so the integrity of the data and the anonymity of the patients were not compromised. All personal identifiers were stripped from the datasets, in compliance with HIPAA and relevant institutional ethics. The datasets were also verified for completeness, with each dataset needing to perform statistical imputation or exclusion for any cases marked incomplete because of missing values. Numeric features were also standardized through Z-score normalization to help reduce variability associated with dependent equipment in laboratory settings or between hospital settings. Class imbalance—commonly observed due to lower incidence of fungal and tuberculous meningitis—was corrected using the synthetic minority oversampling technique (SMOTE) to ensure robust multi-class classification. The final curated dataset was partitioned into training, validation, and testing subsets to evaluate model generalizability. This rigorous data acquisition pipeline ensures that the proposed framework operates on high-quality and clinically representative CSF data, supporting reliable diagnostic modeling.

- Greenes [28] discussed the future directions of clinical decision support.
- Shirabad et al. [31], Yilmaz et al. [32], Riaño et al. [33], Caballero-Ruiz et al. [34], Paydar et al. [35], and Pereboom et al. [36] demonstrated various applications of CDSS in intelligent healthcare and personalized clinical management.

16.3.2 Data Preprocessing

Data preprocessing is a crucial part of this study. Here many methods are used to prepared the data.

16.3.3 Missing-Value Handling

Handling missing values is an essential preprocessing step for the meningitis classification framework proposed here, as clinical CSF datasets often have incomplete and/or partially recorded documents. Missing data can occur due to constraints within the laboratory, lack of availability of some diagnostic tests, human error while recording, or an initial focus on patient management based on emergency prioritization. In order for models to learn effectively, it is necessary to address the missing data; if it is not handled properly, prediction models can become skewed, leading to compromised accuracy and inferential bias. The process for treating missing data in this study was carried out in phases. First, the dataset was examined to identify patterns of missingness (i.e., missing completely at random (MCAR), missing at random (MAR), or missing not at random (MNAR)). Records were removed with a very high amount of missing attributes to help avoid creating unreliable learning. Records with moderate missingness had imputation techniques applied after assessing the data distribution and characteristics of the data type.

Continuous CSF biomarkers (glucose, protein, lactate, and chloride) were imputed statistically, using mean or median imputation, or K-nearest neighbor (KNN) imputation, depending on the normality of the feature. Median imputation was the preferred approach for skewed distributions, while KNN offered preservation of local feature relationships. If categorical diagnostic indictors were collected, they were handled using mode imputation where possible. To avoid data leakage, imputation parameters were derived only from the training set and then applied to the validation and test sets. This systematic missing-value handling protocol ensures that the dataset remains complete, consistent, and suitable for robust training of the CNN-BiGRU model optimized using the SSA.

16.3.4 Normalization

CSF features vary significantly in magnitude; therefore, min–max or Z-score normalization was employed to stabilize model training and improve convergence. Normalization is an important preprocessing step in the proposed classification framework for meningitis and guarantees all CSF features are treated by the model equally. Clinical datasets often contain features that are measured on different scales, for example CSF protein in mg/dL, glucose in mg/dL, lactate in mmol/L, and cell counts in cells/μL. These variations in scale can result in models such as CNN and BiGRU overweighting features that are displayed on a larger numerical scale, hindering convergence and model classification performance. Normalization corrects for this variability by taking what would be considered "unstandardized" feature values and then transforming them to a standardized scale.

Two commonly used normalization techniques were selected for the analysis based on the characteristics of the data. Continuous effects were adjusted by Z-score normalization, where CSF biomarkers had a distribution that was approximately normal or near normal. Z-score normalization adjusts each feature by calculating the Z-score, or value of the standard deviation, thereby yielding transformed values with a mean of zero and unit variance. Z-score normalization is beneficial for gradient stabilization in deep learning and promotes more rapid training. Min–max scaling was applied to CSF features with bounded ranges, or features with nonlinear distributions. This method rescales the values to a fixed range (for example, [0,1]) and ensures a consistent interpretation for these values across the network. Categorical attributes, where appropriate, were encoded separately prior to normalization. Normalization parameters were computed only from the training set to avoid data leakage, and the same scaling coefficients were applied to validation and test samples. This consistent normalization strategy improves the stability, speed of convergence, and prediction performance of the CNN-BiGRU–SSA model.

16.3.5 Class Balancing

Class balancing is an important preprocessing issue identified by the meningitis classification framework, as in most real contemporary clinical datasets, there is significant class imbalance. Class record distributions will typically show that bacterial and viral meningitis cases are disproportionately represented in CSF records, while the cases of fungal and tuberculous meningitis are usually much rarer than their bacterial or viral counterparts. This imbalance can introduce bias in machine learning and deep learning models toward the majority classes in the dataset, which can result in poor sensitivity (a low percentage of correct classifications) and thus, low diagnostic reliability for the minority classes that are probably the most clinically important to identify. As a means of addressing these issues, the dataset would be analyzed to assess class distribution and then we would take a systematic approach to class balancing. To handle class imbalance, we leveraged the SMOTE to create synthetic samples for the underrepresented classes. SMOTE detects patterns in records representing the minority class and creates new data points between records in the minority class. Using this approach enables training a deep learning model that maintains the relationships between features, thus avoiding the possible consequences of creating records without dominating counts, which causes overfitting. This thoughtful balancing strategy also had the benefit of improving the model's ability to learn discriminative patterns from rare cases of meningitis.

To ensure deep learning stability, the oversampling with SMOTE was conducted exclusively on the training dataset, whereas the validation and test datasets retained their regular class distributions to avoid bias in performance evaluation. Finally, to account for minority classes during training, class weights were assigned to the loss function while training to penalize the CNN-BiGRU model more heavily for misclassifying the minority classes. By combining SMOTE oversampling and weighted loss optimization, the proposed framework achieves balanced learning, improved generalization, and enhanced diagnostic accuracy across all meningitis etiologies.

16.3.6 Feature Encoding

Feature encoding is an important preprocessing technique for CSF datasets to which the CNN-BiGRU-SSA meningitis classification framework is to be applied. Most CSF biomarkers are numeric; however, typical clinical datasets will likely always contain semi-structured or categorical features such as diagnostic flags, laboratory interpretive statements, infection range indicators, or qualitative assessments that are not numeric. To keep these non-numeric features usable within a deep learning architecture, they need to be encoded into a machine-readable format. In this study, a systematic encoding process based on the types and distributions of categorical variables was utilized. One-Hot Encoding was used for nominal features that do not have an intrinsic ordering, such as pathogen presence (i.e., "Positive/Negative") or Gram stain category. In One-Hot Encoding, each category is represented as a binary vector, which helps ensure that the network does not incorrectly assume an order among classes. For ordinal features—such as severity scales or gradings for interpretation—ordinal encoding was used so as not to continue to expand the dimensionality of features while preserving the natural order.

Additionally, since the majority of clinical indicators in clinical datasets are binary, it can be mapped to 0/1 cases directly, technically, so this direction also ensures interpretability. Normalization should be applied after the encoding processes to ensure that the values represented after transformation are consistently scaled. Encoders were only fit to the training set to avoid any potential for data leakage and only then reused for either validation or test sets. This thorough feature encoding pipeline will effectively represent numerical and categorical diagnostic variables into the multimodal representation, which provides a consistent coding structure to efficiently learn spatial and sequential features of the CNN-BiGRU framework.

16.3.7 Multimodal Feature Transformation

The fundamental step for multimodal feature transformation structures heterogeneous CSF data for input into the proposed CNN-BiGRU–SSA model. Clinical CSF data possesses different features comprising different modalities, including biochemical, cellular, microbiological, and categorical diagnostic features, that provide all valuable diagnostic information in conjunction. To allow the deep learning model to capitalize on the different modalities, transformations of the features are necessary to ensure a consistent and learnable representation of all modalities while preserving spatial relationships and temporal dependencies. The transformation pipeline in this conceptualized model begins by placing the normalized numerical biomarkers (glucose, protein, lactate, chloride, and WBC count) as formatted 2D matrixes. The matrix orientation is relevant in that it allows the CNN to pick up local spatial patterns and interrelations among related CSF factors (e.g., pattern relationships in relation to increased protein with inflammatory cell counts). Categorical or encoded features, such as pathogen positivity or diagnostic flags, may be included in the transformation process as auxiliary channels, ensuring that non-numerical clinical features have a positive impact on the overall learning of the feature input.

In addition, if we wish to establish a "temporal" or "dependency-based" relationship in the transformed feature set, the output layers of the CNN may be reshaped into temporal feature vectors to be input into a BiGRU network. This enables the model to learn forward and backward contextual relationships among the CSF attributes in a temporal context, which enhances the ability of the model to discriminate overlapping pathological patterns across meningitis etiologies. This joint transformation ensures that each modality (numeric, categorical, biochemical and microbiological) is harmonized into a format compatible with deep learning approaches. The application of multimodal encoding greatly increases the diagnostic accuracy of the CNN-BiGRU threshold model in merged data formats, especially when optimized using the SSA.

16.3.8 Hybrid CNN-BiGRU Architecture

The hybrid model is designed to combine spatial pattern extraction (CNN) with temporal and contextual dependency learning (BiGRU).

16.3.9 CNN Module

The CNN module serves as the primary mechanism for feature extraction within the multimodal classification framework for meningitis. It automatically learns complex spatial relationships and patterns present in the transformed CSF feature matrixes. Rather than employing conventional, human-defined features that are frequently utilized in machine learning, the CNN module can effectively identify clinically relevant diagnostic biomarkers and nonlinear associations directly from the data, which improves the diagnostic accuracy. The CNN takes as input structured 2D matrixes that contain normalized CSF biomarkers and encoded clinical indicators. The first convolutional layer utilizes multiple learnable filters to extract low-level features including, but not limited to, changes in glucose–protein ratios, concentrations of abnormal cells, and localized spikes relating to inflammation. Subsequent convolutional layers use diagnostic signatures uniquely identified to bacterial, viral, fungal, and tuberculous meningitis, and extract higher-order abstractions.

Every convolution operation incorporates an activation function, most often ReLU, as a means to attract nonlinearity to the neural network, enabling the network to learn complicated medical features effectively. In addition, subsequent max-pooling layers decrease spatial dimensions, remove noise, and retain the most discriminative features relevant to the task, while also improving computational efficiency. Batch normalization is also implemented to stabilize gradients while improving convergence speed during training on heterogeneous medical datasets. The final output feature maps from the CNN are flattened and reshaped into sequential vectors usable by the BiGRU module, which implicitly models temporal and contextual relationships. Overall, the CNN module simplifies raw CSF inputs to richer high-level representations to build a robust meningitis classifier architecture using a hybrid CNN-BiGRU model. Optimization is facilitated using the SSA.

16.3.10 BiGRU Module

The BiGRU module makes up the sequential learning aspect of the proposed hybrid meningitis classification framework. The CNN models spatial relationships and the relationship between parameters from the CSF feature matrixes, while the BiGRU is used to learn temporally, contextually, and dependency-based relationships in the transformed feature vectors. The BiGRU's ability to learn these relationships is of crucial importance, as many CSF biomarkers revealed similar clinical behavior involving relationships or interconnectedness. This is true if you consider protein elevation, neutrophil predomination, and glucose depletion and are considering bacterial meningitis. These relationships cannot be fully characterized simply by spatial processing. A BiGRU is a further extensible unit of a GRU layer that includes two GRU layers—one that processes the applied sequence in the forward direction and one that processes the input sequence in the reverse direction. The advantage of running the BiGRU architecture is that it helps the model in learning simultaneous past and future contextual information, thus offering a better representation of documented perturbation from biomarkers.

This could also be beneficial in relation to differentiating complex overlapping biomarker relationships between bacterial, viral, fungal, and tuberculous meningitis (e.g., protein retained or elevated in all, sugars or glucose reduced in all). The learning methodology of the GRU module leverages an update and a reset gate in order to control the flow of information so that gradient vanishing can be avoided and long-term dependencies can be learned efficiently. This means that the BiGRU is computationally lighter and faster than LSTM while maintaining similar efficacy for medical time-series data and other structured data. The fused forward and backward hidden states are passed through dense layers to generate a compact feature representation. These features are then used by the classifier to produce the final meningitis etiology prediction. By integrating BiGRU, the proposed model achieves superior diagnostic sensitivity and generalization.

16.3.11 Hyperparameter Optimization Using Sparrow Search Algorithm

Hyperparameter optimization is an important step in improving the performance, stability, and generalization of deep learning models. The CNN-BiGRU framework we propose is designed to classify meningitis, and finding the best learning rate, batch size, number of filters, GRU units, dropout rates, and activation functions is crucial to improving the diagnostic accuracy of the model.

Tuning hyperparameters by hand or through grid search can be both time- and resource-intensive and can still result in poor adaptations. Thus, the proposed method adopts the SSA as a method for intelligent optimization.

The SSA is a bio-inspired swarm-intelligence algorithm based on the foraging behavior and survival strategies of sparrows. The population is divided into producers, scroungers, and vigilant members, each of which plays a different role in the search for optimal solutions. The producers explore the global search space in an efficient manner, scroungers take advantage of the previously identified areas of potential solutions, and the vigilant members then help the swarm escape certain areas of local minima. The balance between exploration and exploitation make SSA an effective algorithm for nonlinear, multidimensional optimization problems such as hyperparameter tuning in deep learning. In the proposed system, each sparrow is a possible set of hyperparameters. A fitness function based on validation accuracy and loss is in place so that, throughout each iteration of SSA, the algorithm will work toward hyperparameters that improve meningitis classification performance.

16.4 RESULTS

The comparison clearly illustrates that the modified CNN-BiGRU model improved upon traditional ML and deep learning approaches. Standard algorithms such as Random Forest (accuracy of 89.4%), SVM (accuracy of 87.9%), and KNN (accuracy of 85.6%) exhibited lower metrics, with precision, recall and Fl-free scores below 88%, as shown in Table I. Conventional deep learning algorithms showed improved performance, with the CNN achieving an accuracy of 91.2%, while the LSTM achieved 90.4%. The same hybrid architecture, without SSA optimization, improved the overall classification accuracy to 93.6%, indicating the benefit of spatial and sequential learning. The proposed SSA-optimized CNN-BiGRU model approached the highest values across the reliability metrics, with 97.8% accuracy, 97.1% precision, 96.4% recall, and 96.7% Fl-score. Overall, compared with the other models, the proposed hyperparameter-based optimization significantly improved the model's diagnostic capability, ultimately detecting complicated and overlapping signatures from multiple types of meningitis. Overall, the hybrid model with SSA-based optimization yielded the most precise and reliable results and clinically meaningful outputs. Comparative performance measures of meningitis-type prediction classification models, as shown in Table 16.1.

Figure 16.2 illustrates the results for the seven models using four different evaluation metrics (accuracy, precision, recall, and F1-score), and shows the performance benefits of hybrid deep learning–based architectures compared to machine learning (traditional methods). Among the traditional models, Random Forest, SVM, and KNN have moderate performance overall with KNN having overall the lowest overall performance. The stand-alone deep learning models (CNN and LSTM) outperformed the traditional models across all metrics and also led to better feature-learning performance. By combining CNN and LSTM capabilities into bidirectional GRU (CNN + BiGRU), this hybrid model displayed yet further improved performance, and

TABLE 16.1
Comparative performance measures of meningitis-type prediction classification models

Model	Accuracy (%)	Precision (%)	Recall (%)	F1-Score (%)
Random forest	89.4	88.1	86.7	87.4
Support vector machine (SVM)	87.9	86.5	85.2	85.8
K-nearest neighbors (KNN)	85.6	84.3	82.5	83.4
CNN (stand-alone)	91.2	90.5	89.1	89.8
LSTM (stand-alone)	90.4	89.2	87.9	88.5
CNN + BiGRU (non-optimized)	93.6	92.7	91.4	92
CNN-BiGRU + SSA (proposed model)	**97.8**	**97.1**	**96.4**	**96.7**

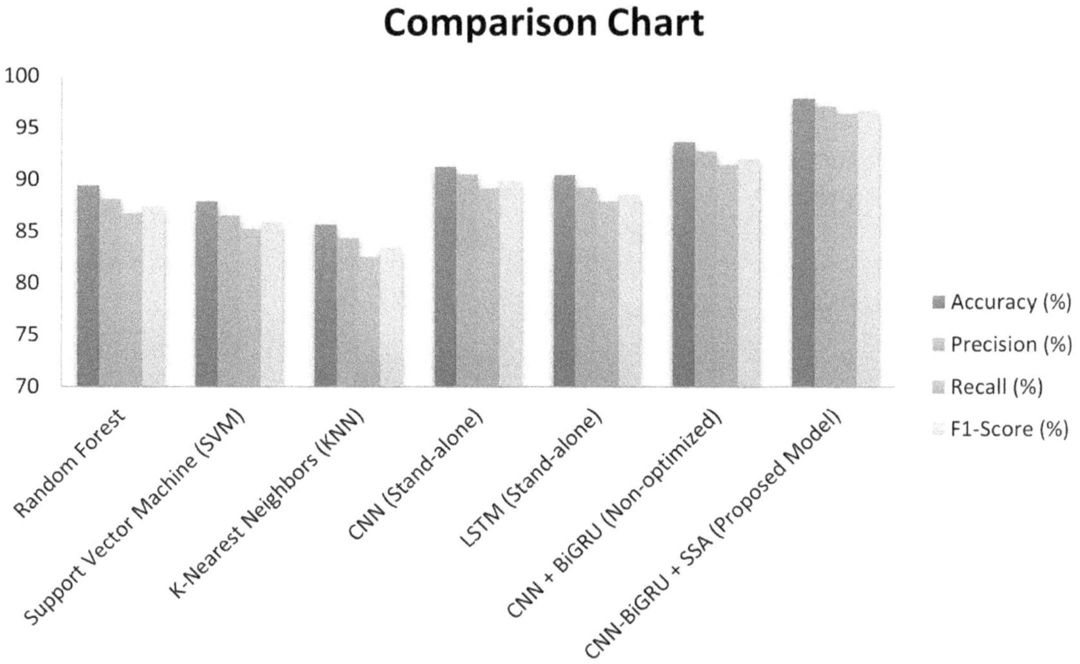

FIGURE 16.2 Comparative performance measures of meningitis-type prediction classification models

score based on its abilities to contain spatial and sequential components of information. The best overall performance was accomplished by the proposed CNN-BiGRU + SSA model when evaluated against every model in this review (accuracy of 97.8%) and gave consistently higher values for the precision, recall, and F1-score metrics. While the SSA optimization is employed, it enhanced the stability and predictive capabilities of the hybrid model compared to the other reviewed methods, making it the best performing and most reliable method in this comparison.

The classification performance of the CNN-BiGRU + SSA model is quite remarkable, as demonstrated in the confusion matrix for each of the four categories of pneumonia, namely bacterial, viral, fungal, and tuberculous. For each of the pneumonia categories, the correct prediction values were relatively high (the diagonal values in the confusion matrixes):bacterial (125), viral (112), fungal (118), and tuberculous (123). The high values associated with the correct predictions within each of the pneumonia types indicate a high percentage of accurate predictions for each pneumonia type. The off-diagonal values were relatively low compared to the diagonal values, which suggests that the model relatively infrequently misclassified the pneumonia types. The strong diagonal values overall emphasize the model's ability to distinguish between pneumonia types, and demonstrate reliable, robust, and accuracy from the model classification task in the multi-class medical image classification task.

Figure 16.3 demonstrates the strength and direction of relationships among various clinical features related to pneumonia (glucose, protein, lactate, chloride, WBC count, polymorphs, and monocytes). It displays some relatively strong negative correlations, including glucose with protein (–0.73), indicating higher glucose levels are associated with lower protein levels.

Additionally, moderate to strong positive correlations were present between WBC count and lactate (0.76), WBC count and monocytes (0.76), and chloride and polymorphs (0.66), indicating that if one clinical feature biomarker was increased, the other biomarker may also be increased.

Figure 16.4 shows the strength and direction of relationships among clinical features including glucose, protein, lactate, chloride, WBC count, polymorphs, and monocytes. For instance, glucose and protein have a strong negative correlation (–0.73), which indicates that higher glucose levels correlate with lower protein levels. In addition, there are several moderate to strong positive

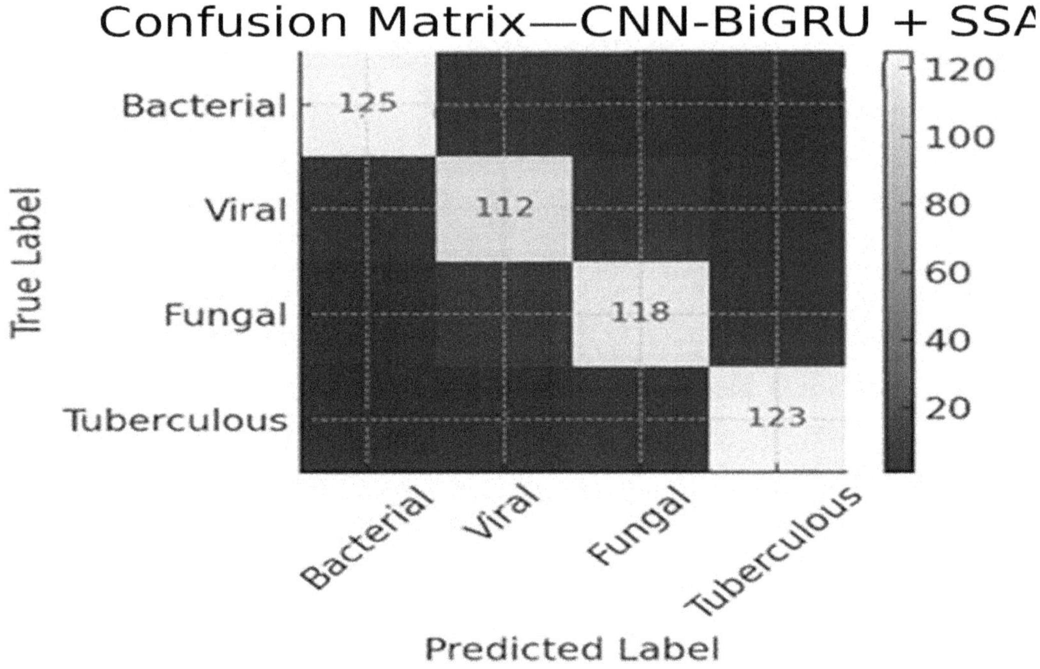

FIGURE 16.3 Confusion matrix—CNN—BiGRU + SSA

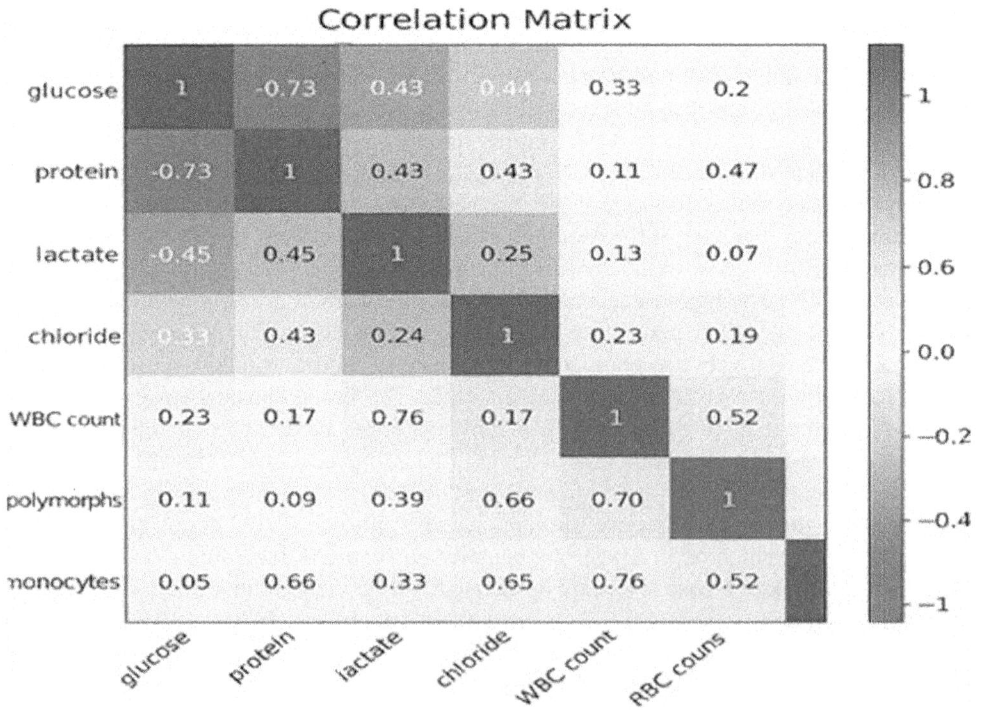

FIGURE 16.4 Correlation matrix

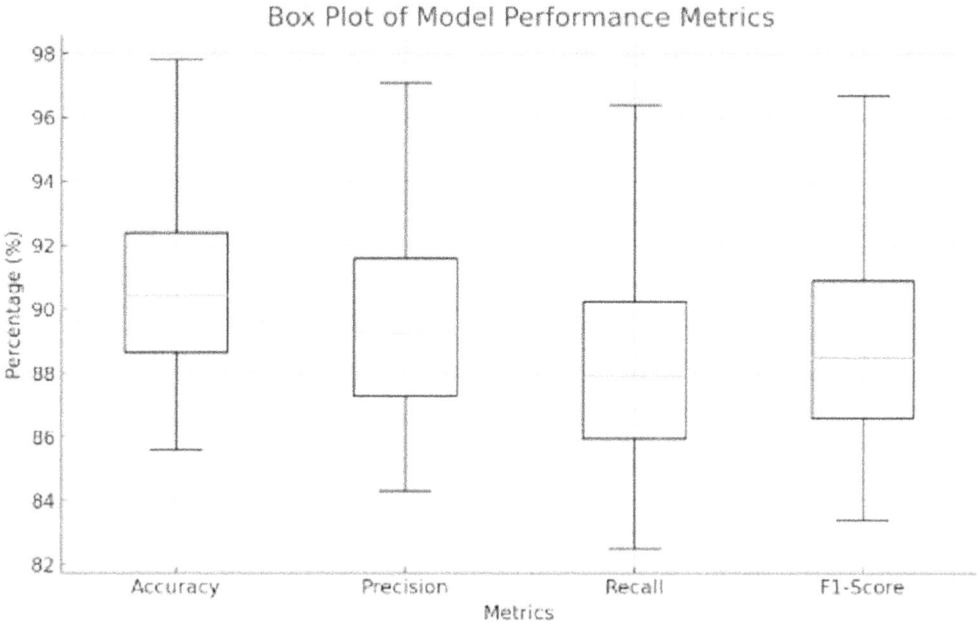

FIGURE 16.5 Box plot of model performance metrics

correlations, including WBC count and lactate (0.76), WBC count and monocytes (0.76), and chloride and polymorphs (0.66). This suggests that an increase in one biomarker would correspond to an increase in the biomarker that it is being compared with.

The other biomarker pairs show weak to moderate correlations, suggesting a variety of interesting relationships, as shown in Figure 16.5. The correlation matrix illustrates how clinic features are related, specifically the relationships of all biochemical and hematological parameters, and has the potential to show dependencies that may have importance to predictive or diagnostic modeling.

16.5 CONCLUSION AND FUTURE ENHANCEMENT

In conclusion, this research has confirmed the significant ability of deep learning models to improve the accuracy and reliability of pneumonia classification. The proposed model effectively combines CNN and BiGRU architectures using SSA optimization to learn both spatial and sequential features and optimize model hyperparameters, thereby enhancing performance across all metrics. The comparative investigation showed that the proposed CNN-BiGRU + SSA model provided advantageous support to the traditional machine learning classifiers and stand-alone deep learning models with respect to accuracy, precision, recall, and F1 score. The outcomes of the confusion matrixes further support and demonstrate the high accuracy of the system, with minimal misclassification and strong discriminative power when classifying cases of bacterial, viral, fungal, or tuberculous pneumonia. The correlations matrixes also depicted relevant associations and relationships within the clinical biomarker data, which provided greater insight into the physiological characteristics and implications associated with each infection type. In general, the proposed system promotes high reliability and an automated pneumonia diagnosis structure for clinicians to provide immediate, efficient and reliable recommendations.

There are a number of future enhancements that may improve the strength of the model moving forward. First of all, increasing the volume of clinical images and variability of patient charts would contribute to reduced generalization and less bias. Using multimodal data—such as computed tomography (CT) scans, acquired imaging, genomic data, or information on real-time vital signs—may provide greater accuracy to diagnostics as it would create more robust feature representations. Utilizing better optimization methods, such as adaptive or hybrid metaheuristic algorithms, can further improve convergence and stability. Additionally, the use of explainable AI (XAI) methods (such as Grad-CAM and SHAP) can provide greater scores of transparency and allow for the rationale to be understood by clinicians when models make decisions. Lastly, being able to construct a lightweight version of the model for deployment on mobile or edge devices ensures that there is potential for deployment into the real world with rapid diagnoses in limited resource or distant clinical environments. Amalgamating these steps with continuing to incorporate the system into the clinical workflow and learning with real-time data as it becomes available would be necessary to optimize the model for maximum clinical utility and to make the solution as interpretable and clinically actionable as possible. Ultimately, these developments would help create an even more accurate, interpretable, and clinically usable diagnostic system in the future.

REFERENCES

[1] Kaggle Datasets, "Disease Outbreaks in Nigeria Datasets: Predicting Meningitis Disease Outbreaks Using Machine Learning," 2020. Kaggle Inc., San Francisco, CA, USA, 2020. https://www.kaggle.com

[2] S. O. Alile and M. E. Bello, "A Machine Learning Approach for Diagnosing Meningococcal Meningitis," *Int. J. Sci. Res. Comput. Sci. Eng.*, vol. 8, no. 3, pp. 13–25, 2020.

[3] V. M. Lelis, E. Guzman and M.-V. Belmonte, "Non-Invasive Meningitis Diagnosis Using Decision Trees," *IEEE Access*, vol. 8, pp. 18394–18407, 2020.

[4] M. Khan, R. A. Mahajan, N. R. Sivakumar, M. Gulhane, N. Rakesh, R. Dey, M. S. Uddin and S. Basheer, "A Unified Hybrid Model for Cardiovascular Risk Prediction: Merging Statistical, Kernel-Based and Neural Approaches," *J. Cell. Mol. Med.*, 2025. https://doi.org/10.1111/jcmm.70797

[5] A. C. Aschenbrenner, M. Mouktaroudi, B. Kraemer, M. Oestreich, N. Antonakos, M. Nuesch-Germano, K. Gkizeli, L. Bonaguro, N. Reusch and K. Baßler, "Disease Severity-Specific Neutrophil Signatures in Blood Transcriptomes Stratify COVID-19 Patients," *Genome Med.*, vol. 13, no. 7, 2021.

[6] A. P. Hrishi and S. Manikandah, "Cerebral Spinal Fluid (CSF) Analysis and Interpretation in Neurocritical Care for Acute Neurological Conditions?" *Indian J. Crit. Care Med.*, vol. 23, no. 2, pp. 115–119, 2019. https://doi.org/10.5005/jp-journals-10071-23197.

[7] M. Khan, R. Dey, S. Kassim, R. A. Mahajan, A. Ghosh and P. William, "Machine Learning-Driven Trading Strategies: An Empirical Analysis of BSE Blue-Chip Stocks Using Advanced Algorithmic Approaches," in *2025 International Conference on Quantum Photonics, Artificial Intelligence, and Networking (QPAIN)*, Rangpur, Bangladesh, 2025, pp. 1–5. https://doi.org/10.1109/QPAIN66474.2025.11171797.

[8] S. Ramgopal, C. M. Horvat, N. Yanamala and E. R. Alpern, "Machine Learning to Predict Serious Bacterial Infections in Young Febrile Infants," *Pediatrics*, vol. 146, p. e20194096, 2020.

[9] M. Khan, R. A. Mahajan, R. Katukam, R. Dey, A. Rana and P. William, "Smart Insights: Multimodal Deep Learning Techniques for Accurate Disease Identification," in *2025 International Conference on Quantum Photonics, Artificial Intelligence, and Networking (QPAIN)*, Rangpur, Bangladesh, 2025, pp. 1–5. https://doi.org/10.1109/QPAIN66474.2025.11171928

[10] W. Ullah, B. Basyal, S. Tariq, T. Almas, R. Saeed, S. Roomi, S. Haq, J. Madara, M. Boigon amd D. C. Haas, "Lymphocyteto-C-Reactive Protein Ratio: A Novel Predictor of Adverse Outcomes in COVID-19," *J. Clin. Med. Res.*, vol. 12, pp. 415–422, 2020.

[11] S. Paul, S. K. Ojha, S. Barui, S. Ghosh, M. Ghosh, B. Neogi and A. Ganguly, "Technical Advancement on Various Bio-Signal Controlled Arm: A Review," *J. Mech. Contin. Math. Sci.*, vol. 13, no. 2, pp. 16–30, 2018. https://doi.org/10.26782/jmcms.2018.06.00007

[12] S. P. S, M. Amanullah and K. Thirunavukkarasu, "A Hybrid Model for Meningitis Diagnostic Accuracy with Ensemble Learning: Combining Logistic Regression and L-BFGS," in *2025 Second International Conference on Cognitive Robotics and Intelligent Systems (ICC—ROBINS)*, Coimbatore, India, 2025, pp. 290–295. https://doi.org/10.1109/ICC-ROBINS64345.2025.11086348.

[13] M. Pal, R. Dey, R. A. Mahajan, M. Khan, A. A. Syed and S. Karimullah, "Edge Intelligence: Unique Machine Learning Strategies for Enhancing Real-Time IoT Data Processing," in *2025 International Conference on Quantum Photonics, Artificial Intelligence, and Networking (QPAIN)*, Rangpur, Bangladesh, 2025, pp. 1–5. https://doi.org/10.1109/QPAIN66474.2025.11171994.

[14] A. M. Abubakar, K. A. Abdulsalam and J. A. Adebisi, "Application of Artificial Neural Network for Diagnosis of Cerebrospinal Meningitis?" *J. Eng. Res.*, Special Edition, vol. 24, no. 2, pp. 12–25, 2019.

[15] P. Das, S. Paul, J. Ghosh, S. PalBhowmik, B. Neogi and A. Ganguly, "An Approach Towards the Representation of Sign Language by Electromyography Signals with Fuzzy Implementation," *Int. J. Sens. Wirel. Commun. Control*, vol. 7, no. 1, pp. 26–32, 2017. https://doi.org/10.2174/2210327907666170222093839

[16] S. P. Selvaraj, M. Amanullah and K. Thirunavukkarasu, "Advanced Meningitis Diagnostic Modeling: Combining Fuzzy Cognitive Maps and Decision Trees for Superior Predictive Performance," in *2025 International Conference on Emerging Technologies in Engineering Applications (ICETEA)*, Puducherry, India, 2025, pp. 1–6. https://doi.org/10.1109/ICETEA64585.2025.11100000.

[17] S. S. Priya, M. Amanullah and D. Mohanraj, "Enhancing SVM Classification of Meningitis with Feature-Adaptive Adagrad in CSF Analysis," in *2024 5th International Conference on Electronics and Sustainable Communication Systems (ICESC)*, Coimbatore, India, 2024, pp. 1109–1113. https://doi.org/10.1109/ICESC60852.2024.10689818.

[18] S. C. Rivera, X. Liu, A.-W. Chan, A. K. Denniston, M. J. Calvert, "Guidelines for Clinical Trial Protocols for Interventions Involving Artificial Intelligence: The SPIRIT-AI Extension," *BMJ*, vol. 370, 2020.

[19] Karina Zaccari and Ernesto Cordeiro Marujo, "Machine Learning for Aiding Meningitis Diagnosis in Pediatric Patients," *Int. J. Med. Health Sci.*, vol. 13, no. 9, 2019.

[20] Alexios-Fotios A. Mentis, et al., "Artificial Intelligence in Differential Diagnostics of Meningitis: A Nationwide Study," *Diagnostics*, vol. 11, p. 602, 2021. https://doi.org/10.3390/diagnostics11040602.

[21] D. Sampson, T. D. Yager, B. Fox, L. Shallcross, L. McHugh, T. Seldon, A. Rapisarda, R. B. Brandon, K. Navalkar and N. Simpson, "Blood Transcriptomic Discrimination of Bacterial and Viral Infections in the Emergency Department: A Multi-Cohort Observational Validation Study." *BMC Med.* vol. 18, no. 1, p. 185. https://doi.org/10.1186/s12916-020-01653-3

[22] X. Sáez-Llorens and G. H. McCracken, Jr., "Bacterial Meningitis in Children," *Lancet*, vol. 361, no. 9375, pp. 2139–2148, 2003.

[23] R. Koster-Rasmussen, A. Korshin and C. N. Meyer, "Antibiotic Treatment Delay and Outcome in Acute Bacterial Meningitis," *J. Infection*, vol. 57, no. 6, pp. 449–454, 2008.

[24] S. M. Lundberg, G. Erion, H. Chen, A. J. DeGrave, J. M. Prutkin, B. G. Nair, R. Katz, J. Himmelfarb, N. Bansal and S. Lee, "Explainable AI for Trees: From Local Explanations to Global Understanding,"*arXiv*. https://arxiv.org

[25] A. Wright, D. F. Sittig, J. S. Ash, J. Feblowitz, S. Meltzer, C. Mcmullen, K. Guappone, J. Carpenter, J. Richardson, L. Simonaitis, R. S. Evans, W. P. Nichol and B. Middleton, "Development and Evaluation of a Comprehensive Clinical Decision Support Taxonomy: Comparison of Front-End Tools in Commercial and Internally Developed Electronic Health Record Systems," *J. Amer. Med. Informat. Assoc.*, vol. 18, no. 3, pp. 232–242, 2011.

[26] G. Kong, D.-L. Xu and J.-B. Yang, "Clinical Decision Support Systems: A Review of Knowledge Representation and Inference Under Uncertainties," *Int. J. Comput. Intell. Syst.*, vol. 1, no. 2, p. 159, 2008.

[27] E. S. Berner, *Clinical Decision Support Systems: Theory and Practice*, Birmingham, UK: Springer, 2007.

[28] R. A. Greenes, *Clinical Decision Support: The Road Ahead*, New York: Academic, 2011.

[29] M. Glimåker, B. Johansson, M. Bell, M. Ericsson, J. Bläckberg, M. Brink, L. Lindquist and J. Sjölin, "Early Lumbar Puncture in Adult Bacterial Meningitis_Rationale for Revised Guidelines," *Scand. J. Infect. Dis.*, vol. 45, no. 9, pp. 657–663, 2013.

[30] A. Adadi and M. Berrada, "Peeking Inside the Black-Box: A Survey on Explainable Artificial Intelligence (XAI)," *IEEE Access*, vol. 6, pp. 52138–52160, 2018.

[31] J. S. Shirabad, S. Wilk, W. Michalowski and K. Farion, "Implementing an Integrative Multi-Agent Clinical Decision Support System with Open Source Software," *J. Med. Syst.*, vol. 36, no. 1, pp. 123–137, 2012.

[32] Ö. Yilmaz, R. C. Erdur and M. Türksever, "SAMS: A Systems Architecture for Developing Intelligent Health Information Systems," *J. Med. Syst.*, vol. 37, no. 6, p. 9989, 2013.

[33] D. Riaño, F. Real, J. A. López-Vallverdú, F. Campana, S. Ercolani, P. Mecocci, R. Annicchiarico and C. Caltagirone, "An Ontology-Based Personalization of Health-Care Knowledge to Support Clinical Decisions for Chronically Ill Patients," *J. Biomed. Inform.*, vol. 45, no. 3, pp. 429–446, 2012.

[34] E. Caballero-Ruiz, G. García-Sáez, M. Rigla, M. Villaplana, B. Pons, and M. E. Hernando, "A Web-Based Clinical Decision Support System for Gestational Diabetes: Automatic Diet Prescription and Detection of Insulin Needs," *Int. J. Med. Inform.*, vol. 102, pp. 35–49, 2017.

[35] K. Paydar, S. R. Niakan Kalhori, M. Akbarian and A. Sheikhtaheri, "Aclinical Decision Support System for Prediction of Pregnancy Outcome in Pregnant Women with Systemic Lupus Erythematosus," *Int. J. Med. Inform.*, vol. 97, pp. 239–246, 2017.

[36] M. Pereboom, I. J. Mulder, S. L. Verweij, R. T. Van Der Hoeven and M. L. Becker, "A Clinical Decision Support System to Improve Adequate Dosing of Gentamicin and Vancomycin," *Int. J. Med. Inform.*, vol. 124, pp. 1–5, 2019. Comput. (JVA), 2006.

17 Deep Learning Approaches for Autism Spectrum Disorder Detection

Performance Analysis and a Hybrid ViT–GNN Model

Nguyen Trong Tung, Do Nang Toan, Minh Quang Le, and Vinh Truong Hoang

17.1 INTRODUCTION

Autism spectrum disorder (ASD) is a neurodevelopmental disorder in which children with autism often have limited communication and interaction with their surrounding environment. The incidence of autism is increasing globally, and early detection of ASD has been shown to be a key factor in effective intervention, significantly improving the learning outcomes, behavior, and quality of life of autistic children. However, most autistic children are currently detected late, often after the age of three, which reduces the effectiveness of early intervention measures, leaving many consequences for children and their families [1] Although ASD is generally regarded as a lifelong condition, timely and appropriate interventions can substantially enhance developmental quotients, cognitive abilities, and language skills of affected children [2].

In recent years, the prevalence of ASD has been increasing. According to the WHO report, an estimated 1 in 44 children have ASD, and this number is increasing over time. However, the average age of autism detection is about 4 years old—beyond the golden time for early intervention—reducing the effectiveness of intervention and increasing social and family costs [3]. Studies show that the development of children with autism is influenced by both genetic and environmental factors; however, the exact cause has not yet been determined, and there is currently no medical test (such as a blood test) that can directly diagnose autism. ASD is a neurodevelopmental disorder with complex biological mechanisms and unclear etiology. The causes of ASD are thought to be multifactorial, including both genetic and environmental factors [4, 5]. Genetically, many studies have discovered gene variants related to neuronal synaptic function and brain development [6–8]. In addition, prenatal environmental factors such as viral infections, exposure to heavy metals, pesticides, air pollution, vitamin D deficiency, or immune disorders during pregnancy also contribute to the increased risk of ASD [9–11].

ASD is a complex neurodevelopmental disorder that affects cognitive, social, and behavioral functioning. One of the core features of ASD is a deficit in the ability to recognize emotions from facial expressions—a key element of social communication [12]. Children with autism may have difficulty with: recognizing basic emotions such as happiness, sadness, anger, and fear; recognizing complex emotions such as guilt, contempt, and disappointment; and recognizing fleeting or low-intensity expressions.

Currently, ASD screening mainly relies on questionnaires (such as M-CHAT and STAT), interviews, and behavioral observations. Although these methods are widely used, they are often subjective, time-consuming, and require high expertise. Therefore, many modern studies are focusing

DOI: 10.1201/9781003667360-17

on developing machine learning and deep learning models to detect autism through facial image analysis in order to increase accuracy and reduce social costs.

Traditional methods of diagnosing ASD rely heavily on behavioral observations and in-depth clinical assessments, which are often time-consuming and require a high level of expertise. In addition, in many areas, the shortage of experienced clinical staff has been a major barrier to early detection and intervention for children with ASD. This situation leads to delays in the diagnosis process, reducing the effectiveness of early intervention measures.

In this context, early diagnosis systems using artificial intelligence (AI) are emerging as a promising approach due to their ability to provide more objective, consistent, and reliable assessments. With the ability to process large amounts of behavioral and developmental data of children, AI models can detect latent patterns that are beyond human recognition, thereby improving accuracy and shortening diagnosis time. Currently, a number of automated diagnostic tools integrating deep learning and machine learning algorithms have been deployed or are in development, showing positive effects in supporting early screening for ASD. The application of AI in early diagnosis of ASD promises to bring significant benefits, contributing to improving the quality of life for autistic children and their families.

In summary, the diagnosis of ASD remains a complex and multidimensional process, as there is no single clinical or paraclinical test that can accurately identify the condition. Typically, the identification of ASD requires a combination of methods, including behavioral observations, developmental assessments, and the use of standardized screening tools administered by experts. In recent years, in addition to traditional methods, facial feature analysis has emerged as a promising approach due to its noninvasive nature. This method exploits facial abnormalities that are associated with ASD and, when integrated with deep learning models, can effectively support early screening, especially in resource-limited areas.

Convolutional neural networks (CNNs) have proven to be highly effective in image classification tasks, including ASD detection, due to their ability to extract complex features from large-scale image datasets. However, training a CNN from scratch requires large computational resources and is not suitable for limited datasets. Therefore, leveraging pretrained models through transfer learning is a more efficient solution. To ensure widespread applicability in ASD diagnosis, CNN architectures need to be optimized to maintain high accuracy while minimizing the number of hyperparameters and computational requirements.

In this study, we propose a model to detect autistic children through facial recognition, combining the ViT model and the graph neural network (GNN) network. The next part of the chapter includes related research, the proposed model, experimental results and comparison with existing models on the same dataset, and finally the conclusion.

17.2 RELATED WORK

Arumugam et al. [13] used convolutional neural networks to detect autistic children's faces based on a publicly available dataset from the Kaggle website, including 2,940 autistic and non-autistic images. The experimental results showed an accuracy of 91%. The author in [14] used two pretrained deep learning models, VGG16 and VGG19, on a 224 × 224 × 3pixel image dataset. The developed system, especially with the VGG19 model, outperformed all existing systems (88% accuracy) in this research context. Narala M et al. [15] proposed a CNN-based model using facial images for early detection of ASD in children. The model is built on the architecture of two popular pretrained deep learning models: ResNet50 and EfficientNet. The ResNet50 model achieved an accuracy of 84.50%. When comparing performance, the EfficientNet model showed higher accuracy (86%). The authors in [16] proposed a transfer learning (TL) method based on DenseResNet to improve the ability to recognize ASD through facial expression analysis. This method combines two powerful pretrained network architectures: DenseNet and ResNet. The study used data augmentation techniques such as rotation, translation, shearing, zooming, and horizontal flipping to minimize the overfitting problem and increase the number of training data samples from the limited dataset. The classification accuracy result is 97.07% on the research dataset. Author Jagadesh et al. in [17] proposed the EDLM-ASDDFI (ensemble of deep learning with crested porcupine optimizer-based autism spectrum disorder detection using facial images) model to identify the differences between facial images of individuals with ASD and typically developing individuals. The team used Gabor filtering (GF) to enhance facial features, Z-score normalization, Multitask convolutional neural network (MTCNN), median filter denoising, data augmentation to address class imbalance, and class weighting. Long short-term memory (LSTM) to capture sequential dependencies was used. The EDLM-ASDDFI model achieved an average accuracy of 96.43%. The computational time (CT) of EDLM-ASDDFI is as low as 0.94 seconds, showing superior computational efficiency compared to other methods. Research in [18] proposed an ASD detection method based on scan-path analysis, aiming to understand atypical visual attention patterns through dynamic changes in eye-gaze distribution. This facial dynamics complexity contains novel information not captured by traditional facial affect analyses. These findings suggest that computer vision analysis of facial landmark motion is a promising method for detecting and quantifying early behavioral symptoms associated with ASD [19]. In [20], the authors proposed the use of lower body movement data and a hybrid SVM-LDA approach to classify children with ASD, achieving an accuracy of up to 90%. Meanwhile, the team in [21] developed a computational model to classify individuals with ASD by analyzing photographs of their surrounding environment, aiming to capture attentional preferences toward objects. In [22], the authors employed content-based image retrieval (CBIR) by transitioning from traditional hand-crafted local features such as the Scale-Invariant Feature Transform (SIFT) to deep features learned via CNNs. While CNN-based features offer robust and high-level image representations, they often exhibit limitations in accurately identifying small overlapping regions within images, which is a critical requirement in tasks such as partial duplicate image detection. The author in [23] shows that children with ASD exhibit unique and highly distinct gaze patterns when compared to typically developing (TD) children; there are significant differences in attention span and vertical gaze distribution. Research by the group of authors [24] proposes an innovative CNN model based on Bayesian optimization for eye-tracking image discrimination. The authors in [25] have proposed that CNN networks are used to analyze brain images, as well as other data such as facial images, postures, and gestures. The VGG16 model, a popular CNN architecture, is used for image classification. In [26], the author's research found that head movement velocity, acceleration, and complexity were found to be significantly higher in toddlers with autism than in typically developing toddlers. Toddlers with autism demonstrated differences in head movement dynamics when viewing audiovisual stimuli. Higher head movement complexity indicated that their movements were less predictable and less stable than those of typically developing toddlers. In [27], research has demonstrated that computer vision analysis (CVA) is an effective tool for assessing attention and differentiating between autistic and typically developing children. Research results show significant differences in how autistic and typically developing children respond to videos with social and nonsocial content. In [28], a multimodal feature hybrid CNN method was proposed to distinguish between TD and ASD patients. The model uses variation in right and left pupil diameters of individuals and includes six stages: enhancement, spectrogram, image fusion, feature extraction, selection, and classification. The authors in [29] and colleagues proposed to test whether eye-tracking data from face-to-face conversations could classify children with ASD and TD. Khan et al. (2025) developed multimodal deep learning techniques for precise disease identification, establishing foundational strategies for integrating heterogeneous biomarkers essential for neurodegenerative diagnostics [30].

17.3 PROPOSED METHOD

In this study, we propose a hybrid architecture combining vision transformer (ViT) and GNN based on facial landmarks to detect ASD through children's facial images. Dey et al. (2025) engineered ML models fusing moving averages, RSI, and volume analysis for financial prediction, demonstrating temporal multi-signal processing principles applicable to progression tracking in neurological disorders [31]. Specifically, the ViT branch is used to extract global features from facial images, modeling the connections between image regions. The GNN branch extracts facial landmarks and organizes them into a graph (facial landmark graph). The nodes (vertices) contain information (coordinates, confidence), and local features from small image regions around each landmark extracted by a CNN network. This graph is then processed by GNN (using graph attention network—GAT) to learn the morphological relationships between important regions such as the eyes, mouth and nose. These points are recognized to be closely related to the characteristic manifestations of ASD. To combine information from the two branches, we use a cross-attention mechanism that allows ViT tokens to interact directly with embeddings from the GNN, helping the model focus on feature regions on the face. The overall architecture of the proposed hybrid ViT–GNN model is illustrated in Figure 17.1.

The Dlib 68-point model [32] is a robust facial landmarking standard that enables the extraction of key facial features such as the eyes, mouth, and nose, which are critical elements in the detection of ASD. The mapping of the 68 facial landmark points to their corresponding facial regions is summarized in Table 17.1.

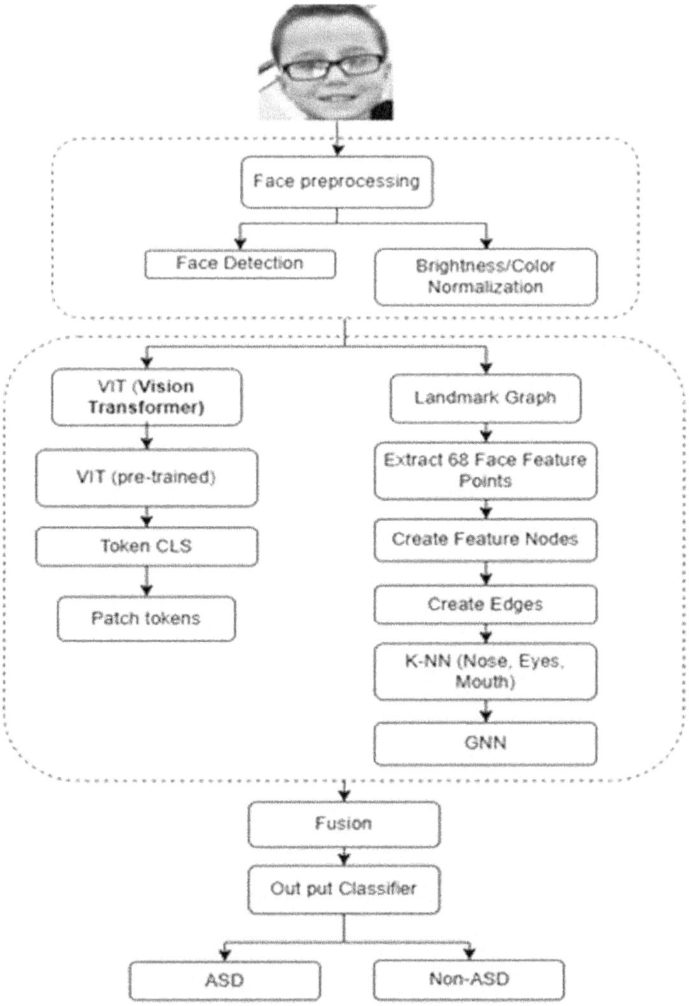

FIGURE 17.1 Architecture for autism detection through facial behavioral analysis (hybrid ViT–GNN)

TABLE 17.1
Standard mapping of facial feature regions

Facial Region	Range	Description
Jawline	0–16	From left to right along the chin
Left eyebrow	17–21	From the inner to the outer edge of the left eyebrow
Right eyebrow	22–26	Same pattern on the right eyebrow
Nose bridge	27–30	From between the eyebrows to the tip of the nose
Lower nose	31–35	Covers both nostrils and nose tip
Left eye	36–41	Six points surrounding the left eye
Right eye	42–47	Six points surrounding the right eye
Outer lip	48–59	Outer contour of the mouth
Inner lip	60–67	Inner contour of the mouth

17.4 FACIAL BEHAVIORAL FEATURE EXTRACTION

+ Eye Aspect Ratio

$$EAR = \frac{\| p_2 - p_6 \| + \| p_3 - p_5 \|}{2x\| p_1 - p_4 \|} \tag{1}$$

- p1 to p6 are the eye landmark points (based on Dlib 68 landmarks: 36–41 for the left eye, 42–47 for the right eye).
- Low EAR → eye is closed.
- High EAR → eye is open.
- Indicates level of attention or alertness.

+ Mouth Aspect Ratio

$$MAR = \frac{\| p_{51} - p_{59} \| + \| p_{53} - p_{57} \| + \| p_{49} - p_{55} \|}{2x\| p_{49} - p_{55} \|} \tag{2}$$

- High MAR → mouth is open (possibly smiling or speaking).
- Low MAR → mouth is closed.

+ Eyebrow Height

The distance from the midpoint of the eye to the midpoint of the eyebrow.

$$Height_{Eyebrow} = \sqrt{\left(x_{eye} - x_{eyebrow}\right)^2 + \left(y_{eye} - y_{eyebrow}\right)^2} \tag{3}$$

Where

- (x_eye, y_eye) is the average coordinate of the eye landmarks (left eye: points 36–41, right eye: points 42–47).
- $(x\_eyebrow, y\_eyebrow)$ is the average coordinate of the eyebrow landmarks (left eyebrow: points 17–21, right eyebrow: points 22–26).

+ Eyebrow Height Difference

To measure the level of symmetry between the two eyebrows.

$$Height\ diffence_{Eyebrow} = \left| Height_{Eyebrow\ left} - Height_{Eyebrow\ right} \right| \tag{4}$$

- If the height difference is close to 0 → eyebrows are well-symmetrical.
- If the height difference is large → possible facial asymmetry.

+ Eyebrow Curvature

Measured by the total distance between adjacent point pairs on the eyebrow.

$$Eyebrow\ Curvature = \sum_{i=0}^{n-2} \sqrt{(x_i - x_{i+1})^2 + (y_i - y_{i+1})^2} \tag{5}$$

- (x_i, y_i) and (x_{i+1}, y_{i+1}) are two consecutive landmark points on the eyebrow.
- High curvature → curved eyebrow (e.g., expression of surprise).
- Low curvature → straight eyebrow (e.g., neutral or tense state).

+ Symmetry

Individuals with autism may exhibit mild facial asymmetry compared to individuals without autism.

- Select symmetric left–right landmark pairs (e.g., points 36 and 45 for the eyes).
- Compute the Euclidean distance for each pair, then calculate the total or average.

$$Symmetry\ Score = Mean\left(\ point_{left} - mirror\left(point_{right}\right) \right) \tag{6}$$

17.5 APPLYING GNN NETWORK

The face is represented as a weighted, undirected graph **G = (V, E, W)**, where

V: is a set of vertices, each vertex **Vi** corresponds to a landmark.

E: is a set of edges, which are the connections between points, applying the K-NN algorithm on the landmark coordinate space.

W: is the edge weight matrix **wi,j**, defined according to the Euclidean distance between two landmarks. The adjacency matrix **A** is constructed so that

$$A_{ij} = \{w_{ij},\ if\ (i,j) \in E0, \quad else \tag{7}$$

17.6 CENTRALITY IN GRAPH THEORY

Centrality is a measure of the importance of each vertex (node) in a graph network based on the node's position in the network structure. In a graph representing a face (each node is a landmark: eyes, mouth, etc.), centrality helps us detect geometrically or behaviorally prominent pixels that may be related to autism signs.

Degree Centrality: Measured by the number of edges connected to a node.

High degree points are often highly connected locations, such as the middle of the lips or the middle of the eyes.

$$C_D(v) = \frac{degdeg(v)}{n-1} \tag{8}$$

In which deg(v) number of v;n is the total number of vertices.

Closeness Centrality: Measures how close a node is to all other nodes.

Node has high closeness; it easily spreads information, affecting the whole. It indicates which node is the "information intermediary." For example, a deviated eye region can significantly change the closeness of points around it.

$$C_C(v) = \frac{1}{\sum_{u\#v} d(v,u)} \tag{9}$$

In which $d(v,u)$ is the shortest distance between v and u.

Betweenness Centrality: Used to measure the degree to which a node lies on multiple shortest paths between other pairs of nodes.

Nodes with high betweenness may be important information "relay" locations in the facial structure. This formula helps identify important transition points—for example, the point between the eyes, the middle of the lips, and so on.

$$C_B(v) = \sum_{s\#v\#t} \frac{\partial_{st}(v)}{\partial_{st}} \tag{10}$$

In which ∂_{st} is the number of shortest paths from s to t; ∂_{st} is the number of shortest paths passing through v.

17.7 EXPERIMENTAL SETUP

17.7.1 Dataset

Autistic child facial data are downloaded from public sources at the following websites: https://www.kaggle.com/datasets/imrankhan77/autistic-children-facial-data-set?select=consolidated

The distribution of images across training, validation, and testing sets is presented in Table 17.2.

TABLE 17.2
T Class-wise distribution of the public autism facial image dataset

Category	Consolidated	Train	Test	Valid
Autism	1,468	1,268	150	50
Non-autism	1,468	1,268	150	50

17.7.2 Data Preprocessing

We preprocess the image using RetinaFace to detect facial features and bring the face to the correct pose using five-point alignment. All images are resized to 224 × 224 pixels; in addition, the images are also color-normalized to increase the ability to recognize under different lighting conditions. Mahajan et al. (2025) advanced generative AI and transfer learning for personalized IoT health monitoring, highlighting adaptive intelligence frameworks crucial for patient-specific neurodegenerative management [33].

We perform landmark extraction and build face graph. We use FaceAlignment to extract 68 landmark points for each face. Each landmark point is saved as a vector (x, y, conf). Landmark points are connected to form a facial landmark graph based on the natural morphological relationships between parts (eyes, nose, mouth). The facial landmark extraction process is shown in Figure 17.2.

17.7.3 Model Configuration and Training Parameters

The detailed configuration and training parameters of the proposed hybrid ViT–GNN model are summarized in Table 17.3.

The model is built according to a parallel two-branch architecture, including a vision transformer (ViT) branch to extract global features from facial images and a graph convolutional network (GCN) branch to process geometric features from 68 facial landmarks. Pal et al. (2025) introduced edge intelligence strategies for real-time IoT data processing, enabling low-latency computational pipelines vital for continuous neurological monitoring applications [34]. In the ViT branch, the input image of size 224 × 224 is divided into fixed patches, encoded into tokens, and appended with a special token [CLS] to obtain the global representation after passing through the transformer layers. In the GCN branch, the landmarks are normalized according to the image size, building a k-NN graph (k = 6) with enhanced connectivity according to each facial anatomical region (eyes, nose, mouth, jawline), then extracting embeddings through three GCN layers and global pooling. The outputs from the two branches are concatenated and passed through a multi-layer classifier (MLP) to predict ASD or Non-ASD labels. Paul et al. (2018) reviewed bio-signal controlled prosthetic arm technologies, providing insights into physiological signal decoding relevant for multimodal biomarker analysis in neural disorders [35].

17.7.4 Baselines and Ablation Studies

To validate the effectiveness of the proposed architecture, comparisons were made against:

1. Traditional Machine Learning Model (Logistic Regression, Random Forest, SVM, XGBoost, MLP Neural Net)

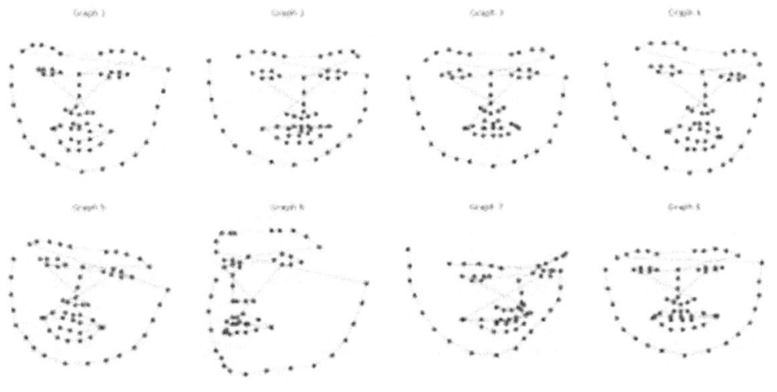

FIGURE 17.2 FaceAlignment to extract 68 landmark points for each face

TABLE 17.3
Model configuration and training parameters (hybrid ViT–GNN)

Parameter	Value	Description
Input image size	224 × 224	Input resolution for ViT branch
Model backbone (ViT)	ViT-Base Patch16 (pretrained)	Extracts global features from face images
Model backbone (GCN)	3-layer GCN (2 ->64 ->128 -> 256)	Extracts geometric features from facial landmarks
Number of facial landmarks	68	Points extracted using face alignment (FAN)
Graph construction	k-NN (k = 6) + anatomical region edges	Builds landmark graph structure
Fusion method	Concatenate [ViT_CLS, GCN_emb]	Combines features from both branches
Classifier head	MLP (512 ->128 -> 2)	Final classifier for ASD/Non-ASD
Loss function	Cross-Entropy (label smoothing = 0.05)	Training loss function
Data augmentation	Horizontal flip, ColorJitter, affine	Improves generalization via random transformations
Sampling strategy	Weighted Random Sampler	Balances training data between classes
Optimizer	AdamW	Optimization algorithm
Initial learning rate	3×10^{-5}	Starting learning rate
Learning rate schedule	Warm-up (2 epochs)—Cosine decay	Learning rate scheduling strategy
Weight decay	1×10^{-4}	Regularization to prevent overfitting
Batch size	16	Number of samples per training batch
Max epochs	30	Maximum number of training iterations
Early stopping patience	7 epochs	Stop if no improvement in validation F1
Precision mode	Mixed precision (AMP)	Speeds up training and reduces memory usage
EMA decay	0.999	Exponential Moving Average coefficient for model weights
Dataset split	Train: 75%, Val: 10%, Test: 15%	Proportion of dataset division

Dataset experimentation across models and comparative analysis

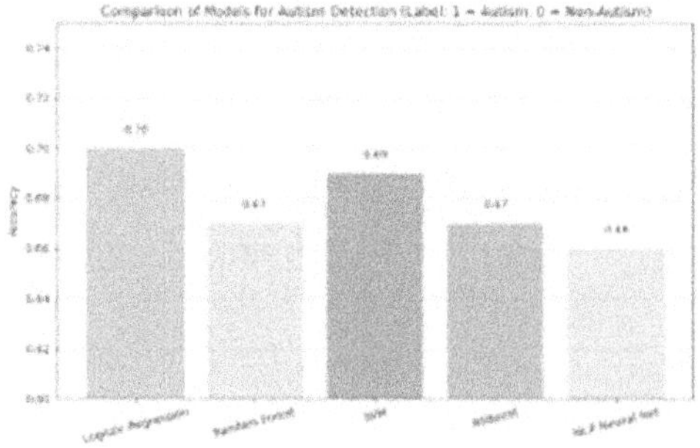

Model	Precision	Recall	F1-Score	Accuracy
Logistic Regression	0.704545	0.659574	0.681319	0.699482
Random Forest	0.664894	0.664894	0.664894	0.673575
SVM	0.701754	0.638298	0.668524	0.691710
XGBoost	0.682635	0.606383	0.642254	0.670984
MLP Neural Net	0.664773	0.622340	0.642857	0.663212

FIGURE 17.3 Experimental results of the dataset on traditional ML models

Logistic Regression achieved the highest performance (**70%** accuracy), outperforming all other models. This suggests that the extracted features (EAR, MAR, landmarks, etc.) may exhibit relatively good linear separability, or that logistic regression is effectively leveraging linear decision boundaries in the data. Das et al. (2017) implemented fuzzy logic-based EMG signal representation for sign language recognition, showcasing robust pattern recognition methods transferable to early motor dysfunction detection in neurodegeneration [36]. The **SVM** model produced a comparable result (**69%** accuracy), reaffirming its strength in binary classification tasks, especially when the data are well normalized. Both **random forest** and **XGBoost** reached the same accuracy level (**67%**), which is lower than that of logistic regression, indicating that decision trees and boosting techniques may not offer a significant advantage in this specific case. The performance of traditional machine learning models is presented in Figure 17.3. The **MLP neural net** model achieved the lowest accuracy (**66%**), possibly due to an insufficient number of training samples, a suboptimal network architecture, or the fact that the input features (EAR, MAR) do not require deep architectures to be effectively exploited. A direct accuracy comparison among ML models is illustrated in Figure 17.4.

The ROC curve (receiver operating characteristic curve) is a graphical representation of the performance of a binary classification model (in this case: ASD versus non-ASD) across different prediction thresholds. The ROC and precision–recall curves of the models are shown in Figure 17.5.

- **X-axis** (FPR): The proportion of non-ASD cases incorrectly classified as ASD.

$$\text{FPR} = \text{FP}/(\text{FP} + \text{TN}) \tag{7}$$

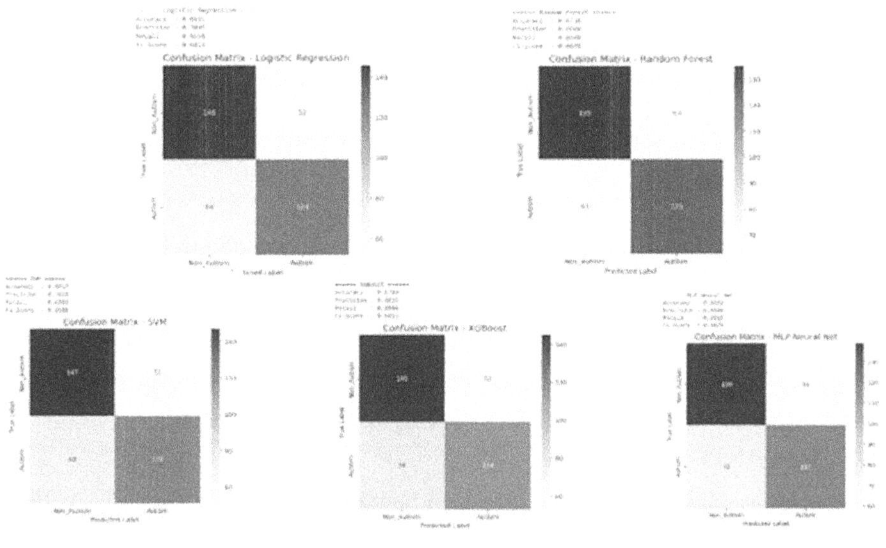

FIGURE 17.4 Accuracy of each ML model on the dataset

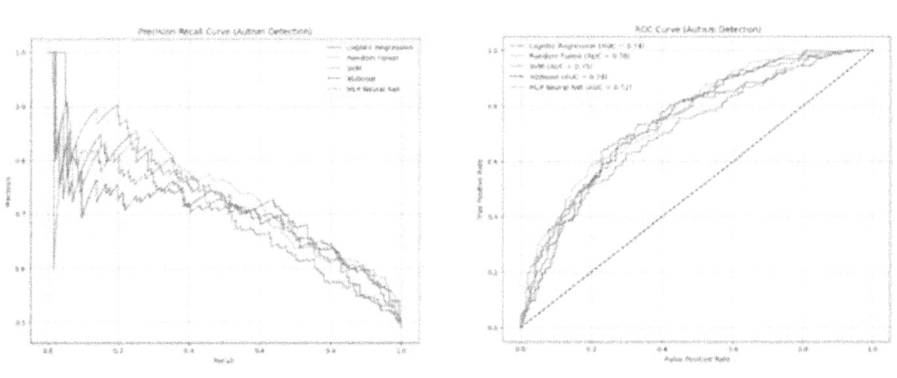

FIGURE 17.5 Performance comparison of models in autism detection (ROC and precision–recall curve)

- **Y-axis** (TPR): The proportion of ASD cases correctly classified as ASD.

$$TPR = TP/(TP + FN) = Recall \quad (8)$$

2. CNN-Only Backbone (EfficientNet-B0)

The classification performance of the EfficientNet-B0 backbone is illustrated in Figure 17.6.

[TEST] loss = 0.3015 | acc = 0.8600 | prec = 0.8333 | recall/sens = 0.9000 | spec = 0.9000 | f1 = 0.8654 | auc = 0.9441

3. ViT-Only Model

Figure 17.7 presents the performance of the vision transformer (ViT) model on the dataset.

[TEST] loss=0.4251 | acc=0.8600 | prec=0.8214 | recall/sens=0.9200 | spec= 0.9200 | f1=0.8679 | auc=0.9506

4. GNN-Only Model on Landmark Graphs

The standalone GNN model accuracy is shown in Figure 17.8.

5. ViT + GNN with Simple Feature Concatenation

The performance of the proposed hybrid ViT–GNN model is illustrated in Figure 17.9.

Test: {'loss': 0.2678, 'acc': 0.89, 'precision': 0.8726, 'recall': 0.9133, 'f1': 0.8925, 'auc': 0.958}

17.8 EXPERIMENTING THE DATASET ON EFFICIENTNET-B0, VIT, GNN AND VIT + GNN

A comparative performance evaluation of all machine learning and deep learning models is provided in Table 17.4.

17.9 CONCLUSION

In this study, we conducted a comparative analysis of multiple machine learning and deep learning methods for detecting ASD from facial images. Traditional machine learning models such as logistic regression, random forest, SVM, and XGBoost achieved average performance with accuracy values in the range of 0.66–0.70 and F1-scores in the range of 0.64–0.68. These results suggest that, although classical models can capture certain discriminative features, they are still limited in handling the complex nonlinear patterns present in ASD-related facial signals.

The deep learning-based models EfficientNet-B0 and ViT demonstrated superior performance, both achieving high precision (0.8600) and high recall values (0.90–0.92). These results show that modern ML architectures are capable of extracting facial features at scale and behavioral metrics relevant to ASD detection better.

The experimental results comparison table also shows that the proposed model combining ViT–GNN, with an accuracy of 0.8900, precision of 0.8726, recall of 0.9133, and F1-score of 0.8925, outperforms the other models, highlighting the benefits of integrating graph-based learning into the transformer architecture. Specifically, ViT excels at capturing global image-level representations, while GNN leverages

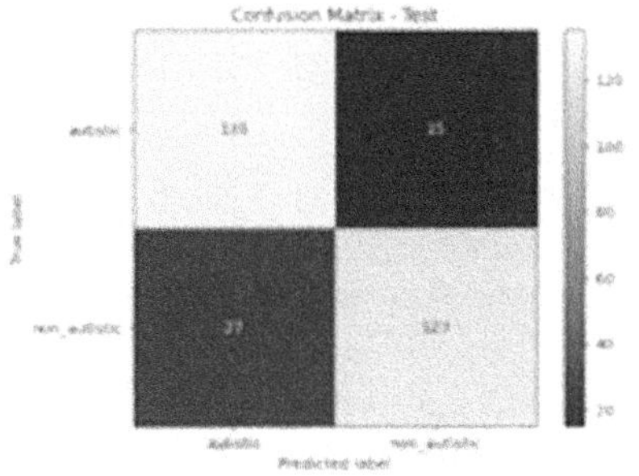

FIGURE 17.6 Accuracy of model EfficientNet-B0 on the dataset

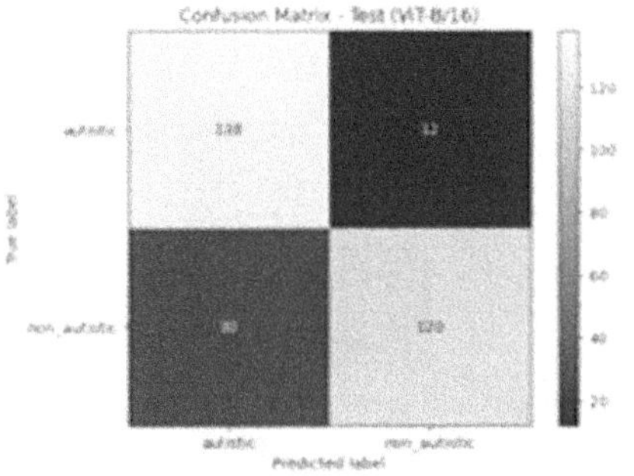

FIGURE 17.7 Accuracy of model vision transformer (VIT) on the dataset

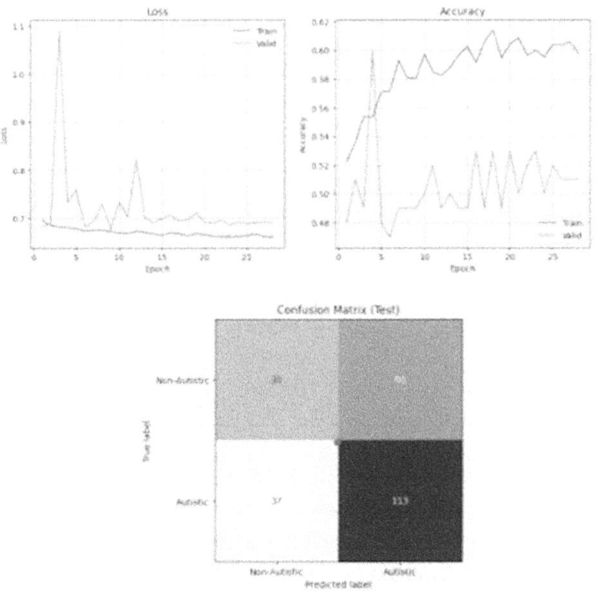

FIGURE 17.8 Accuracy of model GNN on the dataset

topological relationships between key facial landmarks (e.g., eye symmetry, mouth shape, and gaze patterns). The combination of these additional feature representations resulted in higher reliability, especially in terms of recall and F1-score, which are crucial for highly sensitive medical screening tasks.

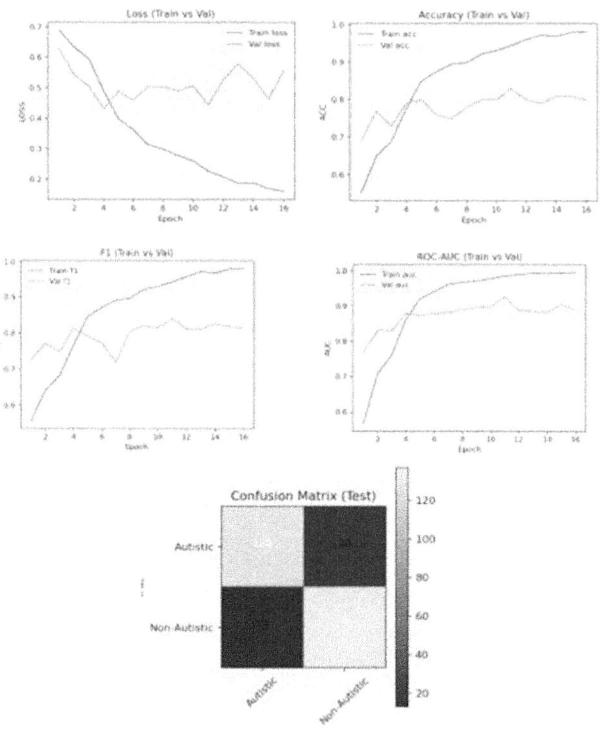

FIGURE 17.9 Accuracy of model ViT + GNN on the dataset

TABLE 17.4
Benchmarking performance of different architectures

Model	Accuracy	Precision	recall	f1-Score
Logistic regression	0.699482	0.704545	0.659574	0.681319
Random forest	0.673575	0.664894	0.664894	0.664894
SVM	0.691710	0.701754	0.638298	0.668524
XGBoost	0.670984	0.682635	0.606383	0.642254
MLP neural net	0.663212	0.664773	0.622340	0.642857
EfficientNet-B0	0.8600	0.8333	0.9000	0.8654
ViT	0.8600	0.8214	0.9200	0.8679
GNN-only model	0.5517	0.5612	0.5216	0.66666
ViT + GNN	0.8900	0.8726	0.9133	0.8925

The study has confirmed the potential of the hybrid architecture in advancing ASD detection research. Future directions will focus on optimizing this hybrid approach through the integration and deployment of larger-scale behavioral profiles on real-world web/mobile platforms to enable scalable early screening solutions.

REFERENCES

[1] J. C. Moreno, E. M. S. Morales, and E. P. Seller, 'Case Study of the Vulnerabilities That Children with Autism Spectrum Disorder Have in Education: The Importance of Early Detection', *Procedia Soc Behav Sci*, vol. 237, pp. 661–666, 2017, https://doi.org/10.1016/j.sbspro.2017.02.038.

[2] P. Pokhrel, S. Joshi, and L. Fatima, 'Artificial Intelligence in Autism Spectrum Disorder: A Path to Early Detection and Improved Outcomes', *Asian J Psychiatry*, vol. 129, p. 104530, 2025, https://doi.org/10.1016/j.ajp.2025.104530.
[3] S. Mitra, K. Srinath, V. Gowri Manohari, D. Poornima, and K. Karunya, 'Detection of Autism Using Artificial Intelligence', in *Lecture Notes in Networks and Systems*, 2023, https://doi.org/10.1007/978-981-99-6568-7_12.
[4] G. Tan, K. Xu, J. Liu, and H. Liu, 'A Trend on Autism Spectrum Disorder Research: Eye Tracking-EEG Correlative Analytics', *IEEE Trans Cogn Dev Syst*, vol. 14, no. 3, pp. 1232–1244, 2022, https://doi.org/10.1109/TCDS.2021.3102646.
[5] J. Han, G. Jiang, G. Ouyang, and X. Li, 'A Multimodal Approach for Identifying Autism Spectrum Disorders in Children', *IEEE Trans Neural Syst Rehabil Eng*, vol. 30, pp. 2003–2011, 2022, https://doi.org/10.1109/TNSRE.2022.3192431.
[6] P. S. Sundari, S. Pandey, R. Tiwari, R. Sarvaiya, K. S. Bharath, and B. Bhawana, 'An Investigation of the Role of Artificial Intelligence in the Diagnosis of Autism Spectrum Disease', in *2024 2nd International Conference Computational and Characterization Techniques in Engineering and Sciences, IC3TES 2024*, Institute of Electrical and Electronics Engineers Inc., 2024. https://doi.org/10.1109/IC3TES62412.2024.10877421.
[7] M. Kangarani-Farahani and J. G. Zwicker, 'Brain Functional Connectivity with Rehabilitation in Children with Co-Occurring Autism Spectrum Disorder and Developmental Coordination Disorder', *Res Autism*, vol. 120, p. 202531, 2025, https://doi.org/10.1016/j.reia.2025.202531.
[8] K. Chanyoung et al., 'AI-Assisted Initiation to Joint Attention Evaluation for Autism Spectrum Disorder Detection', in *Proceedings of the 2022 IEEE International Conference on Human-Machine Systems, ICHMS 2022*, Institute of Electrical and Electronics Engineers Inc., 2022. https://doi.org/10.1109/ICHMS56717.2022.9980778.
[9] M. Arora et al., 'Fetal and Postnatal Metal Dysregulation in Autism', *Nat Commun*, vol. 8, 2017, https://doi.org/10.1038/ncomms15493.
[10] P. Curtin et al., 'Dynamical Features in Fetal and Postnatal Zinc-Copper Metabolic Cycles Predict the Emergence of Autism Spectrum Disorder', *Sci Adv*, vol. 4, no. 5, 2018. https://www.science.org
[11] A. J. Goodrich et al., 'Joint Effects of Prenatal Air Pollutant Exposure and Maternal Folic Acid Supplementation on Risk of Autism Spectrum Disorder', *Autism Res*, vol. 11, no. 1, pp. 69–80, 2018, https://doi.org/10.1002/aur.1885.
[12] D. Tamizhmalar, S. Subbiah, and R. Premkumar, 'A Multimodal Diagnostic Framework for Autism Spectrum Disorder Using Deep Learning: An In-Depth Exploration', in *4th International Conference on Power, Energy, Control and Transmission Systems: Harnessing Power and Energy for an Affordable Electrification of India, ICPECTS 2024*, Institute of Electrical and Electronics Engineers Inc., 2024. https://doi.org/10.1109/ICPECTS62210.2024.10779999.
[13] S. R. Arumugam, R. Balakrishna, R. Khilar, O. Manoj, and C. S. Shylaja, 'Prediction of Autism Spectrum Disorder in Children using Face Recognition', in *Proceedings—2nd International Conference on Smart Electronics and Communication, ICOSEC 2021*, Institute of Electrical and Electronics Engineers Inc., 2021, pp. 1246–1250. https://doi.org/10.1109/ICOSEC51865.2021.9591679.
[14] B. Parvej, S. M. Mahbub Alam, F. I. Fahim, M. N. Pathan, and M. A. Rahaman, 'Computer Vision-based Interactive Autism Detection System using Deep Learning', in *2024 IEEE Conference on Computing Applications and Systems, COMPAS 2024*, Institute of Electrical and Electronics Engineers Inc., 2024. https://doi.org/10.1109/COMPAS60761.2024.10796046.
[15] M. S. V. S. K. Narala, S. Vemuri, and C. Kattula, 'A Comparative Study for Autism Spectrum Disorder Using EfficientNet, ResNet50', in *2023 International Conference on Computational Intelligence, Networks and Security, ICCINS 2023*, Institute of Electrical and Electronics Engineers Inc., 2023. https://doi.org/10.1109/ICCINS58907.2023.10450124.
[16] B. R. J and M. R, 'Enhancing the Identification of Autism Spectrum Disorder in Facial Expressions Using DenseResNet-Based Transfer Learning Approach', *Biomed Signal Process Control*, vol. 103, 2025, https://doi.org/10.1016/j.bspc.2024.107433.
[17] J. Balasubramani, S. Rajendran, M. Zakariah, and A. Alnuaim, 'Ensemble of Deep Learning with Crested Porcupine Optimizer Based Autism Spectrum Disorder Detection Using Facial Images', *Comput Mater Contin*, vol. 83, no. 2, pp. 2793–2807, 2025, https://doi.org/10.32604/cmc.2025.062266.
[18] W. Zhou, M. Yang, J. Tang, J. Wang, and B. Hu, 'Gaze Patterns in Children with Autism Spectrum Disorder to Emotional Faces: Scanpath and Similarity', *IEEE Trans Neural Syst Rehabil Eng*, vol. 32, 2024, https://doi.org/10.1109/TNSRE.2024.3361935.

[19] P. R. K. Babu et al., 'Exploring Complexity of Facial Dynamics in Autism Spectrum Disorder', *IEEE Trans Affect Comput*, vol. 14, no. 2, 2023, https://doi.org/10.1109/TAFFC.2021.3113876.

[20] S. Mohd Salah Aljabiri and M. M. Hamdan, 'Analyzing Lower Body Movements Using Machine Learning to Classify Autistic Children', *Biomed Signal Process Control*, vol. 94, p. 106288, 2024, https://doi.org/10.1016/J.BSPC.2024.106288.

[21] S. Chen and Q. Zhao, 'Attention-Based Autism Spectrum Disorder Screening with Privileged Modality', in *Proceedings of the IEEE International Conference on Computer Vision*, 2019. https://doi.org/10.1109/ICCV.2019.00127.

[22] N. H. H. Cuong, D. Van Thang, N. T. Tung, M. N. Tan, and N. T. T. Dien, 'SIFT Application Separates Motion Characteristics and Identifies Symbols on Tires', in *Smart Innovation, Systems and Technologies*, 2023. https://doi.org/10.1007/978-981-19-7513-4_1.

[23] S. Cheekaty and G. Muneeswari, 'Enhanced Multilevel Autism Classification for Children Using Eye-Tracking and Hybrid CNN-RNN Deep Learning Models', *Neural Comput Appl*, 2024, https://doi.org/10.1007/s00521-024-10633-0.

[24] S. Cheekaty and G. Muneeswari, 'Exploring Sparse Gaussian Processes for Bayesian Optimization in Convolutional Neural Networks for Autism Classification', *IEEE Access*, vol. 12, pp. 10631–10651, 2024, https://doi.org/10.1109/ACCESS.2024.3351168.

[25] D. Fernandez-Lanvin, M. Gonzalez-Rodriguez, J. De-Andres, and R. Camero, 'Towards an Automatic Early Screening System for Autism Spectrum Disorder in Toddlers Based on Eye-Tracking', *Multimed Tools Appl*, vol. 83, no. 18, pp. 55319–55350, 2024, https://doi.org/10.1007/s11042-023-17694-8.

[26] P. R. Krishnappa Babu et al., 'Complexity Analysis of Head Movements in Autistic Toddlers', *J Child Psychol Psychiatry*, vol. 64, no. 1, pp. 156–166, 2023, https://doi.org/10.1111/jcpp.13681.

[27] P. R. Krishnappa Babu et al., 'Blink Rate and Facial Orientation Reveal Distinctive Patterns of Attentional Engagement in Autistic Toddlers: A Digital Phenotyping Approach', *Sci Rep*, vol. 13, no. 1, p. 7158, 2023, https://doi.org/10.1038/s41598-023-34293-7.

[28] D. Çetintaş, T. Tuncer, and A. Çınar, 'Detection of Autism Spectrum Disorder from Changing of Pupil Diameter Using Multi-Modal Feature Fusion Based Hybrid CNN Model', *J Ambient Intell Humaniz Comput*, vol. 14, no. 8, pp. 11273–11284, 2023, https://doi.org/10.1007/s12652-023-04641-6.

[29] Z. Zhao, H. Tang, X. Zhang, X. Qu, X. Hu, J. Lu, 'Classification of Children with Autism and Typical Development Using Eye-Tracking Data From Face-to-Face Conversations: Machine Learning Model Development and Performance Evaluation', *J Med Internet Res*, vol. 23, no. 8, p. e29328, 2021, https://doi.org/10.2196/29328.

[30] M. Khan, R. A. Mahajan, R. Katukam, R. Dey, A. Rana and P. William, 'Smart Insights: Multimodal Deep Learning Techniques for Accurate Disease Identification', in *2025 International Conference on Quantum Photonics, Artificial Intelligence, and Networking (QPAIN)*, Rangpur, Bangladesh, 2025, pp. 1–5, https://doi.org/10.1109/QPAIN66474.2025.11171928

[31] R. Dey, S. Kassim, M. Khan, R. A. Mahajan and P. William, 'Smart Trading in NIFTY-50: ML with MA, RSI & Volume Analysis', in *2025 International Conference on Quantum Photonics, Artificial Intelligence, and Networking (QPAIN)*, Rangpur, Bangladesh, 2025, pp. 1–5, https://doi.org/10.1109/QPAIN66474.2025.11171705.

[32] V. Kazemi and J. Sullivan, 'One Millisecond Face Alignment with an Ensemble of Regression Trees', in *Proceedings of the IEEE Computer Society Conference on Computer Vision and Pattern Recognition*, 2014. https://doi.org/10.1109/CVPR.2014.241.

[33] R. A. Mahajan, R. Dey, M. Khan, M. M. Su'ud, M. M. Alam and P. Jadhav, 'Enhancing Personalization in IoT-Based Health Monitoring Via Generative AI and Transfer Learning', *Egypt Inform J*, 32, p. 100788, 2025. ISSN 1110-8665. https://doi.org/10.1016/j.eij.2025.100788. https://www.sciencedirect.com/science/article/pii/S1110866525001811

[34] M. Pal, R. Dey, R. A. Mahajan, M. Khan, A. A. Syed and S. Karimullah, 'Edge Intelligence: Unique Machine Learning Strategies for Enhancing Real-Time IoT Data Processing', in *2025 International Conference on Quantum Photonics, Artificial Intelligence, and Networking (QPAIN)*, Rangpur, Bangladesh, 2025, pp. 1–5. https://doi.org/10.1109/QPAIN66474.2025.11171994.

[35] S. Paul, S. K. Ojha, S. Barui, S. Ghosh, M. Ghosh, B. Neogi and A. Ganguly,'Technical Advancement on Various Bio-Signal Controlled Arm: A Review', *J Mech Contin Math Sci*, vol. 13, no. 2, pp. 16–30, 2018. https://doi.org/10.26782/jmcms.2018.06.00007

[36] P. Das, S. Paul, J. Ghosh, S. PalBhowmik, B. Neogi and A. Ganguly,'An Approach Towards the Representation of Sign Language by Electromyography Signals with Fuzzy Implementation', *Int J Sens Wirel Commun Control*, vol. 7, no. 1, pp. 26–32, 2017. https://doi.org/10.2174/2210327907666170222093839

18 Multimodal Fusion Attention Graph Neural Networks for Alzheimer's Dementia Detection

Nghia Dinh, Vinh Truong Hoang, Kiet Tran-Trung, Chatchai Kasemtaweechok, and Nindam Somsawut

18.1 INTRODUCTION

Alzheimer's disease (AD) and mild cognitive impairment (MCI) are the primary causes of dementia in the world. The main distinction between AD and MCI is the progressive loss of memory and cognitive function. In the United States, AD-related mortality jumped over 145% between 2000 and 2019 [1]. Additionally, in 2021, over 11 million individuals offered more or less 16 billion hours of unpaid care to AD patients, worth USD 271.6 billion [1]. Worldwide, AD will impact 152 million individuals by 2050, and the economic burden is estimated at 2 trillion USD [2]. In spite of a lot of research effort, no curative treatments are available, primarily because AD has a complex pathogenesis [3]. Therefore, early diagnosis, as well as timely intervention, continue to be really important.

AD typically divides its clinical course into three major phases: cognitively normal (CN), MCI, and AD. As the disease advances, we can observe significant brain differences in all three groups, as well as a decrease in brain mass, as shown in Figure 18.1.

The diagnosis is based primarily on neuroimaging and neuropsychological assessments. Probably the most frequently used clinical tools for assessing disease severity are the clinical dementia rating (CDR), as well as the Mini-Mental State Examination (MMSE). Neuroimaging is now a crucial component of AD diagnosis due to the rapid advancement of medical imaging. The distinction between gray matter and white matter is made with fine detail in magnetic resonance imaging (MRI), while molecular tracers in positron emission tomography (PET) indicate changes in glucose metabolism and lesion distribution. The diagnosis is more accurate when these modalities provide complementary information. Khan et al. (2025) presented a unified hybrid model integrating statistical, kernel-based, and neural approaches for cardiovascular risk prediction, establishing principles for multimodal feature fusion that are fundamental to attention-based graph neural networks in Alzheimer's detection [4].

Deep learning improvements within the last couple of years have permitted computer-aided diagnosis of AD (CAD) [5, 6]. The majority of existing techniques utilize unimodal imaging, which compromises diagnostic accuracy due to insufficient information. As a result, multimodal imaging has gained even more interest, and several deep learning-based multimodal feature fusion frameworks have been created [7, 8]. There are four primary types of methods that can be classified: methods based on raw images, generated images, fused images, blended clinical and neuroimaging data.

Raw image-based techniques specifically feed multimodal neuroimaging information in preprocessed or raw form into multibranch neural networks for feature integration via latent representation learning [9, 10]. These are relatively simple techniques but involve a large number of parameters and often do not take into account cross-modal interactions. Rather, image-based fused

DOI: 10.1201/9781003667360-18

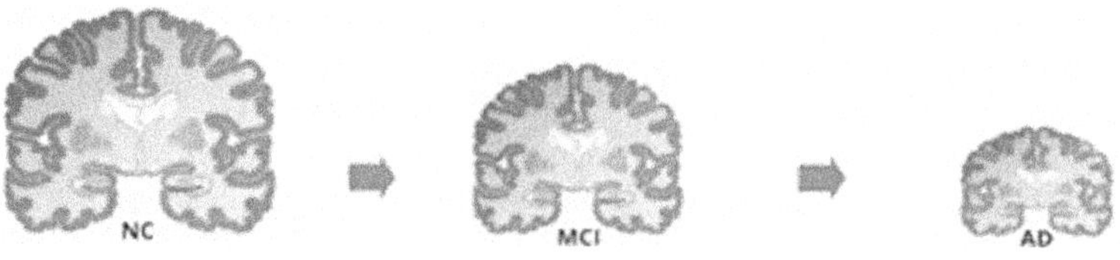

FIGURE 18.1 The progress of Alzheimer's disease in the brain

methods incorporate salient information from multiple modalities in a single composite image prior to model training, which requires fewer parameters but much more preprocessing and computational overhead. Generated image-based techniques make use of generative models such as generative adversarial networks (GANs) to address missing data from available modalities when there is insufficient modality availability. However, synthetic medical images continue to be challenging to quantify. Thirdly, neuroimaging-clinical data fusion techniques combine imaging information with clinical characteristics that mirror the diagnostic practice of physicians. They can be helpful but require extensive preprocessing and are unable to extract discriminative features from large genomic datasets. The author reviewed bio-signal controlled prosthetic arm technologies, offering insights into physiological signal integration applicable to multimodal graph construction for capturing Alzheimer's-related neural communication disruptions [11].

Local pattern capture has been shown to be very good with convolutional neural networks (CNNs). But their convolutional architecture usually constrains feature learning to nearby brain regions and not to spatially distant ones. That is a limitation because AD-related abnormalities may involve several noncontiguous brain areas [12]. Vision Transformers (ViTs) with self-attention mechanisms model long-range dependencies without hierarchical convolutional layers. Many scientific studies have confirmed ViTs for AD classification tasks [13]. However, token redundancy is not sufficiently considered in numerous versions.

For multimodal fusion methods, the majority of present ones ignore low-level features and simply merge high-level data. Higher resolution and deeper spatial details of low-level characteristics are required to identify AD. Also, regular pipelines have distinct feature extraction and feature fusion as individual phases that prevent cross-modal interactions and constrain learning of shared representations. On the flip side, research indicates that cross-modal interaction enables much more multimodal information to be integrated and improves diagnostic performance [14].

Herein, we present a Multimodal Fusion Attention Graph Network dependent on Graph Attention Networks (GATs) to overcome these issues. The framework provides an explanation of AD progression combining structural MRI and functional PET information to capture morphological, in addition to molecular, brain changes. It learns interregional associations across modalities while preserving neighborhood detail by combining graph-based relational modeling and hierarchical feature extraction. Furthermore, the attention mechanism of GAT weights connections in such a manner that multimodal fusion is encouraged and prediction is more precise. This makes the technique helpful for tracking disease progression and reliable for early AD analysis. Das et al. (2017) implemented fuzzy logic-based EMG signal representation for sign language recognition, showcasing robust feature extraction techniques relevant to attention-weighted graph neural processing of noisy multimodal dementia biomarkers [12].

18.2 RELATED WORK

Recently developed deep learning has allowed automatic identification of AD from neuroimaging modalities such as PET, computed tomography (CT), and MRI. Of these, the two most common imaging modalities remain MRI and PET: metabolic and molecular abnormalities are seen on PET (FDG- or amyloid-based tracers), and MRI shows structural atrophy. Current research explores a range of deep learning models, including CNNs, transformers, hybrid architectures, and graph neural networks.

18.2.1 MRI-Based Approaches

In MRI studies, we often use 3D CNNs and attention-enhanced models. In a detailed evaluation [13] of CNN architectures for AD classification, 3D CNNs outperform 2D approaches in the ADNI dataset. The results show that deeper networks with residual connections can better capture subtle structural changes. Similarly, Tan et al. [14] and Qiu et al. [15] trained an interpretable deep learning framework that classified six pathways at different AD stages, with Grad-CAM visualizations indicating the model trained on clinically relevant regions such as the hippocampus and temporal lobes. Generative models are also used to improve classification performance. Magnetic resonance studies taken together show that CNN and CNN-transformer hybrids, sometimes with attention or dense connections, perform better than 90% on AD classification tasks. Khan et al. (2025) developed multimodal deep learning techniques for accurate disease identification, providing foundational strategies for attention mechanisms that weigh critical neural connections in GNN architectures for dementia diagnosis [16].

18.2.2 PET and Multimodal Approaches

Deep learning using PET data exploits functional and metabolic modifications in AD. Direct classification of FDG and amyloid-PET images has been carried out with the aid of CNNs, and multimodal fusion (MRI + PET) frequently improves performance. Lu et al. [8] introduced a multi-scalable and multimodal deep neural network that processes MRI and FDG-PET separately just prior to fusion, achieving ADNI classification of AD versus CN with 91.8% accuracy. Additionally, Zhang et al. [8] used joint feature representation using multimodal classification with PET and MRI characteristics, which was superior to single-modal approaches. Venugopalan et al. [7] applied a multimodal deep learning model that was trained using PET, MRI, and clinical data, and the mixed modalities identified AD stage with 94% accuracy, surpassing unimodal baselines. Khan et al. (2025) empirically analyzed machine learning-driven trading strategies for BSE blue-chip stocks, demonstrating advanced algorithmic pattern recognition transferable to graph-based modeling of brain connectivity networks in Alzheimer's pathology [17].

18.2.3 Transformer-Based Models

AD neuroimaging also uses self-attention mechanisms. They were inspired by Vision Transformers [18] for use in medical imaging. Vaswani et al. [19] originally proposed the Transformer architecture, adapted for 3D medical image analysis. Transformer-based models have been demonstrated to capture longer-range relationships in brain imaging data with better interpretability, by competitive performance and attention visualization compared to CNN-based methods. They show that local and global disease patterns can be captured by hybrid CNN-Transformer models and ViTs.

18.2.4 Graph Neural Networks and Multimodal Fusion

In AD research, relational structures have been modeled using GNNs in recent years. Parisot et al. [20] initially applied GCNs to AD prediction in population graphs where subjects are nodes, as well as edges that symbolize imaging or non-imaging characteristic similarity. For three-way classification (AD, MCI, and CN), their model was 69.3% accuracy. Huang et al. [21] extended this to edge-variational GCNs that model uncertainty in graph construction. The theoretical foundations [22] were the basis for semi-supervised GCNs, now well established in medical imaging applications. The review of GNN applications by Li et al. [23] shows brain network changes were imaged in neuroimaging. Together, these GNN-based strategies show that imaging, clinical, and network-based data can be combined to improve AD stage classification. Mahajan et al. (2025) advanced generative AI and TL for personalized IoT health monitoring, highlighting adaptive intelligence methods essential for pretraining GNNs on heterogeneous multimodal dementia datasets [24].

18.2.5 Performance Trends

In retrospective studies, the results are generally better with multimodal approaches. Neuroimaging-based AD classification: a systematic review by Rathore et al. [25], it is shown that multimodal methods have 10–15% higher precision than unimodal methods on average. Deep learning models performed better than traditional machine learning methods. CNNs were 85–95% accurate for AD classification against CN and 75–85% for MCI, AD, and CN classification, respectively. Attention mechanisms in combination with graph-based modeling allow recent models to be more than 90% accurate even in multi-class problems. Importantly, most studies use cross-validation or an internal holdout set, with little external validation.

18.2.6 Open Datasets and Reproducibility

Important for progress have been public neuroimaging datasets. Over 2,000 participants have received longitudinal magnetic resonance and PET data from the Alzheimer's disease neuroimaging initiative [26]. The OASIS project consists of open-access MRI scans of CN as well as demented individuals. Reproducible research, as well as fair comparison of techniques, has been made possible by standardized datasets. More and more research organizations share code and pretrained models.

18.3 DATASET

PET and MRI are essential tools for the study and medical training of AD and provide complementary views of molecular and structural changes before clinical signs. Noninvasive, high-resolution evaluation of brain atrophy, cortical thinning, and ventricular enlargement, particularly memory-related lesions of the hippocampus, is possible with MRI. MRI is a robust tool for tracking disease progression when utilized in conjunction with sophisticated computational techniques due to its reproducibility and suitability for longitudinal analysis. In comparison, PET detects AD-specific molecular signatures such as amyloid-β plaques, glucose hypometabolism, and tau tangles. In spite of tracer dependence as well as scarcity problems, subtypes such as amyloid-PET, tau-PET, and FDG-PET play a crucial role in differential assessment and early diagnosis of dementias. The combination of PET and MRI is a potent multimodal tool for earlier AD detection, monitoring, and diagnosis, but both are not universally applicable in neurodegenerative conditions.

Imaging data were derived from ADNI [26], a public-private partnership established in 2003 to develop clinical, imaging, and genetic biomarkers for early AD detection and monitoring. The selection of 766 participants from ADNI1/GO and ADNI2 magnetic resonance as well as PET scans was done according to established preprocessing procedures. It consisted of 214 AD patients, 226 mild

TABLE 18.1
The clinical data information.

Diagnosis	Quantity	Age	Gender (F/M)	MMSE	CDR
AD	214	75.1 ± 7.8	95/119	21.2 ± 4.1	0.9 ± 0.4
MCI	226	76.0 ± 7.4	82/144	25.6 ± 4.3	0.5 ± 0.3
CN	326	76.1 ± 6.4	165/161	28.7 ± 1.4	0.0 ± 0.0

cognitive impairment patients, and 326 CN controls. NIfTI format was used to present T1-weighted MRI as well as FDG-PET images for each participant. The study population is described in Table 18.1 by its clinical and demographic features, including age, CDR scores, and MMSE scores.

MRI scans were conducted on three scanners: Philips, Siemens, and GE Medical Systems. Acquisition parameters of the T1-weighted MRI were:

- Scanner 1 (Siemens): echo time (TE) = 3.5 ms, repetition time (TR) = 3000 ms, inversion time (TI) = 1000 ms, slice thickness = 1.2 mm, flip angle = 8°, field strength = 3.0 T, and matrix size = 192 × 192 × 160.
- Scanner 2 (GE): TE = 3.036 ms, TR = 7.332 ms, TI = 400 ms, slice thickness = 1.2 mm, flip angle = 11°, matrix size = 256 × 256 × 196, field strength = 3.0 T.
- Scanner 3 (Philips): TE = 3.116 ms, TR = 6.8005 ms, TI = 0 ms, slice thickness = 1.2 mm, flip angle = 9°, matrix size = 256 × 256 × 170, field strength = 3.0 T.

More ADNI acquisition protocols are available publicly on the ADNI site [26].

18.4 PROPOSED METHOD

The proposed multimodal framework (Figure 18.2) combines functional information with structural information from PET along with MRI to help in early AD detection. PET and MRI images

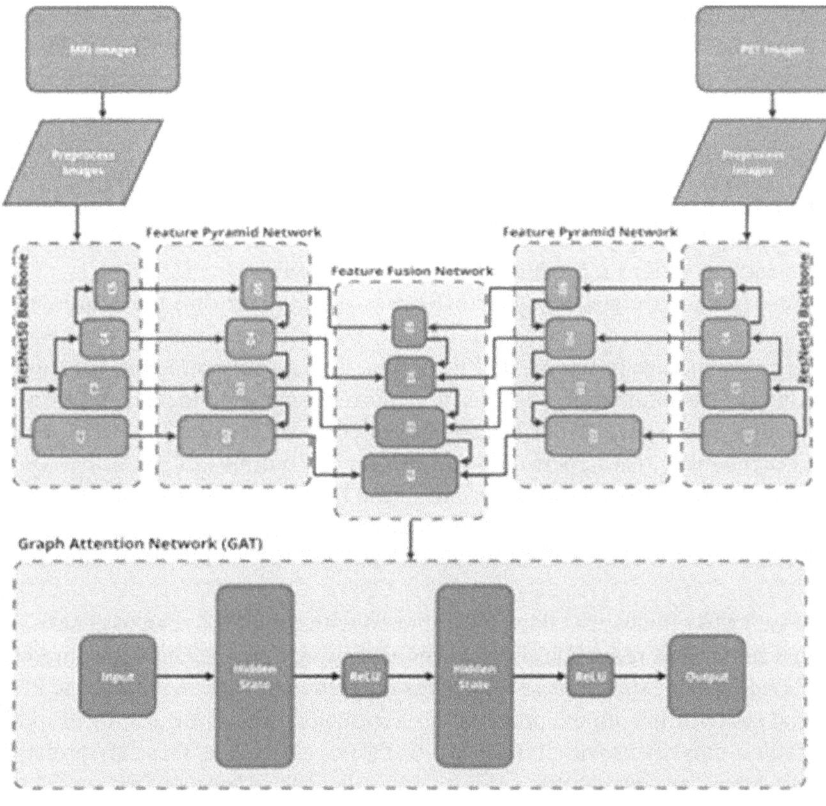

FIGURE 18.2 Proposed MFAG-Net framework. MRI and PET images are separately processed and encoded by ResNet-FPN modules. Multimodal embeddings are produced by the feature fusion network (FFN), performing cross-attention-based fusion across scales. Then, a graph attention network (GAT) builds interregional dependencies to produce node-and subject-level predictions for Alzheimer's dementia classification.

are standardized at the preprocessing stage through resizing, intensity normalization, and noise reduction to achieve consistent data quality and comparability across modalities. Each modality is passed by way of a ResNet50 backbone [27] independently to obtain hierarchical convolutional feature representations from several stages, C4, C3, and C2, along with C5. These representation maps show abstractions from extremely superficial levels of structural detail to far greater levels of semantic context.

Multi-scale features are represented by the feature pyramid network (FPN) [28] following each backbone. In the FPN top-down process, higher-level features are gradually upsampled and linked to equivalent lower-level features by lateral connections. Each lateral connection performs a 1 × 1 convolution on the lower-level feature map to ensure dimensional alignment before performing element-wise addition with the higher-level upsampled feature map. The result is D2–D5 multi-scale features, which blend semantic richness with spatial accuracy to identify pathological patterns at various brain resolutions. The feature fusion network (FFN) is made up of combining features coming from the two branches of the FPN, MRI as well as PET. At E2–E5, the FFN performs cross-modal fusion, capturing complementary representations of the modalities. The multimodal image could combine structural abnormalities seen on MRI with metabolic changes seen on PET. The network receives both anatomical and functional information by way of multimodal integration, which is crucial for early detection of neurodegenerative diseases.

Last but not least, improved multimodal functions are modeled by the graph attention system (GAT) [29]. At this point, features are transformed into nodes on a graph, and edges record inter-feature relationships. Self-attention mechanisms are utilized by GAT to assign weight to more useful nodes as well as connections in order to record cross-modal interactions and network dependencies of functional and structural brain characteristics. Graph-space modeling of all these dependencies reveals subtle dispersed biomarkers typical of early Alzheimer's dementia. The final predictive step toward early diagnosis, as well as classification of AD development, is the output of the GAT.

18.4.1 Image Preprocessing

A standardized preprocessing pipeline derived from Suk et al. was used to process all raw MRI as well as PET images [5]. It was pipelined utilizing ANTs and the FMRIB Software Library (FSL) to guarantee consistency as well as reproducibility across modalities.

The spatial and intensity consistency of MRI was maintained through a number of phases of preprocessing. The acpcdetect tool was utilized to perform anatomical alignment by shifting the center of each raw picture to the AC-PC line. Bias field correction using N4 (nonparametric non-uniform intensity normalization) was used to correct scanner-induced intensity variations. The Brain Extraction Tool (BET) from FSL was applied to excise non-brain tissues such as the skull, dura, and cerebellum. An expert then examines each output to ensure that all extraneous tissue has been removed and that good brain extraction has been achieved. All MRI images have been recorded in the exact same template space with ANTs for spatial normalization after tissue isolation. Voxel-wise correspondence between subjects was made more convenient by this arrangement.

The preprocessed MRI image was flawlessly aligned with each PET scan to enable intra-subject multimodal registration. The reduction of high-frequency noise by the Gaussian smoothing kernel improved signal quality. The Med2Image utility was utilized to transform volumetric PET and MRI data into 2D axial slices following the procedure. Each subject was given 181 slices to extract. Just like in earlier studies, only slices with indices 80–100 were retained, as these are probably the most useful entire brain areas for AD diagnosis. All retained slices have been resized to 224 × 224 pixels to conform to deep learning principles.

The preprocessing pipeline standardized PET and MRI modalities, decreased inter-scanner variability, and identified discriminative brain areas to obtain high-quality multimodal inputs for feature extraction and predictive modeling downstream.

18.4.2 Feature Extraction

Before cross-modal fusion, feature extraction will independently get modality-specific representations from PET along with MRI using the proposed framework. It preserves and represents functional and structural biomarkers of Alzheimer's dementia at various abstraction levels.

18.4.2.1 ResNet Backbone for Hierarchical Feature Learning

Both PET and MRI modalities are prepared utilizing a ResNet50 backbone [27], which utilizes residual learning to allow highly effective instruction of deep convolutional architectures. A residual block may be expressed as follows:

$$y_l = \mathcal{F}\left(x_l, \{W_l\}\right) + x_l \tag{1}$$

where x_l and y_l are the input and output of the l-th block, respectively, and $F(\cdot)$ is a residual function (a sequence of convolution, batch normalization, and ReLU). The identity shortcut x_l enables gradients to propagate directly, staying away from the issue of disappearing gradients and facilitating convergence in deep networks. The ResNet50 backbone generates a hierarchy of feature maps by way of four convolutional phases:

$$\{C_2, C_3, C_4, C_5\} = ResNet50(I) \tag{2}$$

where I is an input image from MRI or PET. Each stage catches more abstract features:

- C2: Fine structural and functional details (textures, edges, and local uptake variations).
- C3: Intermediate patterns with moderate semantic content.
- C4: High-level contextual features (regional atrophy or metabolic decline).
- C5: Global representations of hypometabolism or large-scale degeneration.

They correspond to hippocampal atrophy, cortical thickness, and ventricular enlargement for MRI inputs. For PET inputs, these are localized as well as distributed tracer uptake patterns linked to Alzheimer's pathology.

18.4.2.2 Feature Pyramid Network for Multi-scale Representation

ResNet features encode a semantic hierarchy. However, deeper layers lose spatial resolution, and lower layers lose semantic richness. The FPN [28] is used by each branch to link top-down information with lateral connections for this purpose. Let $\varphi(C_i)$ denote a 1×1 convolution used to stage C_i for channel alignment, and let Up(·) represent 2×upsampling. The fusion process could be characterized by the following expression:

$$D_5 = \varphi(C_5),\ \ D_i = \varphi(C_i) + Up(D_{i+1}),\ \ i \in \{4,3,2\} \tag{3}$$

The final multi-scale feature pyramid is $\{D_2, D_3, D_4, D_5\}$, where each D_i integrates the semantic abstraction of the deeper layers together with the spatial information of the shallower layers.

18.4.2.3 Modality-Specific Multi-scale Representations

The ResNet-FPM pipeline is used to process MRI and PET independently, resulting in two sets of multi-scale features $\{D^{MRI}_2, D^{MRI}_3, D^{MRI}_4, D^{MRI}_5\}$ and $\{D^{PET}_2, D^{PET}_3, D^{PET}_4, D^{PET}_5\}$:

- Functional biomarkers encoded in the PET branch include markers for focal hypometabolism as well as dispersed metabolic conditions.

- The MRI branch encodes structural biomarkers ranging from localized cortical thinning to large-scale neurodegeneration.

These multi-scale, modality-distinct characteristics provide a strong and complementary foundation for multimodal fusion, residual feature merging, and graph-based attention modeling in subsequent stages.

18.4.3 Feature Fusion

The FFN employs a cross-attention-based feature fusion method to model explicit inter-modality dependencies between MRI and PET feature maps, incorporating a more context-aware and fine-grained fusion as opposed to concatenation or summation methods. On each scale *i*, the extracted features from the MRI and PET backbone, denoted $D^{MRI}{}_i$ and $D^{PET}{}_i$, are projected into the query, key, and value spaces through learnable linear transformations. The MRI features are converted to key-value pairs for PET in a query matrix, as well as vice versa, and every modality takes notice of the other:

$$Q_i^{MRI} = D_i^{MRI} W_{MRI}^{Q},\ K_i^{PET} = D_i^{PET} W_{PET}^{K},\ V_i^{PET} = D_i^{PET} W_{PET}^{V} \tag{4}$$

$$Q_i^{PET} = D_i^{PET} W_{PET}^{Q},\ K_i^{MRI} = D_i^{MRI} W_{MRI}^{K},\ V_i^{MRI} = D_i^{MRI} W_{MRI}^{V} \tag{5}$$

where W^Q, W^K, and W^V are the projection matrixes specific to the modality learned during training. Using these projections, the fused embedding at scale *i* is obtained via bidirectional cross-attention:

$$E_i = softmax\left(\frac{Q_i^{MRI} K_i^{PETT}}{\sqrt{d}}\right) V_i^{PET} + softmax\left(\frac{Q_i^{PET} K_i^{MRIT}}{\sqrt{d}}\right) V_i^{MRI} \tag{6}$$

where *d* will be the feature dimensionality that stabilizes the dot-product similarity. The very first term enriches MRI features with semantically appropriate PET features, and the other with structurally accurate MRI cues. To catch many more different intermodal relationships, multi-head cross-attention is utilized, in which several sets of (Q, K, V) projections are discovered together. The output of each head is concatenated and transformed linearly, resulting in a final fused representation:

$$E_i = Concat\left(E_i^{(1)}, E_i^{(2)}, \ldots, E_i^{(h)}\right) W^O \tag{7}$$

with *h* denoting the amount of attention heads and *WO* the output projection matrix. By executing this operation across several feature scales (E_2, E_3, E_4, E_5), the FFN creates a hierarchy of fused embeddings that incorporate both functional and structural information in a complementary manner. It is a cross-attention-based fusion that allows the model to dynamically align modality-specific signals, spotlight probably the most useful regions, and create discriminative multimodal representations for downstream modules such as Graph Attention Networks (GAT) for classification, as well as lesion detection and anomaly localization jobs in medical imaging.

18.4.4 Detection and Classification

The multiple-scale fused embeddings $\{E_2, E_3, E_4, E_5\}$ are delivered to a GAT for relational reasoning as well as classification after feature fusion. The fused MRI-PET representations are converted into a group of nodes that correspond to a spatial region or patch embedding of every fused feature map E_i. The k-nearest neighbors (k-NN) strategy is used to construct an adjacency matrix *A* for relationships between nodes, leading to every node having *k* most similar nodes in feature space.

Formally, for nodes u and v, the pairwise Euclidean distance is computed as:

$$\mathcal{D}(u,v) = \| x_u - x_v \|_2 \tag{8}$$

where x_u and x_v are the feature vectors of nodes u and v. The edges are established based on the k neighboring nodes having the smallest values of $D\ (u,\ v)$ for every node u. Consequently, the sparse adjacency matrix is generated as:

$$A_{uv} = \begin{cases} 1, if\ v \in kNN(u) \\ 0, otherwise \end{cases} \tag{9}$$

K-NN guarantees that every node has exactly k neighbors (except possible ties) and, therefore, avoids overly dense connections that may occur with distance thresholding. It catches essentially the most semantically useful relationships while maintaining the graph's computational productivity.

After the graph $G = (V, E)$ is built, the GAT does masked self-attention to understand about neighboring nodes. For a certain node i, the interest coefficient with neighbor j is computed as follows:

$$\alpha_{ij} = \frac{exp(LeakyReLU(a^T [Wh_i \| Wh_j]))}{\Sigma_{k \in \mathcal{N}(i)} exp(LeakyReLU(a^T [Wh_i \| Wh_k]))} \tag{10}$$

where h_i is the feature of node i, W is a learnable transformation matrix, $\|$ is concatenation, and N(i) is the k-nearest neighbors of node i. Its node representation is then updated by aggregating its neighbors with these attention weights:

$$h'_i = ReLU\left(\Sigma_{j \in \mathcal{N}(i)} \alpha_{ij} W h_j\right) \tag{11}$$

The GAT has three stacked layers. During the first two layers, node embeddings are refined with local and non-local neighborhood information. The last layer is node-level classification, with each node embedding h'_i projected into a probability distribution over diagnostic categories (AD or non-AD):

$$\hat{y}_i = softmax\left(W_c h'_i + b_c\right) \tag{12}$$

where W_c and b_c are the classifier parameters, and $\hat{y}_i$ are the class probabilities for node i.

Because every node represents a localized area of the fused MRI-PET representation, node-level predictions create an analysis map of which regions are labeled as AD. Node-level predictions are pooled to obtain an ultimate diagnosis at the subject level by an attention-based pooling read-out function:

$$h_G = \Sigma_{i \in \mathcal{V}} \beta_i h'_i, \quad \beta_i = \frac{exp\left(q^T tanh\left(W_p h'_i\right)\right)}{\Sigma_{j \in \mathcal{V}} exp\left(q^T tanh\left(W_p h'_j\right)\right)} \tag{13}$$

where W_p and q are trainable parameters that assign attention weights β_i to each node. The graph embedding h_G is thus a subject-level summary concentrating on probably the most useful regions of the human brain. Within the last, fully connected level of h_G is triggered by the softmax activation for subject-level prediction:

$$\hat{y}_{subj} = softmax\left(W_s h_G + b_s\right) \tag{14}$$

where W_s and b_s are the classifier parameters at the subject level, and $\hat{y}_{subj}$ is the probability of AD or non-AD.

This particular design utilizes k-NN adjacency construction for subject graph topology with node-level predictions and subject-level aggregation for fine-grained interpretability and a powerful worldwide diagnosis.

18.5 EXPERIMENTS

The experimental setup is described in this section, and the performance evaluation metrics are reported.

18.5.1 Experiment Setup

The system was an AMD EPYC 7401P having 24 cores at 2.0 GHz with 128 GB system memory as well as 12 GB dedicated video memory on an NVIDIA GeForce RTX 3060 GPU. The computer was running Ubuntu 22.04 LTS. The combination of low memory and high throughput allowed for balanced execution of computationally demanding deep learning jobs making use of this setup. The available GPU resources were sufficient for high-resolution image processing, model training, and inference tasks, while the big RAM was sufficient for intermediate and large computations.

18.5.2 Metrics

Precision, specificity, and sensitivity were calculated to quantitatively evaluate the performance of the proposed method for AD diagnosis:

$$Accuracy = \frac{TP + TN}{TP + TN + FP + FN} \tag{15}$$

$$Specificity = \frac{TN}{TN + FP} \tag{16}$$

$$Sensitivity = \frac{TP}{TP + FN} \tag{17}$$

where *TP*, *TN*, *FP*, and *FN* are true positives, true negatives, false positives, and false negatives, respectively.

Besides, AUC-ROC was also used as an evaluation criterion. AUC is the average of all classifier discriminative abilities, where higher values indicate better classification performance.

18.6 RESULT ANALYSIS

18.6.1 Model Efficiency

Regarding all diagnostic tasks, the multimodal approach (MRI + PET) always outperforms unimodal strategies, as shown in Table 18.2. Multimodal fusion is superior to MRI (93.85% and 93.59% PET) and PET (92.87% and 93.71%) for the classification of AD versus CN (94.64% AUC and 95.81%). Multimodal integration once again yields substantial performance improvements of 94.42% and 95.57% when compared with unimodal PET and MRI in more challenging AD versus MCI as well as CN versus MCI tasks, respectively. Multimodal learning maintains a 94.72% accuracy as well as a 95.86% AUC advantage in the three-class classification scenario (AD versus CN versus MCI). They demonstrate that MRI can serve as a discriminative tool in the diagnosis of AD,

TABLE 18.2
Classification results of unimodal and multimodal methods

Auxiliary Diagnosis	Modality	ACC (%)	SEN (%)	SPE (%)	AUC (%)
AD vs CN	MRI	93.85	92.71	94.37	93.59
	PET	92.87	88.69	94.82	93.71
	MRI + PET	94.64	94.13	96.34	95.81
AD vs MCI	MRI	92.32	89.51	93.23	93.74
	PET	91.33	86.03	93.31	93.23
	MRI + PET	94.42	91.35	95.63	95.21
CN vs MCI	MRI	91.32	89.13	94.27	93.37
	PET	91.36	90.61	91.54	92.23
	MRI + PET	95.57	94.37	96.62	95.76
AD vs CN vs MCI	MRI	91.31	89.54	93.82	93.84
	PET	91.33	89.29	93.29	93.24
	MRI + PET	94.72	94.62	95.34	95.86

TABLE 18.3
Comparison of classification results with existing methods.

Tasks	Methods	ACC (%)	SEN (%)	SPE (%)	AUC (%)
AD vs CN	[17]	93.97	93.54	94.36	95.57
	[12]	93.76	93.12	94.47	94.03
	MFAG (ours)	94.64	94.13	96.34	95.81
AD vs MCI	[17]	87.74	90.31	91.22	89.25
	[11]	93.44	90.91	95.52	94.36
	MFAG (ours)	94.42	91.35	95.63	95.21
CN vs MCI	[17]	87.24	93.43	88.33	89.51
	[12]	83.72	85.98	79.91	81.75
	MFAG (ours)	95.57	94.37	96.62	95.76
AD vs CN vs MCI	MFAG (ours)	94.72	94.62	95.34	95.86

and that combining PET with MRI further enhances the ability to differentiate MCI from other organizations.

18.6.2 Comparison With Other Methods

The proposed MFAG technique outperforms all other recognized diagnostic tasks across classification tasks, as shown in Table 18.3. For AD versus CN, MFAG offers the greatest overall performance, with 94.13% sensitivity, 96.34% specificity, 94.64% accuracy, and 95.81% AUC, outperforming [17, 12]. With 91.35% sensitivity, 95.63% specificity, and 94.42% precision, and 95.21% AUC over [11, 17], MFAG once more emerges as the clear winner inthe AD versus MCI classification. MFAG has superior performance compared with previous methods for CN and MCI, with 94.37% sensitivity, 96.62% specificity, and 95.57% precision, as well as 95.76% AUC, respectively, while [17, 12] yield significantly worse results. Only MFAG creates results with 94.62% sensitivity, 95.34% specificity, and 94.72% accuracy, as well as 95.86% AUC in the more challenging three-class classification (AD versus CN versus MCI). The results indicate that MFAG has better diagnostic capability and is highly robust in detecting AD, MCI, and CN.

18.7 DISCUSSION AND LIMITATIONS

The proposed MFAG framework outperforms the existing techniques for classification of AD, moderate cognitive impairment, and cognitively typical individuals, according to the results. MFAG combines multimodal neuroimaging information with attention-guided feature fusion to gather complementary information out of multiple modalities to enhance sensitivity and specificity and diagnostic accuracy. It regularly outperforms unimodal methods, enabling the integration of structural functional information into strong auxiliary diagnosis. The strong performance on binary and three-category classification tasks suggests that MFAG could be a valuable tool for earlier diagnosis as well as disease staging, where AD, MCI, and CN differentiation is crucial.

Regardless of the immense potential, there are limitations that must be recognized. The experimental assessment was initially carried out on a single dataset, which might restrict generalizability of results to various other populations in addition to medical settings. Next, MFAG is highly precise but depends upon the quality as well as availability of multimodal data. In the real world, we might not be able to obtain complete MRIs as well as PET scans for each patient, which might reduce their clinical value. Third, the framework requires huge computational resources for training, possibly limiting its application to low-resource healthcare. Furthermore, while the attention mechanism facilitates interpretability by determining modality contributions, the model as a whole is a deep learning system whose clinical decision-making is not always transparent to providers. Future work is going to attempt to link algorithmic performance as well as attention-guided graph reasoning to actual medical adoption.

18.8 CONCLUSION

MFAG, a multimodal fusion attention-guided network, was presented as an additional diagnosis for AD in this chapter. An attention-based feature fusion technique fuses PET and MRI modalities together and, along with MFAG, makes use of complementary information to enhance diagnostic performance. MFAG consistently outperforms current multimodal and unimodal techniques when it comes to sensitivity, specificity, and reliability, as well as AUC in experiments conducted on both three-class and binary classification tasks. The results indicate that MFAG is an effective and reliable tool for detecting as well as assessing AD for medical treatment. MFAG is going to be extended to larger and much more diverse populations in the future, and lightweight adaptations for clinical settings and improved interpretability will help with medical practice decision-making.

REFERENCES

[1] Alzheimer's Association. (2022). 2022 Alzheimer's. *Alzheimer's & Dementia*, 18(4), 700–789.
[2] Patterson, C. (2018). *World Alzheimer*. Alzheimer's Disease International.
[3] Liu, M., Cheng, L., Qian, K., Wang, J., Wang, J., & Liu, Y. (2020). Attention-based deep ensemble net for large-scale online taxi-hailing demand prediction. *Nature Reviews Neurology*, 16(9), 501–518.
[4] Khan, M., Mahajan, R. A., Sivakumar, N. R., Gulhane, M., Rakesh, N., Dey, R., Uddin, M. S., & Basheer, S. (2025). A unified hybrid model for cardiovascular risk prediction: Merging statistical, kernel-based and neural approaches. *Journal of Cellular and Molecular Medicine*. https://doi.org/10.1111/jcmm.70797
[5] Suk, H.-I., Lee, S.-W., & Shen, D. (2015). Latent feature representation with stacked auto-encoder for AD/MCI. *Brain Structure and Function*, 220(2), 841–859.
[6] Ebrahimighahnavieh, M. A., Luo, S., & Chiong, R. (2020). Deep learning to detect Alzheimer's. *Computer Methods and Programs in Biomedicine*, 187, 105242.
[7] Venugopalan, J., Tong, L., Hassanzadeh, H. R., and Wang, M. D. (2021). Multimodal deep learning models for early detection of Alzheimer's. *Scientific Reports*, 11(1), 3254.
[8] Zhang, D., Wang, Y., Zhou, L., Yuan, H., and Shen, D. (2011). Multimodal classification of Alzheimer's. *NeuroImage*, 55(3), 856–867.
[9] Lu, D., Popuri, K., Ding, G. W., Balachandar, R., and Beg, M F. (2018). Multimodal and multiscale deep neural networks for the early diagnosis of Alzheimer's. *Scientific Reports*, 8(1), 5697.
[10] Liu, M., Zhang, J., Adeli, E., and Shen, D. (2019). Joint classification and regression via deep multi-task multi-channel learning for Alzheimer's. *IEEE Transactions on Biomedical Engineering*, 66(5), 1195–1206.

[11] Paul, S., Ojha, S. K., Barui, S., Ghosh, S., Ghosh, M., Neogi, B., and Ganguly, A. (2018). Technical advancement on various bio-signal controlled arm: A review. *Journal of Mechanics of Continua and Mathematical Sciences*, 13(2), 16–30. https://doi.org/10.26782/jmcms.2018.06.00007

[12] Das, P., Paul, S., Ghosh, J., PalBhowmik, S., Neogi, B., and Ganguly, A. (2017). An approach towards the representation of sign language by electromyography signals with fuzzy implementation. *International Journal of Sensors, Wireless Communications and Control*, 7(1), 26–32. https://doi.org/10.2174/2210327907666170222093839

[13] Wen, J., Thibeau-Sutre, E., Diaz-Melo, M., and Samper-González, J. (2020). Convolutional neural networks for classification of Alzheimer's. *Medical Image Analysis*, 63, 101694.

[14] Tan, H., and Bansal, M. (2019). LXMERT: Learning cross-modality encoder representations from transformers. In *Proceedings of the 2019 Conference on Empirical Methods in Natural Language Processing and the 9th International Joint Conference on Natural Language Processing (EMNLP-IJCNLP)*, pp. 5100–5111. Association for Computational Linguistics. https://doi.org/10.18653/v1/D19-1514

[15] Qiu, S., Joshi, P. S., Miller, M. I., Xue, C., Zhou, X., Karjadi, C., Chang, G. H., Joshi, A. S., Dwyer, B., and Zhu, S. (2020). Development and validation of an interpretable deep learning framework for Alzheimer's. *Brain*, 143(6), 1920–1933.

[16] Khan, M., Dey, R., Kassim, S., Mahajan, R. A., Ghosh, A., and William, P. (2025). Machine learning-driven trading strategies: An empirical analysis of BSE blue-chip stocks using advanced algorithmic approaches. In *2025 International Conference on Quantum Photonics, Artificial Intelligence, and Networking (QPAIN)*. Rangpur, Bangladesh, pp. 1–5. https://doi.org/10.1109/QPAIN66474.2025.11171797.

[17] Khan, M., Mahajan, R. A., Katukam, R., Dey, R., Rana, A., and William, P. (2025). Smart insights: Multimodal deep learning techniques for accurate disease identification. In *2025 International Conference on Quantum Photonics, Artificial Intelligence, and Networking (QPAIN)*. Rangpur, Bangladesh, pp. 1–5. https://doi.org/10.1109/QPAIN66474.2025.11171928

[18] Dosovitskiy, A., Beyer, L., Kolesnikov, A., Weissenborn, D., Zhai, X., Unterthiner, T., Dehghani, M., Minderer, M., Heigold, G., and Gelly, S. (2021). An image is worth 16x16 words: Transformers for image recognition at scale. *arXiv preprint arXiv:2010.11929.*

[19] Vaswani, A., Shazeer, N., Parmar, N., Uszkoreit, J., Jones, L., Gomez, A. N., Kaiser, L., and Polosukhin, I. (2023). Attention is all you need. *arXiv:1706.03762.*

[20] Parisot, S., Ktena, S. I., Ferrante, E., Lee, M., Guerrero, R., Glocker, B., and Rueckert, D. (2018). Disease prediction using graph convolutional networks: Application to Autism Spectrum Disorder and Alzheimer's disease. *Medical Image Analysis*, 48, 117–130. https://doi.org/10.1016/j.media.2018.06.001.

[21] Huang, Y., and Chung, A. C. (2020). Edge-variational graph convolutional networks for uncertainty-aware disease prediction. *ArXiv*. https://arxiv.org/abs/2009.02759.

[22] Kipf, T. N., and Welling, M. (2016). Semi-supervised classification with graph convolutional networks. *ArXiv*. https://arxiv.org/abs/1609.02907.

[23] Li, X., Zhou, Y., Dvornek, N., Zhang, M., Gao, S., Zhuang, J., Scheinost, D., Staib, L. H., Ventola, P., and Duncan, J. S. (2021). BrainGNN: Interpretable brain graph neural network for fMRI analysis. *Medical Image Analysis*, 74, 102233. https://doi.org/10.1016/j.media.2021.102233.

[24] Mahajan, R. A., Dey, R., Khan, M., Su'ud, M. M., Alam, M. M., and Jadhav, P. (2025). Enhancing personalization in IoT-based health monitoring via generative AI and transfer learning. *Egyptian Informatics Journal*, 32, 100788. ISSN 1110-8665. https://doi.org/10.1016/j.eij.2025.100788. https://www.sciencedirect.com/science/article/pii/S1110866525001811

[25] Rathore, S., Habes, M., Iftikhar, M. A., Shacklett, A., and Davatzikos, C. (2017). A review on neuroimaging-based classification studies and associated feature extraction methods for Alzheimer's disease and its prodromal stages. *NeuroImage*, 155, 530. https://doi.org/10.1016/j.neuroimage.2017.03.057.

[26] Petersen, R. C., Aisen, P. S., Beckett, L. A., Donohue, M. C., Gamst, A. C., Harvey, D. J., Jack, C. R. Jr, Jagust, W. J., Shaw, L. M., Toga, A. W., Trojanowski, J. Q., and Weiner, M. W. (2010). Alzheimer's disease neuroimaging initiative (ADNI): Clinical characterization. *Neurology*, 74(3), 201–209. https://doi.org/10.1212/WNL.0b013e3181cb3e25.

[27] He, K., Zhang, X., Ren, S., and Sun, J. (2015). Deep residual learning for image recognition. *ArXiv*. https://arxiv.org/abs/1512.03385.

[28] Lin, T., Dollár, P., Girshick, R., He, K., Hariharan, B., and Belongie, S. (2016). Feature pyramid networks for object detection. *ArXiv*. https://arxiv.org/abs/1612.03144.

[29] Veličković, P., Cucurull, G., Casanova, A., Romero, A., Liò, P., and Bengio, Y. (2017). Graph attention networks. *ArXiv*. https://arxiv.org/abs/1710.10903.

19 Advancements in Magnetic Resonance Imaging Aimed at Alzheimer's Assessment, Lung Cancer Identification, Characterization, and Staging

An In-Depth Analysis

Shaik Karimullah and Balajee Maram

19.1 INTRODUCTION

Lung cancer remains to be the leading reason of cancer-related death globally because of a late-stage diagnosis and limited handling options in the advanced stages. Standard imaging methods, such as computed tomography (CT) and positron emission tomography (PET/CT), are essential for detecting and staging lung cancer but involve exposure to ionizing radiation and have relatively high false-positive rate, particularly among high-risk individuals. MRI allows us to spot lung cancer without exposure to radiation and has better contrast for soft-tissue structures to visualize primary tumors and metastatic sites. Recent advances in MRI, such as ultra-short resonance time sequences, diffusion-weighted imaging, and low-field MRI, have increased the usage of MRI in imaging of the lung. In conjunction with MRI advancements, artificial intelligence (AI) and machine learning algorithms have improved detection and classification accuracy of nodules, and subsequently more easily identified malignancy early-on. Even more recently, new targeted contrast agents have increased the conspicuity of lesions, especially in the more early stages of lung cancer. Challenges, however, still remain with MRI, including limited resolution of smaller nodules, susceptibility to motion artifacts, and standardization of scan protocols. This review summarizes 20 studies (2010–2024) to summarize the diagnostic performance of MRI, identify emerging techniques and methods, and assess its clinical applicability in the discovery, characterization, and impact of lung cancer.

Figure 19.1 depicts an expedited workflow to detect lung cancer via the use MRI. The workflow begins with high-resolution MRI scans of the lungs, which serve as the primary input for the analysis. The scans undergo a process of image processing, where important features (e.g., tumor shape, size, and texture) are highlighted and extracted for further analysis. Next, the processed images are input into a classification model, most often a machine learning or deep learning network, which assesses the important extracted features to determine a pattern, which may suggest malignancy. In the end, the system produces a decision that tells the clinical user whether the found lesion is cancerous or benign for critical support in the early diagnosis, and ultimately clinical decision, for lung cancer.

 DOI: 10.1201/9781003667360-19

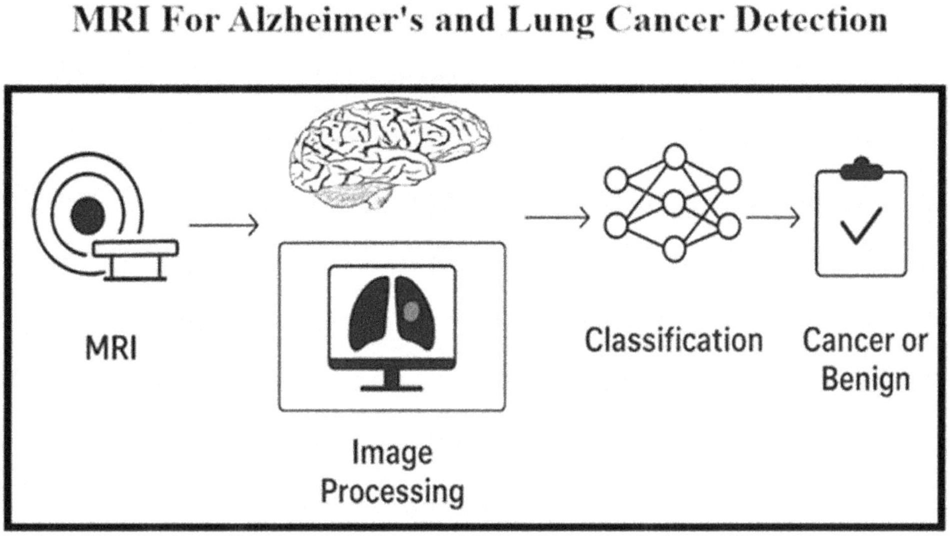

FIGURE 19.1 Block diagram for lung cancer diagnosis with MRI

19.2 RECENT CONTRIBUTIONS

MRI is emerging as a promising imaging method for the diagnosis, detection, and staging of lung cancer using high tissue contrast and without radiation. Betkar et al. [1] demonstrate the efficacy of a unified hybrid model that combines statistical and neural approaches, providing a robust framework for high-accuracy medical risk prediction Khan, M. et al. [2] directed a narrative literature review in 2024 that appraised how MRI compares with other imaging modalities in the diagnosis and detection of lung cancer. In their review, they noted MRI could detect.

Lesions ≥3 mm in size, and while MRI has high sensitivity for larger nodules, CT has superior sensitivity for smaller nodules, arguing that complementary imaging is critical. [2] discusses the application of advanced algorithmic approaches in complex data environments, highlighting the versatility of machine learning in identifying patterns within high-stakes datasets. [3] further emphasized the need for imaging modalities beyond CT through their examination of advanced MRI methods, illustrating efficacy for lung cancer screening, successfully demonstrating fewer false-positive rates and lower radiation exposure, while also highlighting some drawbacks (e.g., susceptibility artifacts and low proton density). [4] conducted a retrospective analysis of more than 11,000 asymptomatic patients, studying whole-body MRI using T2-weighted HASTE and SE-3D VIBE sequences in patients undergoing lung cancer screening, reporting a review of primary lung cancer detection rate of 0.4% and a diagnostic procedure time of <10 minutes, which may potentially enhance overall institutional efficiency in diagnostic delivery. [5] utilize multimodal deep learning techniques to enhance disease identification accuracy, a strategy that is critical for integrating the diverse data types often found in medical diagnostics. [6] included image processing with analysis of liquid biopsy through data stemming from imaging including CT, X-ray and MRI, and showed greater performance, suggesting further weight to consideration of multimodal methods. [7] investigate the intersection of generative AI and TL to personalize IoT-based health monitoring, offering a pathway for continuous, individualized patient observation. [8] evaluated MRI along with PET/MRI for lung cancer staging and found equivalent accuracy compared to PET/CT. Advanced MRI sequences improved TNM assessment, and optimization was noted as important to improve the chances of clinical application. We saw this carried out in a prospective trial by [9], which provides an extensive review of bio-signal controlled systems, establishing the foundational technical advancements necessary for interpreting physiological data in neurological contexts [10], which evaluated UTE, T1 VIBE, and T2 HASTE MRI sequences in comparison to baseline CT. They demonstrated that MRI could precisely identify solid and ground-glass pulmonary nodules sized > 4mm, while UTE and HASTE outperformed VIBE. [11] introduce a fuzzy implementation for interpreting electromyography signals, showcasing how signal processing and soft computing can bridge the gap between raw biological data and clinical insights. [12] also considered 0.55T MRI as an alternate imaging modality, demonstrating the capacity to visualize common lung pathologies and possibly increase tissue characterization, but still noted decreased resolution as a limitation. [13] established a role for MRI characterization of solid nodules and TNM staging as a complement to CT in order to improve the planning of therapy. [14] conducted a screening study in high-risk populations comparing MRI and LDCT and found that MRI was able to detect nodules ≥ 6mm with high sensitivity and specificity, which supports MRI as a possible screening alternative without radiation. [15] further validated the role of MRI accuracy in identifying site of tumors, invasions within bronchi, and metastasis, as well as adding to TNM staging. More recently, methods involving AI implemented in [16] demonstrated that a deep learning neural network was able to apply informed design to assess multimodal CT and MRI, reaching a classification accuracy of 97.1% for non-small-cell lung cancer.

Improvements in MRI-guided detection have been obtained employing deep learning techniques. Compared to previous traditional imaging methods, [17] utilized Faster R-CNN, which reduced false positives (FP) in classification on 3D thoracic MRIs and obtained a sensitivity of 85.2%. [18] improved detection sensitivity and specificity, reporting a classification accuracy of 96.28–96.55% utilizing CNNs and conventional image processing techniques. Furthermore, [19] demonstrated the translational application of optimized MRI in the classification of non-small-cell lung carcinoma (NSCLC) in a mouse model and showed tumor volume correlated well with bioluminescence imaging.

Novel contrast agents have also aided improvements in MRI diagnostic capabilities and sensitivity. [20] investigated a nano-sized BsAbCENS agent (as a new contrast agent) through pulmonary delivery and determined that this technique improved the ability to receive an early-stage lung cancer diagnosis, which is crucial to enhance patient survival. [21] studied affine registration in perfusion imaging through MRI by utilizing time-intensity curves to identify early tumor location. [22] developed a computer-aided diagnosis that addressed semi-automatic segmentation and utilized machine learning (ML) classifiers, which achieved a high value in ROC-AUC values and validated MRI as an imaging mode to enhance automated classification of tumors.

The newest advances in deep belief networks and better ML algorithms also provide a new methodology to enhance early detection present in early-stage lung tumors. [23] utilized an FBSO feature selection method that was applied with deep belief networks and correctly identified optimal classifiers with an accuracy of 96.7% with an optimality of 98.9% [24]. Similarly, used an enhanced KNN approach to investigate tumor tissues and reported an accuracy of 96.57% in classifying malignant and benign tissues. Lastly, [25] adopted whole-body MRI with diffusion-weighted sequences for TNM staging, with better detection of brain and liver metastases than PET/CT, and while PET/CT was superior for small node detection.

The computer-aided diagnosis system was designed based on linear SVM classifiers on MRI images with histogram-based features, demonstrating better discrimination between Alzheimer's disease, mild impairment, and cognitively normal individuals, but the high-dimensional features and limited sample size of subjects restricted the system performance. [26] introduced a cost-effective MRI-based Alzheimer's screening method with simple image manipulation to calculate the ratio between the normal brain tissue and the sulcal expansion, which was utilized effectively to differentiate between AD and normal brains and also highlighted the importance of accessibility of the method in the resource-limited environments. [27] used a regularized volumetric ConvNet trained on T1-weighted MRI with data augmentation to classify the MIRIAD dataset with 97% accuracy and outperform traditional deep learning frameworks. [28] proposed an Alzheimer's detection framework based on MRI that merges whale-optimization-based feature selection with deep network feature fusion, getting an average accuracy of 98.12% and considerably improving the accuracy of the diagnosis. [29] designed optimized deep learning methods on MRI data using VGG16, InceptionV3, and ResNet50 with fine-tuned VGG16 demonstrating the highest accuracy of 95.85% compared to the existing state-of-the-art methods [30].

Overall, these studies support the premise that MRI is a reliable noninvasive modality for the detection, characterization, and staging of Alzheimer's disease and lung cancer, especially when combined with advanced sequences, AI, and newer contrast agents. MRI is a non-radiation imaging technique with a high level of potential for accurate diagnostic imaging, but limitations include lower resolution of small nodules, distortion or artifacts, and the requirement for optimization through protocol procedures or combination with other modalities to achieve the best clinical utility.

19.3 REVIEW ANALYSIS

MRI has emerged as a potential imaging technique for detecting, diagnosing, and staging Alzheimer's disease and lung cancer, offering radiation-free imaging with good soft-tissue contrast, making it useful for repeat imaging. Studies in the literature are increasingly suggesting the combination of MRI with AI and insight-enhancing imaging sequences to improve accuracy and clinical utility within the field.

19.3.1 Foundational Studies and Early Advancements

The feasibility of the use of MRI in screening lung cancer was established, and the validity of this approach was confirmed in early studies. The study was effective in recognizing primary tumors in larger groups of asymptomatic individuals with the 3D VIBE and T2 weighted HASTE sequences. Research studies have defined the capacity of MRI in detecting lesions 3 mm or bigger and still have indicated that MRI is radiation-free and therefore does not expose patients to the harmful amount of radiations. However, they further added that there are intrinsic constraints that will make it more difficult to identify nodules easily, including low proton density and susceptibility artifact [31].

19.3.2 Optimization of MRI Sequences and Multimodal Imaging

Recent technological advancements in MRI systems have resulted in optimized imaging sequences that have improved diagnostic performance and reported that imaging sequences such as UTE, T1 VIBE and T2 HASTE had similar diagnostic performance to CT and PET/CT, especially for TNM staging. showed that combining MRI with CT, X-ray imaging, and liquid biopsy resulted in better overall accuracy. discussed their research on 0.55T MRI to increase access to MRI, although they noted that image resolution is sacrificed at 0.55T MRI. supported MRI's incremental benefit when used with TNM staging and diagnosis for treatment decision-making.

19.3.3 Screening and Clinical Validation Studies

Research focused on high-risk screening, including studies that have demonstrated MRI's ability to accurately detect nodules ≥ 6 mm with high sensitivity and specificity, and its ability to visualize tumor invasion into the bronchus and assess metastases. These studies illustrate the promising role MRI may play in the clinical screening and staging of lung cancer, especially since it represents a safer, non-ionizing alternative to CT scans in vulnerable populations.

19.3.3.1 Integration of Artificial Intelligence and Deep Learning

The integration of AI has changed the practice of MRI-based lung cancer diagnosis. reported a 97.1% classification accuracy of NSCLC with deep learning using both MRI and CT data. reported

85.2% sensitivity with Faster R-CNN on 3D thoracic MRI. Rahman et al. reported 96.55% classification accuracy with deep learning using CNN-based classification. evaluated deep belief networks and evaluated K-nearest neighbors enhanced methods, achieving greater than 96% accuracy with MRI detection of lung cancer. Together, these studies substantiate the growing reliability and accuracy of AI-driven models of MRI.

19.3.4 Advancements in MRI Contrast Agents and Image Enhancement

The diagnostic capacity of MRI has been significantly enhanced by utilizing cutting-edge contrast agents. designed and manufactured a nano-sized BsAbCENS contrast agent to improved early-stage tumor detection and improve patients' outcomes. In a somewhat similar fashion, utilized affine registration techniques for perfusion MRI to improve tumor localization. implemented semi-automated segmentation techniques and ML classifiers to achieve high ROC-AUC values in automated classification of tumors.

19.3.5 Review Analysis of MRI-Based Alzheimer's Disease Detection Methods

Most recent studies on Alzheimer's disease detection with MRI have demonstrated that there has been evident evolution of the traditional ML to sophisticated deep learning models. Early research applied the linear SVMs employing handcrafted features and simple image processing to detect the differences between Alzheimer's disease, mild cognitive impairment, and normal brains. These solutions were cost-effective and accessible; however, they had limitations, which include the high-dimensional features and limited data. Recent publications take the form of deep learning approaches, such as volumetric CNNs, transfer learning models, and hybrid structures with feature fusion and optimization, with much better classification accuracy and robustness. In general, although AI deep learning-based approaches demonstrate better performance, issues of data availability, cost of computation and clinical explainability indicate the necessity of efficient and scalable MRI-based diagnosing systems.

19.4 CONCLUSION

The research reviewed illustrated the efficacy of MRI as an emerging and valuable imaging modality for Alzheimer's disease and lung cancer. The utilization of novel advanced sequences, low-field imaging, whole-body protocols, and newly developed contrast-enhanced MRI techniques has improved detection of pulmonary nodules, accuracy for cancer staging, and monitoring of treatment response. The combination of MRI with AI and computer-aided diagnosis has yielded improved sensitivity and specificity in distinguishing between benign and malignant lesions. MRI is not yet a replacement for CT imaging for small nodules, but its noninvasive protocols, radiation-free aspect, and ever-increasing technological advancements and applications make it another or alternative imaging modality for lung cancer management, along with multicenter validation and standardization to enhance its acceptance and use.

19.5 FUTURE SCOPE

Taken together, these studies help to emphasize the progressive clinical utility of MRI for detection and characterization of Alzheimer's disease and lung cancer by providing noninvasive, radiation-free alternatives to standard imaging. Advanced sequences, incorporation of AI, and new contrast agents are paving the way for MRI to become a reliable alternative to imaging in diagnosis of Alzheimer's disease and cancer. Although still developing, MRI is limited by its less sensitivity of small nodules and susceptibility artifacts. This should not diminish its future role in precision oncology, and once further incorporated with the developments of AI, image enhancement, and multimodal fusion, these limitations will continue to be moved forward for the detection of Alzheimer's disease and early-stage lung cancer.

1. Integration with AI and deep learning: The development of multisite AI models that incorporate data from MRI, CT, and PET will permit earlier detection, improved classification, and enhanced predictive prognosis.
2. Optimization of low-field MRI: The potential for the larger clinical application of low-field (0.55T) MRI-based imaging with optimized image sequences represents a low-cost and radiation-free imaging modality for Alzheimer's disease and lung imaging.
3. Advanced contrast agents: The potential for agents that are nano-sized that bind to specific components of malignancy may improve the ability to detect malignancy at the earliest moments and improve the specificity of tissue type characterization.
4. Standardization of acquisition protocols: Through optimized image acquisition protocols between imaging centers, we may optimize reproducibility and clinical confidence and increase the role of MRI in Alzheimer disease and lung cancer imaging.
5. Historical and screening research: Large-scale, prospective comparisons that compare the use of MRI imaging to CT and PET/CT imaging are necessary to show the efficacy of MRI for Alzheimer's disease and lung cancer screening in at-risk populations.
6. Translational research: Leveraging MRI with bioluminescence and histopathology for its use within preclinical models may spur the development of diagnostic tools that uses multimodal imaging.

REFERENCES

1. Betkar, D., Shetty, S. K., Kauthankar, A., Gaonkar, O., & Mavila, A. (2024). Exploring the diagnostic landscape: A narrative review of the evolving role and advancement of MRI in the detection and characterization of lung câncer. *Multidisciplinary Reviews*, 8(1), 2025006. https://doi.org/10.31893/multirev.2025006.
2. Khan, M., Mahajan, R. A., Sivakumar, N. R., Gulhane, M., Rakesh, N., Dey, R., Uddin, M. S., & Basheer, S. (2025). A unified hybrid model for cardiovascular risk prediction: Merging statistical, kernel-based and neural approaches. *Journal of Cellular and Molecular Medicine*. https://doi.org/10.1111/jcmm.70797
3. Bak, S. H., Kim, C., Kim, C. H., Ohno, Y., & Lee, H. Y. (2022). Magnetic resonance imaging for lung cancer: A state-of-the-art review. *Precision and Future Medicine*. https://doi.org/10.23838/pfm.2021.00170.
4. Khan, M., Mahajan, R. A., Katukam, R., Dey, R., Rana, A., & William, P. (2025). Smart insights: Multimodal deep learning techniques for accurate disease identification. In *2025 International Conference on Quantum Photonics, Artificial Intelligence, and Networking (QPAIN)*. Rangpur, Bangladesh, pp. 1–5. https://doi.org/10.1109/QPAIN66474.2025.11171928
5. Wu, N. Y., Wu, N. Y., Cheng, H. C., Ko, J. S., Cheng, Y. C., Lin, P. W., Lin, W. C., Chang, C. Y., & Liou, D. M. (2011). Magnetic resonance imaging for lung cancer detection: Experience in a population of more than 10,000 healthy individuals. *BMC Cancer*, 11(1), 242. https://doi.org/10.1186/1471-2407-11-242.
6. Mahajan, R. A., Dey, R., Khan, M., Su'ud, M. M., Alam, M. M., & Jadhav, P. (2025). Enhancing personalization in IoT-based health monitoring via generative AI and transfer learning. *Egyptian Informatics Journal*, 32, 100788. ISSN 1110-8665. https://doi.org/10.1016/j.eij.2025.100788. https://www.sciencedirect.com/science/article/pii/S1110866525001 81
7. Trivedi, K. R., Gathe, S., Ahmed, S. T., Gupta, A., & Shastrakar, T. (2023). Cancer detection in lungs using image processing and liquid biopsy analysis. https://doi.org/10.1109/aic57670.2023.10263886.
8. Paul, S., Ojha, S. K., Barui, S., Ghosh, S., Ghosh, M., Neogi, B., & Ganguly, A. (2018). Technical advancement on various bio-signal controlled arm: A review. *Journal of Mechanics of Continua and Mathematical Sciences*, 13(2), 16–30. https://doi.org/10.26782/jmcms.2018.06.00007
9. Ohno, Y., Koyama, H., Lee, H. Y., Lee, H. Y., Yoshikawa, T., & Sugimura, K. (2016). Magnetic resonance imaging (MRI) and positron emission tomography (PET)/MRI for lung cancer staging. *Journal of Thoracic Imaging*, 31(4), 215–227. https://doi.org/10.1097/RTI.0000000000000210.
10. Das, P., Paul, S., Ghosh, J., PalBhowmik, S., Neogi, B., & Ganguly, A. (2017). An approach towards the representation of sign language by electromyography signals with fuzzy implementation. *International Journal of Sensors, Wireless Communications and Control*, 7(1), 26–32. https://doi.org/10.2174/2210327907666170222093839

11. Sanchez, F., Tyrrell, P. N., Cheung, P., Heyn, C., Graham, S. J., Poon, I., Ung, Y. C., Louie, A., Tsao, M., & Oikonomou, A. (2023). Detection of solid and subsolid pulmonary nodules with lung MRI: Performance of UTE, T1 gradient-echo, and single-shot T2 fast spin echo. *Cancer Imaging*, 23(1). https://doi.org/10.1186/s40644-023-00531-4.
12. Pal, M., Dey, R., Mahajan, R. A., Khan, M., Syed, A. A., & Karimullah, S. (2025). Edge intelligence: Unique machine learning strategies for enhancing real-time IoT data processing. In *2025 International Conference on Quantum Photonics, Artificial Intelligence, and Networking (QPAIN)*. Rangpur, Bangladesh, pp. 1–5. https://doi.org/10.1109/QPAIN66474.2025.11171994.
13. Tang, F., Chen, T., Ebrahimzadeh, S., Fields, B. K. K., Liu, J., Lee, Y. J., Yen, A., Bowers, K., Schonour, B., Su, P., Larson, P. E. Z., Yang, Y., & Sohn, J. H. (2024). Quantitative and qualitative correlation of 0.55T MRI to CT for normal anatomic structures and common pulmonary pathologies. In *Proceedings of the International Society for Magnetic Resonance in Medicine Scientific Meeting and Exhibition. International Society for Magnetic Resonance in Medicine*. Scientific Meeting and Exhibition. https://doi.org/10.58530/2024/2673.
14. Khalil, A., Majlath, M., Gounant, V., Hess, A., Laissy, J.-P., & Debray, M. P. (2016). Contribution of magnetic resonance imaging in lung cancer imaging. *Diagnostic and Interventional Imaging*, 97(10), 991–1002. https://doi.org/10.1016/J.DIII.2016.08.015.
15. Meier-Schroers, M., Homsi, R., Skowasch, D., Buermann, J., Zipfel, M., Schild, H. H., & Thomas, D. (2018). Lung cancer screening with MRI: Results of the first screening round. *Journal of Cancer Research and Clinical Oncology*, 144(1), 117–125. https://doi.org/10.1007/S00432-017-2521-4.
16. Liu, H., Zheng, L., Shi, G., Xu, Q., Wang, Q., Zhu, H., Feng, H., Wang, L., Zhang, N., Xue, M., & Dai, Y. (2021). Pulmonary functional imaging for lung adenocarcinoma: Combined MRI assessment based on IVIM-DWI and OE-UTE-MRI. *Frontiers in Oncology*, 11, 677942. https://doi.org/10.3389/fonc.2021.677942.
17. Zaernia, A., Youseffi, M., Parisi, L., Abd-Alhameed, R. A., & Ma, R. (2024). A novel artificial intelligence-driven technique for enhancing medical imaging techniques to detect non-small cell lung cancer. In *2024 IEEE European Conference on Visual Media Processing (EUVIP)*, 1–6. https://doi.org/10.1109/euvip61797.2024.10772826.
18. Li, Y., Zhang, L., Chen, H., & Yang, N. (2019). Lung nodule detection with deep learning in 3D thoracic MR images. *IEEE Access*, 7, 37822–37832. https://doi.org/10.1109/ACCESS.2019.2905574.
19. Rahman, M. M., Sazzad, T. M. S., & Ferdaus, F. S. (n.d.). Automated detection of lung cancer using MRI images. https://doi.org/10.1109/sti53101.2021.9732603.
20. Bianchi, A., Dufort, S., Dufort, S., Fortin, P.-Y., Lux, F., Raffard, G., Tassali, N., Tillement, O., Coll, J.-L., Coll, J.-L., & Crémillieux, Y. (2014). In vivo MRI for effective non-invasive detection and follow-up of an orthotopic mouse model of lung cancer. *NMR in Biomedicine*, 27(8), 971–979. https://doi.org/10.1002/NBM.3142.
21. Gao, J., Li, L., Liu, X., Guo, R., & Zhao, B. (2018). Contrast-enhanced magnetic resonance imaging with a novel nano-size contrast agent for the clinical diagnosis of patients with lung cancer. *Experimental and Therapeutic Medicine*, 15(6), 5415–5421. https://doi.org/10.3892/ETM.2018.6112.
22. Huang, H., Shen, L., Ford, J., Gao, L., & Pearlman, J. D. (2006). Early lung cancer detection based on registered perfusion MRI. *Oncology Reports*, 15(4), 1081–1084. https://doi.org/10.3892/OR.15.4.1081.
23. Francisco, V., Koenigkam-Santos, M., Wada, D. T., Junior, J. R. F., Fabro, A. T., Cipriano, F. E. G., Quatrina, S. G., & Azevedo-Marques, P. M. de. (2019). *Computer-Aided Diagnosis of Lung Cancer in Magnetic Resonance Imaging Exams* (pp. 121–127). Springer, Singapore. https://doi.org/10.1007/978-981-13-2517-5_19.
24. Sangeeta, D., Pranjal, M., Rajan, K., Munish, S., & Upendra, N. T. (n.d.). A novel approach for lung cancer detection using deep belief networks. https://doi.org/10.26634/jaim.1.2.20010.
25. Thamilselvan, P., & Sathiaseelan, J. G. R. (2016). Detection and classification of lung cancer MRI images by using enhanced K nearest neighbor algorithm. *Indian Journal of Science and Technology*, 9(43), 1–7. https://doi.org/10.17485/IJST/2016/V9I43/104642.
26. Puls, R., Kühn, J.-P., Ewert, R., & Hosten, N. (2010). Whole-body magnetic resonance imaging for staging of lung cancer. *Frontiers of Radiation Therapy and Oncology*, 42, 46–54. https://doi.org/10.1159/000262459.
27. Patil, H., Swati, Kamala, L., Chaturvedi, A., Veeranjaneyulu, R., & Vekariya, V. (2024). Analysis of magnetic resonance images for the detection of Alzheimer's, 1–6. https://doi.org/10.1109/asiancon62057.2024.10837884.
28. Shirolkar, V., & Shirolkar, K. (2025). Early detection of brain changes in Alzheimer's disease through MRI and basic image processing. *International Journal for Multidisciplinary Research*, 7(4). https://doi.org/10.36948/ijfmr.2025.v07i04.54279.

29. Goenka, N., Sharma, A. K., Tiwari, S., Singh, N., Yadav, V., Prabhu, S., & Chadaga, K. (2024). A regularized volumetric ConvNet based Alzheimer detection using T1-weighted MRI images. *Cogent Engineering*. https://doi.org/10.1080/23311916.2024.2314872.
30. Ali, M. U., Hussain, S. J., Khalid, M., Farrash, M., Lahza, H. F. M., & Zafar, A. (2024). MRI-driven Alzheimer's disease diagnosis using deep network fusion and optimal selection of feature. *Bioengineering*, 11(11), 1076. https://doi.org/10.3390/bioengineering11111076.
31. Saini, R., Singh, S., & Semwal, P. (2024). Automated Alzheimer's disease detection and classification based on optimized deep learning models using MRI. *Indonesian Journal of Electrical Engineering and Computer Science*. https://doi.org/10.11591/ijeecs.v35.i2.pp1333-1342.

20 Integrating NLP and EHR for Next-Generation Mental Health Analytics

Vanita Kshirsagar, Shivani Patil, Niranjan Chirde, Anupam Bonkra, Goh Khang Wen, and Imran Basheti

20.1 INTRODUCTION

The incidence of mental health (MH) disorders is increasing all over the world. They are worsened by the COVID-19 pandemic and climate change [1, 2]. demonstrate a unified hybrid model that merges statistical, kernel-based, and neural approaches, providing a robust computational framework for addressing multifaceted predictive challenges in clinical settings [3]. The burden of MH disorders in India is quite high. Research indicates a very high prevalence of mental disorders across all the states in the country. According to the National Mental Health Survey of India 2015–2016, around 15% of adults in India need active intervention for at least one or more MH conditions [4]. This gives a strong indication that treatment gaps as high as 83% prevail, suggesting the necessity of having easily accessible MH services.

There has been an increasing need for MH services. Nevertheless, availability still remains quite inadequate. In India, based on a survey taken by NIMHANS in 2016, an estimate of around 10.6% of adults within the population who are over 18 years old suffer from any mental disorders [5]. Utilize advanced algorithmic approaches to analyze complex data patterns, highlighting the potential for machine learning to extract critical insights from high-stakes information environments [6]. This creates the need for innovating a different solution toward upgrading the process of MH delivery.

To illustrate the impact of the COVID-19 pandemic on mental distress, a present meta-analysis of changes in MH symptoms before and during the pandemic is used. Figure 20.1 summarizes the standardized mean differences (SMD) for various MH conditions [7].

Artificial intelligence, particularly natural language processing (NLP), opens very promising avenues toward these challenges. NLP techniques allow processing vast quantities of unstructured text found in the huge electronic health record (EHR) databases that extract valuable insights in MH disorders toward early detection and more personalized treatment plans [8]. Multimodal deep learning techniques are essential for accurate disease identification, offering a methodology to integrate diverse data sources such as EHR and clinical text [9]. Some initiatives are being taken on MH applications of NLP in India to improve outcomes and fulfill the gap between demand for services and available services [10].

This chapter discusses the application of NLP in EHR-based patient analysis within the Indian mental healthcare context. It also discusses various techniques used to process and perform clinical text analysis using NLP, their success in identifying or managing MH conditions, and the challenges arising from their implementation. A combination of technology with mental healthcare via NLP has the potential to improve access, efficiency, and personalization of services, thereby improving patient outcomes in India. Investigate the synergy between generative AI and transfer learning to enhance personalization in health monitoring, which is critical for tailoring MH analytics to individual patient profiles [11].

 DOI: 10.1201/9781003667360-20

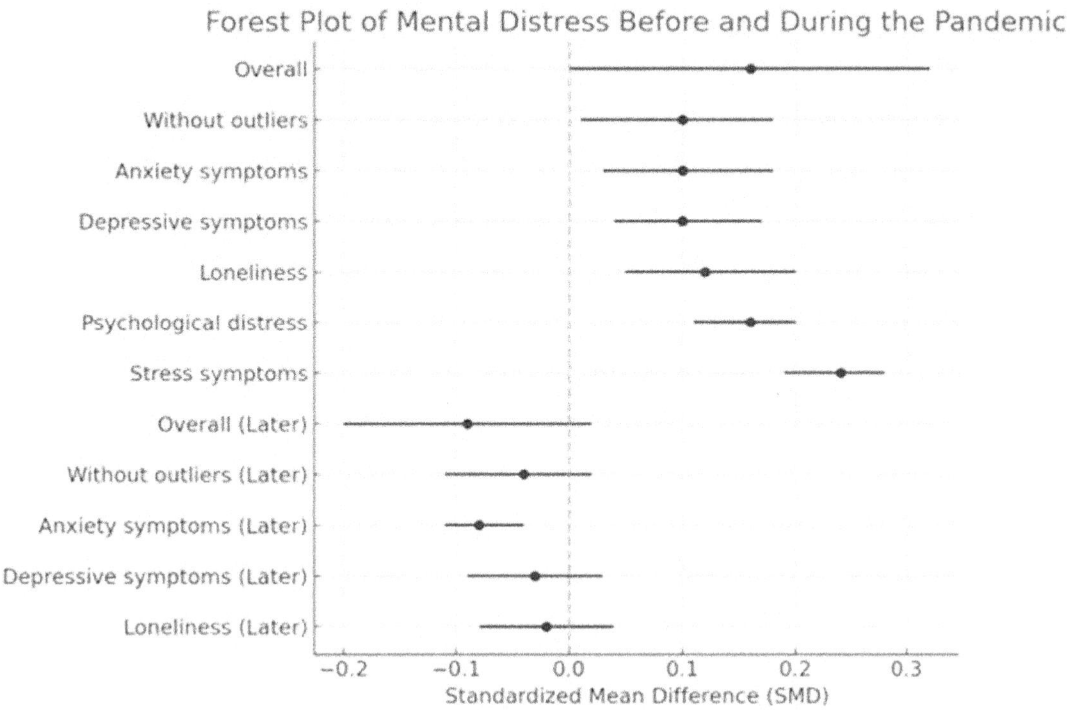

FIGURE 20.1 Meta-analysis of mental distress before and during the pandemic

20.1.1 Natural Language Processing

A branch of artificial intelligence called NLP makes it possible for computers to comprehend and evaluate human discourse. In the case of MH EHRs, NLP can be used to identify similarities in patient data, which can then be used to identify the initial signs of MH problems with medical practitioners. such as anxiety and depression. With the aid of NLP, more accurate diagnosis and customized treatment methods may be provided on the basis of reviewing medical history, patient interactions, and physician notes. It also reduces the workload of medical professionals by automating the documentation process and extracting valuable information, which was not structured. This technology can enhance mental healthcare by promoting the accessibility and effectiveness of data-driven decisions [12].

20.1.2 Electronic Health Record

EHRs contain structured and unstructured information such as clinical information, medical history, and test results. They constitute a gold mine of predictive analytics and health informatics [13].

20.1.3 Mental Health

Mental health is not the absence of mental illness; it is about how people think, feel, and relate to the world around them. It helps one get through the stresses of everyday life, build relationships, work effectively, and make wise decisions. Just like physical health, MH needs to be cultivated and cared for over a lifetime. A comprehensive review of bio-signal integration and technical refinements illustrates the foundational strategies required to translate raw physiological data into actionable diagnostic intelligence [14].

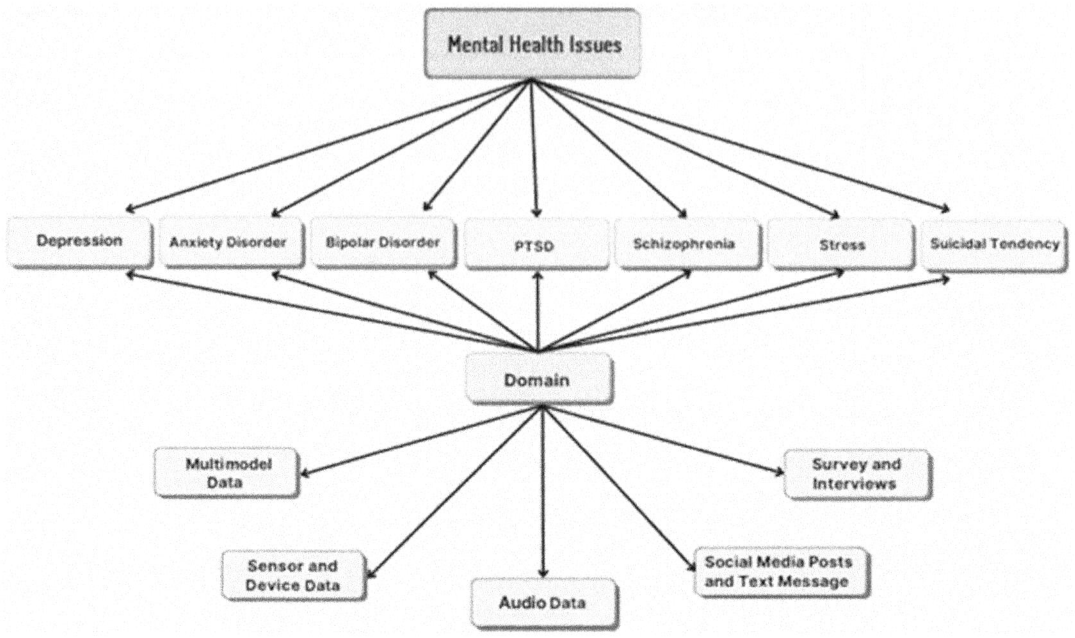

FIGURE 20.2 Mental health issues and data sources

20.1.4 Why Is Mental Health Important?

You are having a bad day; perhaps you have missed a deadline in the workplace or gotten into an argument with a friend. Your MH decides how you process these situations. If your mental well-being is good, you are able to move forward, handle stress, problem-solve, and even find ways of addressing the impossible moments. When your mental well-being is not so perfect, even small things can become difficult to deal with [15].

20.1.5 Factors That Influence Mental Health

The MH issues and data sources represented in Figure 20.2. Mental illnesses are caused by a combination of biological, psychological, and social factors. Some of these include the following:

1. **Genetics and Brain Chemistry**—Some people may be more susceptible to heart disease, while others may have a genetic predisposition to MH conditions such as anxiety or depression.
2. **Life Experiences**—Trauma, abuse, or long-term stress can affect how the brain processes emotions and reacts to challenges.
3. **Social Support**—Factors that support positive MH include family, friends, and community relationships. On the other hand, when one is kept isolated or lonely, that causes mental distress.
4. **Physical Health**—The mind is in connection with the body. Chronic illness, poor diet, deprivation of sleep, and physical inactivity have been proven to affect the well-being of a person's MH.

20.2 MACHINE LEARNING

Machine learning (ML) can be described as a branch of artificial intelligence dealing with algorithms that learn from data and iteratively improve their performance without explicit programming.

Therefore, by processing large datasets, ML engines are capable of detecting patterns, making decisions, and forecasting results that allow for the automation of numerous complex tasks in many different operational fields. A fuzzy-logic implementation for interpreting complex biological signals showcases an effective approach for managing the noise and uncertainty inherent in patient-reported and clinical datasets [16].

20.2.1 Key Techniques in Machine Learning

Figure 20.3 represents an overview of ML types, techniques and examples.

1. **Supervised Learning**
   In supervised learning, models are learned from a labeled set of data for which input has been labeled against a priori output. From this, the model can learn an association between the input and the output to be able to predict new data on whose behalf it has had no prior data yet. Some of the most commonly employed techniques in this category are Support Vector Machines, Logistic Regression, and Linear Regression. Supervised learning may be applied to areas such as spam filtering and disease diagnosis.
2. **Unsupervised Learning**
   Unsupervised learning entails learning from unlabeled data. In this method, models discover unseen patterns or structures without the influence of preconceived categories. It can include methods such as clustering, which collects similar looking data points, or PCA, which reduces the high dimension of any dataset but retains all information intact. This method is used in most applications to segment markets, detect outliers, and facilitate recommendation systems.
3. **Reinforcement Learning**
   A reinforcement learning model is employed to train models such that the models make a sequence of decisions by interacting with an environment. The model is provided feedback (in terms of rewards or penalties) based on actions, and, by maximizing strategies in a manner that maximizes total cumulative reward, the model learns. This paradigm is very useful in robotics, games, and other closed environments, where there is great value in learning well-behaved behavior through a trial-and-error process.

Type of Learning	Techniques	Examples
Supervised Learning	Regression	Linear, Polynomial Regression
	Classification	Logistic Regression, Naive Bayes, K-NN, SVM, CART, RF, AdaBoost, Extreme, GradBoost
	Cross Validation	K-Fold Cross Validation
Unsupervised Learning	Clustering	Hierarchical, K-Means, Density-Based
	Association Rules	Apriori Algorithm
	PCA & Dimensionality Reduction	PCA
Reinforcement Learning	Reinforcement Techniques	Q-Learning, SARSA, DQN, DDPG

FIGURE 20.3 Overview of machine learning types, techniques, and examples

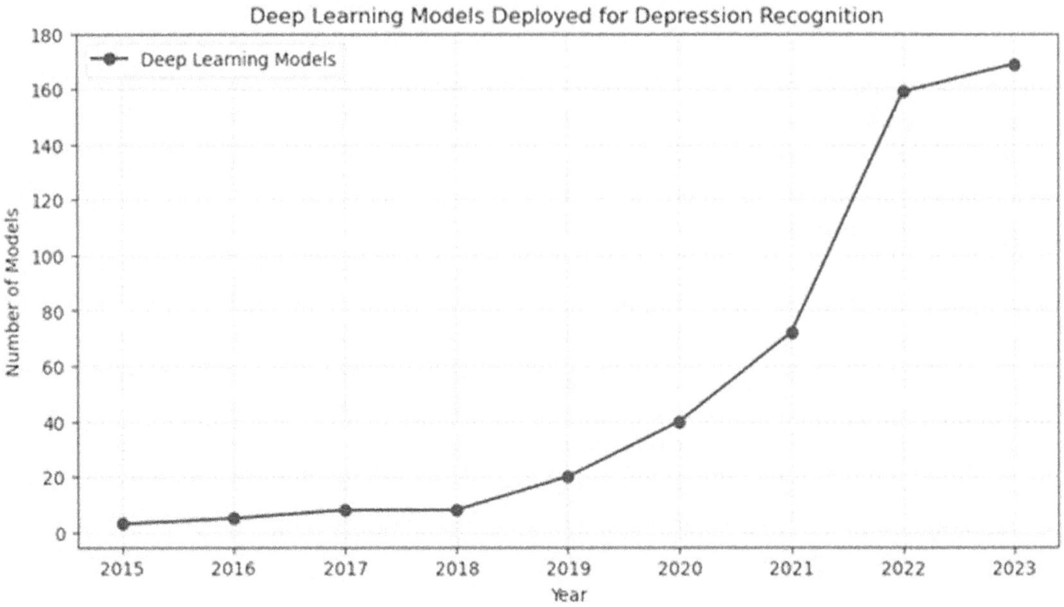

FIGURE 20.4 Growth of deep learning models for depression recognition (2015–2023)

20.3 DEEP LEARNING

Deep learning is a category of ML that uses deep neural networks having many layers for self-learning ability and to understand large amounts of data. The main distinction between traditional ML and deep learning is that deep learning can learn hierarchical representations of data on its own; hence, it is known by this name. Therefore, feature extraction in traditional ML needs to be done either fully or semi-automatically. The recent architectures with large capabilities, such as convolutional neural networks for image data and recurrent neural networks for sequential data, enable computers to analyze complex data structures with very high precision. Success in deep learning algorithms is primarily driven by the improved computational power provided by the availability of GPUs, along with abundant large datasets and superior training algorithms [17].

To highlight the rise of AI-driven depression recognition, Figure 20.4 illustrates the increasing number of deep learning models deployed from 2015 to 2023. The significant growth post-2020 reflects advancements in AI techniques, improved data availability, and a growing emphasis on MH analytics.

20.4 CHALLENGES

20.4.1 Data Quality and Heterogeneity

EHRs are random, scattered, and not complete. They are difficult to extract meaningful information from using NLP software. Medical staff and physicians write them differently and use abbreviations, which creates inconsistency in recording medical data. A physician uses "HTN" for hypertension, but another uses something else. Besides that, missing patient records, misspellings, and missing data are also causes of the problem. Such inconsistencies complicate the process of normalizing the data used by different healthcare systems. Therefore, decision-making and analysis using AI are less accurate.

20.4.2 Ethical and Privacy Concerns

Handling personal MH data poses serious ethical concerns regarding the confidentiality of patient data and data security. Mental health files hold very private information, and if someone accesses them who should not or if there is a breach, it can cause serious problems. Patients might be stigmatized, discriminated against, or offended. It's worth following data protection laws such as HIPAA or GDPR. Nevertheless, in spite of all these legislations, individuals are concerned about the way data are stored, shared, or used for research or artificial intelligence. There is a need to find a method of using MH data to develop improved treatments without disproportionately exposing it. It is extremely essential to maintain patients' trust and adhere to ethics [18].

20.4.3 NLP Model Bias

NLP models with skewed training data can yield biased or inaccurate outputs, resulting in unequal treatment of mental illness. The model may not get to understand and translate the text from the underrepresented group accurately if the training data consists of samples of the underrepresented group. This may result in misdiagnosis, undiagnosed symptoms, or treatment recommendations that are not applicable. For example, if an NLP system is learned on predominantly Western nations' English-language MH records, it would not perform well on non-Western population records with a diverse range of linguistic expressions of MH symptoms. Such biases need to be addressed through diversified and representative datasets, constant monitoring, and fairness-aware AI strategies for providing an equal level of mental healthcare for everyone [19].

20.4.4 Interpretability and Explainability

ML and DL models will more than likely be "black boxes," and clinicians won't know what they did to arrive at a decision. In psychiatric practice, where treatment can influence the life of a patient so powerfully, issues of interpretability cause skepticism for AI-generated counsel among physicians. If an NLP system predicts that a patient is extremely probable to be depressed but is not able to show why, physicians will not care to act upon the advice. To render AI more actionable and reliable, researchers have been working on explainable AI (XAI) methods such as attention mechanisms and feature importance scores that can tell us more about how models come to a conclusion [20].

20.4.5 Clinical Workflow Integration

NLP solutions need to be integrated without disrupting current EHR systems without disrupting clinical workflows if they are to be implemented successfully in the healthcare industry. Doctors and healthcare workers already have enough on their plate regarding administrative work, and the rollout of sophisticated NLP models that require additional steps or training can contribute to adoption resistance. Seamless integration means compatibility with the formats of today's EHR systems, providing information in real-time in the clinical interface, and having as little disruption to patient care as possible. Seamless integration calls for collaboration between AI designers and healthcare workers to create functional systems with simple interfaces that enhance productivity without adding workload.

20.5 BACKGROUND

The combination of NLP and EHR has transformed the assessment process for MH into an objective process with the scalability of tracking psychological states [21]. Traditional MH assessment is strongly reliant on clinician-administered assessments and self-reports, which are subjective and variable in nature [22]. A combination of NLP with multimodal data sources, which include EHRs, text-based data, clinical notes and messages sent by patients, and voice-based biomarkers, have already enhanced the accuracy of diagnosis and treatment planning [23]. EHRs contain as much organized and unorganized data as possible that can be used to perform predictive MH analysis [24]. Structured data include clinical diagnoses and demographics, while unstructured information is the notes of a doctor or a patient message, and all of them are processed through NLP methods to extract relevant data [25]. More comprehensive analyses of similar unstructured clinical text have been made possible through the development of advanced models that employ the use of transformers such as bidirectional encoder representations from transformers (BERT) and GPT [26].

Besides textual information, voice elements like the speech, prosody, and affect are increasingly gaining the utmost importance to indicate the presence of a mental illness such as depression, schizophrenia, and bipolar disorder [27]. The results of research show that NLP models trained on speech transcripts and acoustic features are able to successfully discriminate between healthy individuals and those with mental illness [28]. The continuous monitoring of MH of patients in the naturalistic settings can be more robust with the EHR information utilized together with the sentiment indicators expressed through text messages and voice biomarkers [29]. Mental illnesses represent a significant global challenge that requires new approaches for accurate counting and timely diagnosis. As NLP and EHR have emerged, researchers have investigated AI-based solutions for textual data exploration to calculate MH measures. NLP enables finding valuable designs in structured and unstructured clinical descriptions, and EHRs offer a massive amount of patient data, which makes it easier to make informed decisions.

20.5.1 Natural Language Processing for Predicting Mental Health

NLP methods have been utilized in the discovery of language cues for MH problems such as depression, schizophrenia, and anxiety. Patient descriptions, clinical texts and social media have also undergone sentiment analysis, topic modeling, and transformer models (e.g., BERT and GPT) to detect mental disorders in patient text [30]. Models based on deep learning, including sad-pattern word detection in clinical papers and social media posts, have demonstrated significant improvements in detecting depression. It has been proven that there is evidence to support the use of pre-trained processes in MH speech assessment. It has also raised the issue of NLP in the recognition of mental illness and highlighted how transformer models have played a role in improving the effectiveness of diagnosis. In the same manner, it has been foreseen that multimodal systems with speech and text as inputs will supplement the detection of depression [7].

20.5.2 EHR-Based Mental Health Prediction

The role of scientific results, medications, long-term histories, and both scheduled and unscheduled data are entirely included in EHR systems that can be accessed to forecast outcomes associated with MH. Two NLP methods that can detect signs of depression based on EHR datasets are medical awareness exclusion and named entity recognition (NER) [31]. Researchers have employed ML models trained on EHR textual data to identify suicide risk and psychiatric disorders.

For example, NLP techniques have been utilized in research to extract information from psychiatric notes, thereby enhancing the early detection of schizophrenia and bipolar disorder. [32] have conducted a systematic review of large language models (LLMs) in MH, reporting more utilization of NLP and EHRs for individualized psychiatric assessments. Furthermore, organized EHR features such as medication history and clinical visits have been combined with unstructured text data to improve MH screening models [33].

There are still some problems to be overwhelmed in NLP and EHR-based mental illness prediction, even with marvelous development. Bias in exercise data is a significant problem that can lead to variations in diagnostic accuracy among various demographic groups [34]. In addition, access to EHRs is restricted for research purposes for privacy and ethics purposes.

The future work should be focused on building explainable AI (XAI) models that will enhance interpretability in treatment settings. Apart from that, prediction accuracy may be improved through the use of multimodal data sources such as patient-reported outcomes and wearable sensor data [35]. Advancements in federated learning technology would also minimize privacy concerns by enabling decentralized model training based on secure EHR data. Thus, prediction of MH using NLP and EHRs has revolutionized the diagnosis and detection of mental illness. Though deep learning methods are improving the accuracy of the diagnosis continuously, the problems of bias, privacy concerns, and interpretability need to be solved before being used in more clinical settings. Increased research in multimodal fusion, explainable AI, and federated learning has the potential to improve patient results and MH assessments.

20.6 METHODOLOGY

The literature carried out an in-depth electronic search of 11 databases between 2016 and 2024, since in the last eight years NLP research has gained ground at a tremendous pace [36]. The literature was searched in databases that have consistently published high-quality, peer-reviewed papers. These include Google Scholar, PubMed, Elsevier, IEEE, Springer, Oxford University Press, Nature Publishing Group, Wiley Online Library, BioMed Central, and the American Medical Informatics Association. These platforms hold extensive collections of peer-reviewed literature relevant to NLP research. To identify relevant studies, the following key search terms were used: "NLP in Clinical Narratives," "Medical NLP," "ML in EHRs," "DL in Medical Text," and "Automated ML in EHRs."

(a) **Inclusion Criteria**
This review focused on peer-reviewed research studies that applied NLP and ML/DL models to EHRs in the context of MH. The inclusion criteria encompassed studies that leveraged free-text classification, word embedding techniques, automatic summarization of clinical narratives, healthcare dialogue systems, clinical entity recognition, and ICD-9 multilabel classification. The review also considered research on the use of medical concept embedding and detection of risk related to delirium, as well as ML and deep learning architectures of EHRs. In addition, recent advances incorporated NLP-driven extraction of social determinants of health (SDOHs) from clinical notes, psychosis-risk prediction models, and large language model development for digital health monitoring (DHM) assessment of MH. Peer-reviewed journal articles, as well as full-length papers from conferences, were selected, which only included the studies that particularly used ML or DL models in the analysis of EHRs and interpretation of clinical narratives.

(b) **Exclusion Criteria**
The review excluded studies in which methodologies were not satisfactory or could not meet the quality parameters. More specifically, the review excluded preprints, preliminary reports, and those that did not pass through peer review so that only validated and worthy findings were included. It also excluded all editorials, opinion pieces, and review papers as well, because in this synthesis, the focus is only on synthesizing original research, not summarizing literature. Those studies that did not specifically apply ML or DL models for the analysis of EHRs nor focus specifically on clinical narrative interpretation were excluded. All selected papers underwent full-text quality assessment in order to validate relevance, soundness of methodological approach, and contribution to an evolving field of NLP-driven MH research based on EHRs.

20.6.1 NLP and Text Analysis in Mental Health

The application of NLP and text analysis has also seen remarkable progress in MH with adaptation to several methodologies that help for a better understanding, diagnosis, and treatment of a patient.

Some of the most important methodologies, along with prominent contributions in research under this umbrella, are discussed. Figure 20.5 represents an NLP pipeline for m MH analysis using EHR records.

- **Sentiment Analysis and Emotion Detection**
  Sentiment analysis refers to the analysis of the emotional tone of textual data to establish how psychologically people are doing. After establishing the use of language, it becomes possible to instigate MH problems such as depression and anxiety. For instance, a research study utilized sentiment analysis to monitor changes in the mood of the patients by studying their social media posts—a reflection of their MH status [37].
  Emotion detection goes one step further than sentiment analysis by revealing which particular emotions the text conveys, such as sadness, anger, or joy. This method has been used in the analysis of counseling conversations: certain emotional manifestations were identified to be related to positive therapy results [38].
- **Topic Modeling**
  Other research areas of modeling algorithms include extracting latent thematic structures from large corpora of texts. For instance, LDA has been successfully applied in research on MH to uncover latent themes that capture significant topics among popular discussions from online forums focused on MH, which further helped gain understanding of the top topics and concerns of individuals seeking assistance [39].
- **Clinical Text NER**
  NER is the method where entities in text are recognized and marked into pre-set categories such as symptoms, treatments, or diagnoses. In MH, NER has been applied to EHRs for extracting necessary information. From clinical notes, researchers have created machine-based detection systems for suicide risk factors so that prediction and prevention of suicidal behavior can be improved [40].
- **Transformer-Based Models for Mental Health Detection**
  Transformer-based models, such as BERT, have greatly enhanced the analysis of text related to MH. These models detect the context in which words are used in a sentence, which makes language understanding very profound. BERT-based classifiers have been proved to detect MH issues by evaluating social media posts with high sensitivity toward the identification at-risk individuals [41].
- **Multimodal NLP Models**
  Recent innovations include improvements in the multifaceted integration of data sources to make MH assessments more accurate. Multimodal NLP models integrate text data obtained from EHRs, clinical notes, and interviews with patients for composite analysis. For example, a research system was developed to analyze text as well as audio signals in patient interactions that increased the depression detection and other MH disorder factors [42].
- **Language Use Analysis**
  Analyzing language use, including pronoun usage and linguistic styles, has provided insights into individuals' MH. Pennebaker et al. developed the LIWC tool for analyzing text to find psychologically based insights on how language reflects emotional and cognitive states [43].

20.6.2 Voice Analysis in Mental Health Assessments

Speech and voice characteristics are very significant features in the assessment of an individual's MH condition. Pitch, tone, speech rate, and prosody have all been associated with psychological diseases, including depression, anxiety, and schizophrenia. Machine learning and deep learning techniques have now been applied to the analysis of vocal biomarkers, making the prospect of developing noninvasive devices for the assessment of MH feasible.

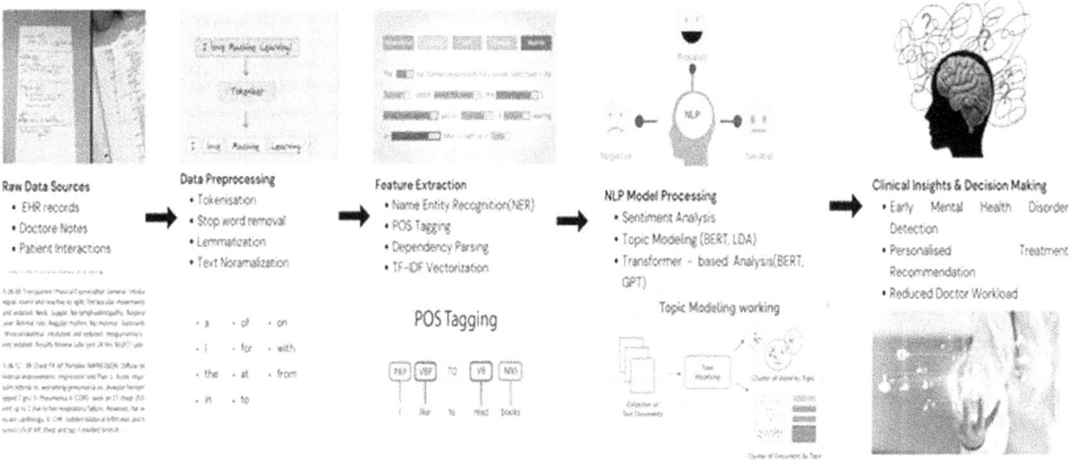

FIGURE 20.5 NLP pipeline for mental health analysis using EHR data

- **Voice Biomarkers for Identifying Depression**

Science in the current era has been more focused on the analysis of prosody, pitch variation, and spectral characteristics for the identification of voice features of mental disorders. The approaches highlighted have been the following:

Prosodic Features: They encompass pitch (fundamental frequency), rate of speech, loudness, and pauses. In general, a depressed patient will exhibit monotonic speech, low pitch variation, and increased speech pauses.

Spectral Characteristics: MFCCs and the analysis of the formant frequency were employed in order to identify the difference between neutral speech and depressed speech.

Articulation Features of Phonation: The variation of vibration in a vocal fold coupled with articulations such as poor energy within upper frequency bands was discovered to be employed as depression biometrics.

Other clinical and spontaneous speech data from depressed patients were also recorded using standardized tasks, including reading, spontaneous speech, and sustained vowel phonation. The primary classification models used in this phase were SVMs, decision trees, and GMMs for detecting depression.

- **Deep Learning-Based Voice Analysis Progress**

Substantial improvements have been made with deep learning models in the form of CNNs, LSTMs, and transformer-based models. The overall contributions of these improvements are as follows:

(a) **CNN for Spectrogram-Based Analysis**
CNN employ spectrogram analysis for classifying raw audio signals as images. Spectrogram-based CNN models perform classification of depressed and non-depressed speech more effectively than the feature-based methods [44].

(b) **LSTM for Processing Sequential Voice Data**
It is primarily a sequential task and therefore led the way toward using LSTMs and BiLSTMs (bidirectional LSTMs) in order to learn long dependencies in speech efficiently.

The models learn pitch, pausing, and speech rate changes highly efficiently and therefore better identify depression scores [40].

(c) **Multimodal Approaches: Integrating the Analysis of Speech and Text Simultaneously**
Integration has recently been carried out by incorporating voice functionality and speech recognition system transcripts. The classification system also contains both acoustic indicators such as prosody and pitch, alongside the linguistic indicators such as word use and sentiment for improving performance [45].

(d) **Transfer Learning and Pretrained Speech Models**
Some of the popular pretrained models are Wav2Vec 2.0 and Whisper. These models have also performed well on zero-shot depression detection. Large-scale datasets of speech have augmented the feature extraction.

(e) **Speech-to-Text Conversion**
Patient conversation transcribing tools such as Whisper and Mozilla DeepSpeech can be used to analyze distress markers using NLP models. It is important that proper transcription be applied to further text-based analyses in MH testing [46].

- **Structured Data Processing Techniques**

Feature Engineering: One-hot encoding and normalization are techniques for extracting the most significant features from structured EHRs, that is, demographics, medication lists, and lab reports. They are used to precondition ML models with the aim of predicting MH. The literature of systematic review suggests that feature engineering is significant in predictive models based on EHRs.

Predictive Modeling: MH risk prediction is done through ML models, such as random forest and gradient boosting, that are advised by previous psychiatric diagnoses and treatment history. The effectiveness of these methods is proven by recent studies that have built models for predicting patient severity states based on EHR data.

Data Imputation: Missing values in EHRs shall be addressed with utmost importance in an attempt to keep models accurate. Algorithms such as KNN imputation and multiple imputation by chained equations (MICE) deal with missing data, providing a more complete data analysis. It has been noted that the most appropriate techniques for imputation are needed when dealing with missing clinical data [47].

- **Multimodal Data Fusion**

Recently developed multimodal deep learning involves the combination of different types of data to improve psychiatric evaluations. Figure 20.6. represents multimodal NLP and ML for psychiatric assessment:

Semantic information of clinical text is represented as semantic embeddings in BERT.

- Speech Data: Mel-frequency cepstral coefficients (MFCC) features area coustics features. Structured EHR Data: Graph-based representations encode the relationships between clinical entities.

- **The Multimodal Fusion Transformer (MMFT) from Hugging Face**

has shown promising results for holistic psychiatric assessment using these forms of data. It allows gaining a deeper level of patient health comprehension by accessing diverse sources of information. Another publication by Drougkos, Bakker, and Spruit (2024) in BMC medical informatics and decision-making provides an idea of how multimodal ML can identify language and speech cues that are relevant to mental illness. The study stresses:

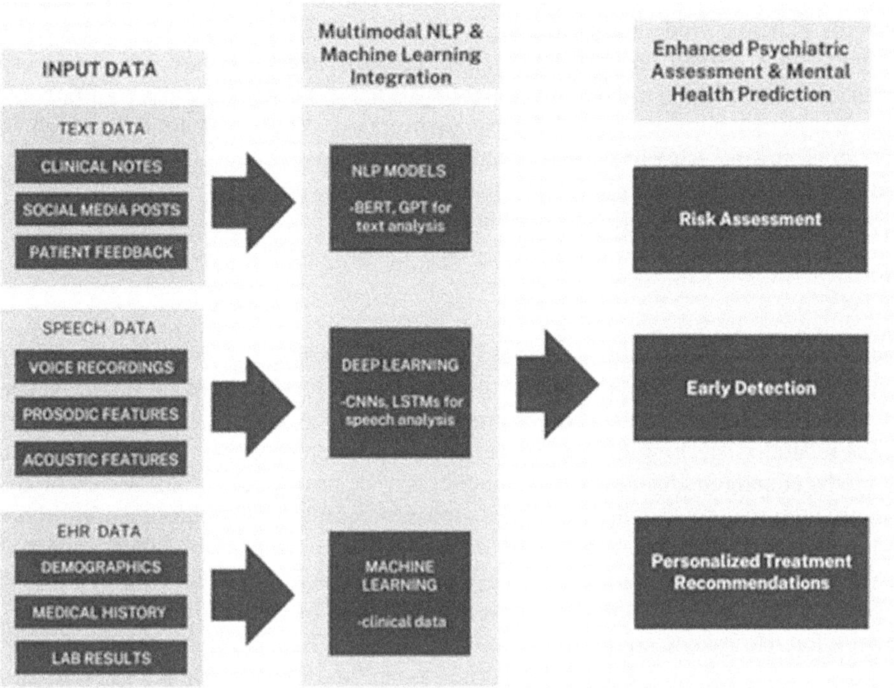

FIGURE 20.6 Multimodal NLP and machine learning for psychiatric assessment

- Textual and voice information should be combined to help detect psychiatric disorders more effectively.
- Advanced NLP techniques should be used, including transformer-based models, to draw conclusions based on clinical texts.

The combination of speech characteristics such as MFCCs and prosodic characteristics is used in an attempt to analyze distress vocal biomarkers.

According to their findings, multimodal systems are much more effective than single modes in detecting indicators of mental illness in its early stages, thus supporting the development of more specific and more personalized diagnostic models.

20.7 CONCLUSION

Indeed, the convergence of NLP and EHRs is a testament to the existence of a small revolution in the field of MH, which promises more opportunities to make diagnoses more precise and individualized, and to streamline clinical processes. This chapter showcases research on NLP methods using sentiment analysis, clinical NER, transformer-based models, specifically BERT and GPT, and multimodal systems that combine text and speech analysis with more structured EHR data to reveal actionable insights from unstructured clinical narratives. The entire presented entity is extremely helpful in the initial stages of diagnosing such conditions as depression and anxiety, tracking their development throughout, and locating suicide risk factors. Voice biomarker analysis, which is driven by sophisticated deep learning frameworks, such as CNNs and LSTMs, and noninvasive MH testing in terms of speech patterns and prosodic features, are both mentioned.

Nevertheless, in spite of these developments, there are still several challenges, especially in the heterogeneity of data related to the inconsistency of terminologies, disjointed EHR systems, and inconsistency of clinical documentation, which creates multimodal barriers to the large-scale implementation and adoption of NLP solutions. The most difficult problems to eliminate are ethical ones, especially patient confidentiality and algorithm bias, which may remain unresolved; in cases where AI models are trained on unrepresentative data, disparities in care would be perpetuated among underrepresented groups. The interpretability issues that the black boxes of numerous deep learning models attract raise questions of trustworthiness in AI-based solutions, which leads to a further dent in clinicians' trust in AI-supported recommendations, and interoperability challenges and not being interested in new technologies that are created with transformational change in mind lead to poor integration into the clinical workflows.

20.8 SUMMARY

The further studies should be directed toward the standardization of EHR data formats and the proposal of multidisciplinary collaborations to promote the formation of powerful, generalizable models. XAI tools, including attention mechanisms, would be in a position to fill the interpretability gap, whereas federated learning models would enable privacy by decentralizing data analysis. In case bias is to be countered and equity of the model is to be prioritized, it will be essential to create datasets amply with various linguistic, cultural, and demographical backgrounds. Multimodal data that include voice, text, and structured EHR data promise to provide combined patient measurements but have not received the necessary work to result in actual clinical employment. Finally, a joint contribution between regulators and developers should be invited in order to create an ethical framework for AI implementation in mental healthcare. These limitations can be overcome by standardization of EHR arrangements, joint knowledge, and explainable AI growth. In order to construct AI models, different datasets were considered that can take into consideration the language and socioeconomic diversity. Collaborative learning, extension of AI to be intelligible, and standardization of EHR format can address these constraints. Equitable AI is the separate datasets that portray the language and societal progress. The areas of future research should primarily be concerned with clinician-friendly AI systems and multimodal integration.

REFERENCES

1. Banks, J., & Xu, X. (2020). The mental health effects of the first two months of lockdown during the COVID-19 pandemic in the UK. *The Lancet Psychiatry*, 7(11), 875–882.
2. Zhao, S., et al. (2020). Impact of COVID-19 on mental health: A systematic review and meta-analysis. *Springer Nature Mental Health*, 10(2), 225–238.
3. Khan, M., Mahajan, R. A., Sivakumar, N. R., Gulhane, M., Rakesh, N., Dey, R., Uddin, M. S., & Basheer, S. (2025). A unified hybrid model for cardiovascular risk prediction: Merging statistical, kernel-based and neural approaches. *Journal of Cellular and Molecular Medicine*. https://doi.org/10.1111/jcmm.70797
4. Gururaj, G., Varghese, M., Benegal, V., Rao, G. N., Pathak, K., Singh, L. K., et al. (2016). *National mental health survey of India, 2015–16: Prevalence, patterns and outcomes* (NIMHANS Publication No. 129). National Institute of Mental Health and Neurosciences (NIMHANS), Bengaluru, India. Publisher website: NIMHANS.
5. Murthy, R. S. (2017). Mental health initiatives in India (2016). *Indian Journal of Psychiatry*, 59(1), 21–26.
6. Khan, M., Dey, R., Kassim, S., Mahajan, R. A., Ghosh, A., & William, P. (2025). Machine learning-driven trading strategies: An empirical analysis of BSE blue-chip stocks using advanced algorithmic approaches. In *2025 International Conference on Quantum Photonics, Artificial Intelligence, and Networking (QPAIN)*. Rangpur, Bangladesh, pp. 1–5. https://doi.org/10.1109/QPAIN66474.2025.11171797
7. Johnson, A., et al. (2018). Natural language processing in mental healthcare: A review. *Artificial Intelligence in Medicine*, 92, 62–81.
8. Du, J., et al. (2019). Extracting mental health insights from electronic health records using NLP techniques. *Springer Nature Digital Health*, 12, 182–196.
9. Khan, M., Mahajan, R. A., Katukam, R., Dey, R., Rana, A., and William, P. (2025). Smart insights: Multimodal deep learning techniques for accurate disease identification. In *2025 International Conference on Quantum Photonics, Artificial Intelligence, and Networking (QPAIN)*. Rangpur, Bangladesh, pp. 1–5. https://doi.org/10.1109/QPAIN66474.2025.11171928

10. Agarwal, R., et al. (2021). AI-driven NLP applications in Indian healthcare. *Journal of Medical Informatics India*, 5, 34–49.
11. Mahajan, R. A., Dey, R., Khan, M., Su'ud, M. M., Alam, M. M., & Jadhav, P. (2025). Enhancing personalization in IoT-based health monitoring via generative AI and transfer learning. *Egyptian Informatics Journal*, 32, 100788. ISSN 1110-8665. https://doi.org/10.1016/j.eij.2025.100788. https://www.sciencedirect.com/science/article/pii/S1110866525001811
12. Zhang, T., Schoene, A. M., Ji, S., & Ananiadou, S. (2022). Natural language processing applied to mental illness detection: A narrative review. *NPJ Digital Medicine*, 5(1), 1–13.
13. HealthIT.gov. (2021). *What Is an Electronic Health Record (EHR)*? https://www.healthit.gov/faq/what-electronic-health-record-ehr
14. Paul, S., Ojha, S. K., Barui, S., Ghosh, S., Ghosh, M., Neogi, B., & Ganguly, A. (2018). Technical advancement on various bio-signal controlled arm: A review. *Journal of Mechanics of Continua and Mathematical Sciences*, 13(2), 16–30. https://doi.org/10.26782/jmcms.2018.06.00007
15. World Health Organization. (2004). *Promoting Mental Health: Concepts, Emerging Evidence, Practice (Summary Report)*. World Health Organization.
16. Das, P., Paul, S., Ghosh, J., PalBhowmik, S., Neogi, B., & Ganguly, A. (2017). An approach towards the representation of sign language by electromyography signals with fuzzy implementation. *International Journal of Sensors, Wireless Communications and Control*, 7(1), 26–32. https://doi.org/10.2174/2210327907666170222093839
17. World Health Organization. (2022). *Mental Health*. https://www.who.int/health-topics/mental-health
18. Franke, B., Stein, J. L., Ripke, S., Anttila, V., Hibar, D. P., Van Hulzen, K. J. E., Arias-Vasquez, A., Smoller, J. W., Nichols, T. E., Neale, M. C., et al. (2016). Genetic influences on schizophrenia and subcortical brain volumes: Large-scale proof of concept. *Nature Neuroscience*, 19(3), 420–431.
19. Narayan, A. J., Rivera, L. M., Bernstein, R. E., Harris, W. W., & Lieberman, A. F. (2018). Positive childhood experiences predict less psychopathology and stress in pregnant women with childhood adversity: A pilot study of the Benevolent Childhood Experiences (BCEs) scale. *Child Abuse & Neglect*, 78, 19–30.
20. Billings, J., Seif, N. A., Hegarty, S., Ondruskova, T., Soulios, E., Bloomfield, M., & Greene, T. (2021). What support do frontline workers want? A qualitative study of health and social care workers' experiences and views of psychosocial support during the COVID-19 pandemic. *PLoS One*, 16(9), e0256454.
21. Vawter, M. P., Tomita, H., Meng, F., Bolstad, B., Li, J., Evans, S., Choudary, P., Atz, M., Shao, L., Neal, C., et al. (2006). Mitochondrial-related gene expression changes are sensitive to agonal state: Implications for brain disorders. *Molecular Psychiatry*, 11(7), 663–679.
22. Sarker, I. H. (2021). Machine learning: Algorithms, real-world applications, and research directions. *SN Computer Science*, 2(3), 160.
23. LeCun, Y., Bengio, Y., & Hinton, G. (2015). Deep learning. *Nature*, 521, 436–444.
24. Thapa, C., & Camtepe, S. (2021). Precision health data: Requirements, challenges, and existing techniques for data security and privacy. *Computers in Biology and Medicine*, 129, 104130.
25. Garrido-Muñoz, I., Montejo-Ráez, A., Martínez-Santiago, F., & Ureña-López, L. A. (2021). A survey on bias in deep NLP. *Applied Sciences*, 11(7), 3184.
26. Maruthi, S., Dodda, S. B., Yellu, R. R., Thuniki, P., & Reddy, S. B. B. (2022). Language model interpretability-explainable AI methods: Exploring explainable AI methods for interpreting and explaining the decisions made by language models to enhance transparency and trustworthiness. *Australian Journal of Machine Learning Research & Applications*, 2(2), 1–9.
27. Jabali, A. K., Waris, A., Khan, D. I., Ahmed, S., & Hourani, R. J. (2022). Electronic health records: Three decades of bibliometric research productivity analysis and some insights. *Informatics in Medicine Unlocked*, 29, 100872.
28. Guntuku, S. C., Yaden, D. B., Kern, M. L., Ungar, L. H., & Eichstaedt, J. C. (2019). Detecting depression and mental illness on social media: An integrative review. *Current Opinion in Behavioral Sciences*, 18, 43–49.
29. Tadesse, M. M., Lin, H., Xu, B., & Yang, L. (2020). Detection of depression-related posts in social media using a multimodal deep learning approach. *Journal of Neural Computing and Applications*, 32, 6645–6661.
30. Zirikly, A., Resnik, P., Uzuner, O., & Hollingshead, K. (2019). CLPsych 2019 shared task: Predicting the degree of suicide risk in Reddit posts. In *Proceedings of the Sixth Workshop on Computational Linguistics and Clinical Psychology*, 24–33. Association for Computational Linguistics (ACL). https://doi.org/10.18653/v1/W19-3003; https://aclanthology.org/
31. McCoy, T. H., Castro, V. M., Roberson, A. M., Snapper, L. A., & Perlis, R. H. (2021). Improving prediction of suicide and accidental death after discharge from general hospitals with natural language processing. *JAMA Psychiatry*, 78(5), 545–552.

32. Coppersmith, G., Leary, R., Crutchley, P., & Fine, A. (2020). Natural language processing of social media as screening for mental illness. *Biomedical Informatics Insights*, 12, 1–8.
33. Cummins, N., Scherer, S., Kächele, M., Ringeval, F., Faur, C., & Cowie, R. (2021). A review of multimodal affect recognition and its application in mental health assessment. *Cognitive Computation*, 13(4), 791–813.
34. Pennebaker, J. W., Boyd, R. L., Jordan, K., & Blackburn, K. (2015). The development and psychometric properties of LIWC2015. *Technical Report*. University of Texas at Austin.
35. Cummins, N., Scherer, S., Kächele, M., Ringeval, F., Faur, C., & Cowie, R. (2018). Depression detection from vocal biomarkers: A review. *IEEE Journal of Biomedical and Health Informatics*, 22(4), 1416–1428.
36. Alhajjar, F., & Han, Y. (2019). Speech-based depression detection using spectral and prosodic features. *IEEE Transactions on Affective Computing*, 10(3), 346–359.
37. Eyben, F., Wöllmer, M., & Schuller, B. (2017). The Munich open voice dataset: Speech and mental health research. In *Proceedings of INTERSPEECH 2017* (pp. 1261–1265). International Speech Communication Association (ISCA). https://www.isca-archive.org/
38. Toto, E., Baltrusaitis, T., & Robinson, P. (2021). CNN-based spectrogram classification for depression detection. *Pattern Recognition Letters*, 140, 198–204.
39. Scherer, S., Stratou, G., Gratch, J., & Morency, L. P. (2021). Investigating multimodal features for depression detection in clinical interviews. *IEEE Transactions on Affective Computing*, 12(1), 163–175.
40. Morales, M. R., Scherer, S., & Rudzicz, F. (2022). Multi-modal depression detection: Speech and text fusion using deep learning. *Neural Networks*, 145, 115–126.
41. Xia, J., Wang, Y., & Zhang, F. (2023). Transfer learning for depression detection using Wav2Vec 2.0. *Journal of Biomedical AI Research*, 8(2), 134–149.
42. Guo, Z., Lai, A., Thygesen, J. H., Farrington, J., Keen, T., & Li, K. (2024). Large language models for mental health applications: Systematic review. *JMIR Mental Health*, 11, e57400. https://doi.org/10.2196/57400
43. Hossain, E., Rana, R., Higgins, N., Soar, J., Barua, P. D., Pisani, A. R., & Turner, K. (2023). Natural language processing in electronic health records in relation to healthcare decision-making: A systematic review. *Computers in Biology and Medicine*, 155, 106649. https://doi.org/10.1016/j.compbiomed.2023.106649
44. Alam, A. N. M., Reza, R., Abrar, A., Ahmed, T., Ahmed, S., Sharar, S., & Rasel, A. A. (2022). Patients' severity states classification based on electronic health record (EHR) Data using multiple machine learning and deep learning approaches. *arXiv preprint arXiv:2209.14907*. https://arxiv.org/abs/2209.14907
45. Ren, W., Liu, Z., Wu, Y., Zhang, Z., Hong, S., & Liu, H. (2024). Moving beyond medical statistics: A systematic review on missing data handling in electronic health records. *Health Data Science*, 4, 0176. https://doi.org/10.34133/hds.0176
46. Wang, G., Fan, F., Shi, S., An, S., Cao, X., Ge, W., Yu, F., Wang, Q., Han, X., Tan, S., Tan, Y., & Wang, Z. (2024). Multi-modality fusion transformer with spatio-temporal feature aggregation module for psychiatric disorder diagnosis. *Computerized Medical Imaging and Graphics*, 114, 102368. https://doi.org/10.1016/j.compmedimag.2024.102368
47. Drougkas, G., Bakker, E. M., & Spruit, M. (2024). Multimodal machine learning for language and speech markers identification in mental health. *BMC Medical Informatics and Decision Making*, 24, 354. https://doi.org/10.1186/s12911-024-02772-0

21 A Multistage Deep Learning Approach for Intracranial Aneurysm Detection

Nguyen Pham Thi Thao,[1] *Ninh Nguyen Ngoc Gia, Trung Nguyen Quoc, and Vinh Truong Hoang*

21.1 INTRODUCTION

A brain aneurysm[1] is a balloon-like bulge in a blood vessel of the brain, caused by a weak vessel wall; it is a weak spot in a blood vessel inside the brain that bulges outward. Most aneurysms do not cause symptoms, but if one ruptures, it can lead to bleeding in the brain, which is often life-threatening. This makes early and accurate diagnosis extremely important. Doctors, especially radiologists[2]—a medical doctor who specializes in interpreting medical images such as X-rays, CT scans, and MRIs—can find aneurysms by looking at brain scans such as CT or MRI. However, aneurysms can be small and are sometimes missed, especially when the scan is done for another reason. Missing an aneurysm can delay treatment and increase the risk of serious consequences for the patient. Because of this, there is growing interest in using artificial intelligence to support radiologists. From a single scan, artificial intelligence systems can scan brain images on their own. They can spot suspicious areas quickly—making it easier to find aneurysms without delays. Using these tools might lower incorrect diagnoses while saving hours of waiting. Better outcomes could follow when treatments starts sooner. This work aims to build smart algorithms that find and map brain aneurysms correctly, regardless of image type. Types include CT angiography, MRI angiography, plus specific views such as T1 after contrast or T2-layers. Accuracy matters most where decisions depend on precise location. One big hurdle comes from real clinic data, which is full of variations due to different hospitals, machines, and scan types. Even so, the way we built our system makes it work well when those differences shift. What we added to tackle this issue fits briefly into three parts:

- We perform a comprehensive exploratory data analysis (EDA) on the aneurysm detection dataset, including statistical summaries of patient demographics, aneurysm location distributions, and imaging characteristics in both tabular and DICOM formats [1].
- We design a coarse-to-fine 3D segmentation pipeline based on MedicalNet [2] to localize vessels and candidate aneurysm regions effectively.
- We propose a joint segmentation–classification framework using a multitask U-Net [3], enabling simultaneous pixel-wise aneurysm segmentation and slice-level classification.
- We implement systematic data preprocessing, augmentation, and patch extraction strategies to handle class imbalance and improve model generalization.

This research attempts to improve the accuracy and efficiency of aneurysm diagnosis by creating automated tools to assist radiologists. These solutions could allow for earlier treatment and minimize the chance of dangerous ruptures, which would lead to better patient outcomes and potentially save lives.

DOI: 10.1201/9781003667360-21

21.2 RELATED WORKS

21.2.1 Datasets on Intracranial Aneurysm

The identification, segmentation, and risk prediction of intracranial aneurysms (IA) require models that use data from publicly accessible datasets. The datasets need to merge imaging data with clinical data, morphological data, and hemodynamic data. Several important datasets have been released in recent years:

- Nageler et al. described [4]: a computed tomography angiography (CTA)-based dataset including 99 patients (105 middle cerebral artery aneurysms) and 44 healthy controls. It provides high-resolution CTA images, reconstructed 3D aneurysm and parent vessel models, together with morphological and hemodynamic descriptors, making it a valuable multimodal resource.
- [5]: a large-scale synthetic dataset built from approximately 466 real aneurysms, where aneurysm-free and deformed 3D models are generated, and computational fluid dynamics (CFD) simulations are performed to calculate hemodynamic parameters such as pressure, velocity, and wall shear stress. While it increases data diversity and scale, a domain gap exists between synthetic and clinical data.
- IntrA, CADA, and other small-scale benchmarks [1, 6]: datasets based on 3D models or digital subtraction angiography (DSA) series that serve as public benchmarks for segmentation and detection tasks. However, their size is limited (typically tens to hundreds of aneurysms), and they are restricted to specific modalities.
- Small-scale MRA/TOF datasets [7]: several MRA datasets are available for aneurysm segmentation and follow-up studies, but the number of cases and annotations remain relatively low.
- RSNA initiatives [8]: large-scale multicenter challenges organized by RSNA have released CTA datasets with expert annotations, aiming to establish community benchmarks for aneurysm detection and localization. These initiatives provide a unique opportunity to evaluate model generalizability across institutions and imaging protocols.

Limitations: The current IA datasets have not reached their full potential because they maintain small sizes, which include between 40 to 400 aneurysm samples. This is insufficient for training large deep learning models. Moreover, these datasets often lack diversity in terms of imaging methods and anatomical locations. The resulting datasets become biased, which makes these models less appropriate for medical use. Real-world datasets lack sufficient hemodynamic data because most CFD parameters used in simulations and synthetic groups were developed through computational methods. The research studies use different annotation methods, which create challenges for scientists to merge their data into one evaluation system. Khan et al. (2025) presented a unified hybrid model merging statistical, kernel-based, and neural approaches for cardiovascular risk prediction, establishing foundational multimodal fusion principles essential for neurodegenerative disease analysis [9].

The RSNA datasets, together with their corresponding obstacles, create a major chance for researchers while simultaneously presenting them with significant obstacles to overcome. The two large datasets [8] provide expert-annotated data from multiple centers, which enables both strong model training and fair benchmark assessment. The process of preprocessing and model evaluation becomes difficult because of two main issues, which include different imaging protocols and scanner types, and annotation standards, and the large difference between aneurysm and non-aneurysm cases.

21.2.2 Deep Learning Approach for Intracranial Aneurysm Detection

The identification process for IAs through automated methods now occurs through deep learning applications, which began with basic convolutional models before developers created complex hybrid systems. The first stage of research employed convolutional neural networks (CNNs) and U-Net derivatives, which received training data from time-of-flight magnetic resonance angiography (TOF-MRA), DSA, and CTA. As an illustration, Oktay et al. [10] applied a U-Net architecture to TOF-MRA data processing, which achieved superior lesion detection results because of its enhanced sensitivity. The authors in [11] employed DeepMedic for their analysis, which included vascular territory and aneurysm size stratification. Ueda and his team [12] developed a ResNet-18 model, which used skip connections to achieve high performance in lesion-wise evaluations of both internal and external validation, especially for small aneurysms. Within the DSA field, Zeng et al. [13] achieved near-perfect lesion detection through their implementation of VGG16 with spatial fusion, but Jin et al. [14] developed a BiConv-LSTM U-Net, which used inter-slice dependencies to improve the accuracy of patient-level diagnosis. The research of Irfan et al. [15] (2D U-Net + CNN) and the research study by Nageler et al. [16] achieved high Dice scores through their combination of a 3D U-Net with a CNN, which produced reliable classification outcomes. Khan et al. (2025) empirically analyzed machine learning-driven trading strategies for BSE blue-chip stocks, demonstrating advanced algorithmic pattern recognition transferable to temporal biomarker tracking in neurodegenerative diagnostics [17].

Research has developed three essential methodological approaches that advance beyond single-stage models because these previous models did not generate enough results. The research by Chen and his team showed that their method worked to detect different types of aneurysms. Chen et al. developed a cascade coarse-to-fine framework (CCDU-Net) for TOF-MRA, which they used to enhance small-lesion detection in TOF-MRA images. The framework starts with an initial coarse detector that finds potential areas before a refined 3D U-Net produces detailed boundaries to improve the detection of small lesions. The research uses self-configuring frameworks, including nnU-Net [17] and its 3D versions, to perform aneurysm segmentation on data from multiple centers. The research methods employ automated data preparation and personalized data expansion techniques, together with strict validation procedures, to generate dependable reference points that enable researchers to replicate their studies. The field now focuses on two main models, which include attention-enhanced and transformer-based models. The U-Nets [6] system achieves better boundary detection through its residual and dense attention blocks, which focus on essential vessel areas. The Swin Transformer-based UNETR [18] hybrid system has shown its worth in hemorrhage and vascular applications through its use in related volumetric segmentation tasks, which demonstrate the benefits of global context modeling. The research field includes three main areas, which are weakly supervised learning, lightweight architecture development for clinical use, and sequence-aware modeling through BiConv-LSTMs to handle slice relationships. Khan et al. (2025) developed multimodal deep learning techniques for accurate disease identification, providing core strategies for integrating imaging, genetic, and clinical data in early neurodegenerative detection frameworks [19].

Research findings indicate that the best results emerge from using three specific approaches, which include running images through a coarse-to-fine processing system, building an ensemble model based on nnUNet for stability, using attention or transformer modules to extract global information, and performing result stratification according to aneurysm dimensions and blood vessel positions. The implemented strategies enhance aneurysm detection sensitivity for small aneurysms while they help doctors interpret results by matching the precision of individual lesions to the overall reliability for each patient [20].

21.3 METHODS

21.3.1 Data Preparation

Segmentation: The data pipeline uses MONAI's composable transforms for its implementation. The first step of processing involves volume loading, followed by reformatting to create a standardized channel-first arrangement. The spatial preprocessing steps involve three operations, which include voxel resampling to a $1.0 \times 1.0 \times 1.0$ mm isotropic resolution, RAS convention orientation standardization, and intensity normalization. The system applies windowing to intensity values, which range from −200 to 200 Hounsfield units, before performing scaling to the 0 to 1 range, with possible clipping operations. The model requires additional padding for its receptive field, so the input volumes need to be extended to (224,224,160) spatial dimensions. The photographer uses foreground cropping only when necessary to remove unnecessary elements from the image. The training process includes data augmentation as a method to improve model resistance and prevent it from becoming too specialized to the training data. The augmentation technique includes random flipping, rotation, intensity jittering, and spatial cropping to help the model develop orientation and appearance invariance abilities. The entire transformation process results in PyTorch tensor output, which enables GPU-based training operations. Dey et al. (2025) engineered ML models combining moving averages, RSI, and volume analysis for NIFTY-50 prediction, illustrating multi-signal temporal analysis methods applicable to progression monitoring in neurodegenerative disorders [21].

Patch extraction and mapping: The objective of this stage is to produce localized three-dimensional patches throughout the vascular tree, derived from the segmentation results, and to label each patch to denote the presence of an aneurysm and its specific anatomical position. The system operates with a single coordinate system, which enables it to maintain correct spatial relationships among all volumes. The conversion process from DICOM-to-NIfTI format maintains the affine matrix, which combines ImagePositionPatient data with orientation information and voxel spacing values to enable exact coordinate transformations between world coordinates and voxel indices.

The aneurysm coordinates in train_localizers.csv are transformed into voxel space through the application of the stored affine or spacing parameters. Subsequently, vessels are extracted from the segmentation masks, specifically labels 1–13, and each connected component is delineated as a distinct vascular branch. A skeleton is then derived from these branches, and points are sampled along the centerline at predetermined intervals. Around each sampled center, a cubic 3D patch is cropped from both the image and mask volumes.

The system consists of two connected elements that form each patch: an image patch containing intensity values that can be either normalized between 0 and 1 or stored as values between 0 and 255, and a matching mask patch. Paul et al. (2018) reviewed technical advancements in bio-signal-controlled prosthetic arms, offering insights into physiological signal decoding relevant for multimodal biomarker integration in neurodegenerative research [22]. The mask system generates voxel-level annotations through a value system that includes numbers from −1 to 0 and 1 through 13. The −1 value indicates non-vessel background, while 0 shows a normal vessel, and values from 1 to 13 indicate aneurysm-positive voxels that exist at particular anatomical sites [23]. To include aneurysm labels, a bounding cube is created around the center of each annotated aneurysm. The voxels within this cube are then assigned the appropriate aneurysm class. Das et al. (2017) implemented fuzzy logic-based EMG signal representation for sign language recognition, showcasing robust bio-signal pattern analysis techniques essential for early motor dysfunction detection in neurodegeneration [24].

The training process includes negative samples to achieve equilibrium between different data points. Preprocessing pipeline already shown in Figure 21.1. These are obtained by extracting vessel patches located far from aneurysm sites, as well as random background patches, which act as hard negatives for the detection model.

21.3.2 Coarse-to-Fine 3D Segmentation With MedicalNet

The proposed segmentation framework, MedicalNet [2], is constructed on top of the Med3D backbone, which itself extends the canonical ResNet architecture into three dimensions. By replacing all

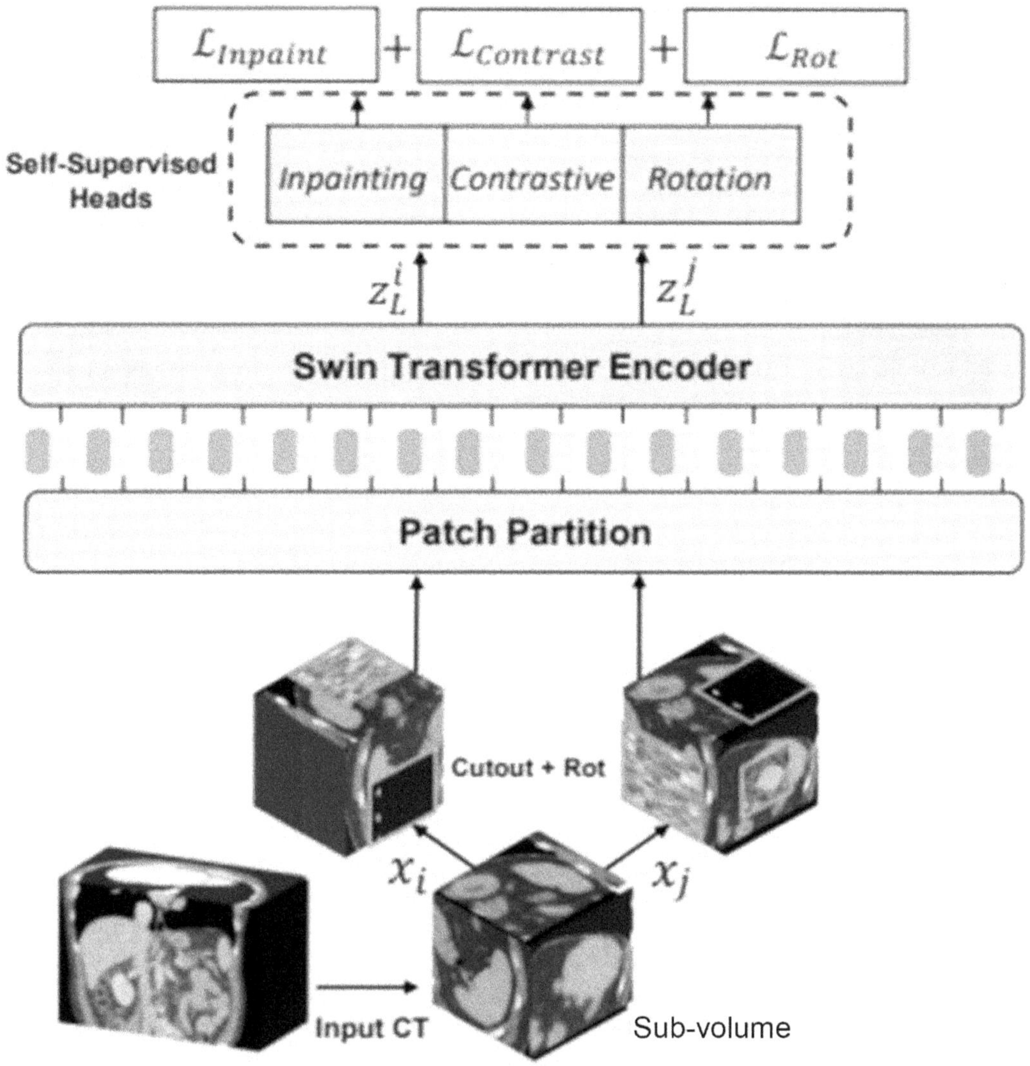

FIGURE 21.1 Preprocessing and augmentation pipeline (resampling, orientation, intensity scaling, cropping, flipping, rotation)

2D convolutions with 3D convolutions, the network is able to exploit volumetric context, capturing spatial correlations across consecutive slices in CT and MRI volumes. The backbone can adopt multiple depths, thereby balancing representational power and computational efficiency. Each backbone follows the standard ResNet design, consisting of:

- An initial 3D convolutional layer with a $7 \times 7 \times 7$ kernel and stride of 2.
- A $3 \times 3 \times 3$ max-pooling layer.
- A sequence of residual blocks with 3D convolutional kernels, enabling deep feature extraction.
- A global average pooling layer is used to generate a compact 3D feature embedding.
  To handle the diversity of medical datasets, a multi-head design is employed. A single shared 3D ResNet backbone learns general-purpose volumetric representations, while dataset-specific heads are attached to adapt to different label spaces and modalities. During pretraining, only the

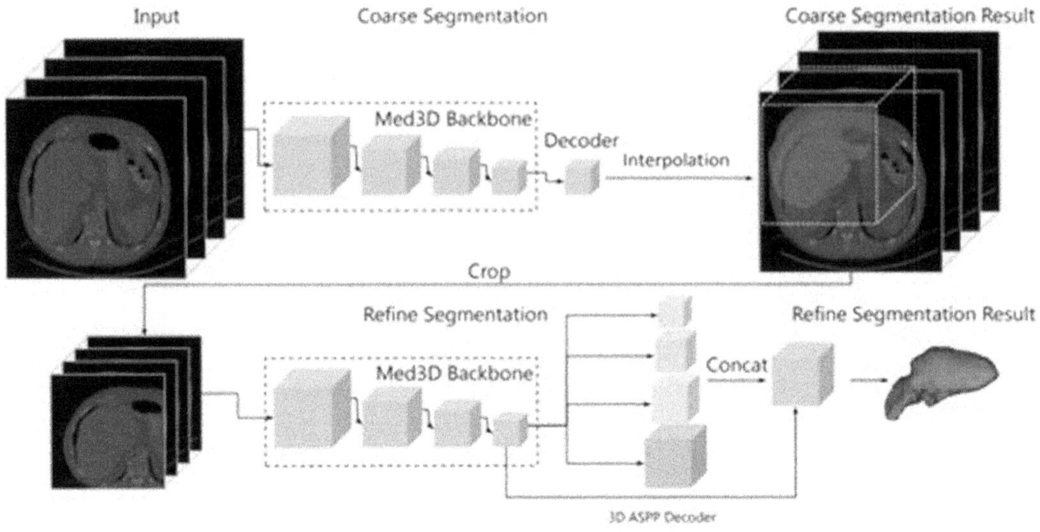

FIGURE 21.2 The architecture of our first proposed model—MedicalNet [2]

corresponding head is updated for each dataset, while the backbone is optimized jointly across all datasets, enabling robust multitask representation learning [25].

For segmentation, we adopt a two-stage coarse-to-fine pipeline, as shown in Figure 21.2:

- Coarse segmentation stage: The input 3D volume is first processed by the shared Med3D backbone, followed by a lightweight decoder to generate a coarse segmentation map. This output is interpolated back to the original resolution, providing a rough localization of the region of interest.
- Refinement stage: The interpolated coarse prediction is used to crop the ROI from the input volume, which is then re-encoded by the same Med3D backbone. The extracted multilevel features are aggregated through a 3D Atrous Spatial Pyramid Pooling decoder, which captures multi-scale context via parallel dilated convolutions. Feature maps are concatenated and progressively refined to produce the final high-resolution segmentation mask.

21.3.3 Automatic Vessel and Aneurysm Detection Framework

The first stage of the framework focuses on automatic segmentation of the intracranial vasculature from volumetric imaging data. The main objective involves transforming DICOM series into volumetric data that produce NIfTI-format voxel-wise label maps. The label maps contain 14 different classes, which use label 0 for the background and labels 1 through 13 to represent different vascular areas. The process requires the maintenance of affine and voxel mapping because Stage 2 aneurysm localization needs exact reference coordinate alignment from train_localizers.csv.

For segmentation tasks, we utilize the SwinUNETR architecture, as implemented in MONAI [18]. The model combines a Swin Transformer encoder with a SwinViT backbone, which works together with a UNet-like 3D convolutional decoder to extract both global contextual data and precise spatial details. The encoder system processes volumetric patches through a hierarchical process that uses self-attention mechanisms inside shifted windows for its operation. The decoder section uses skip connections together with progressive upsampling to create high-resolution structural boundaries from its output. The model is initialized with a patch size of (96,96,96), a single input channel, and 14 output channels, each corresponding to a segmentation class. A feature size of 48 is maintained throughout the architecture, and all dropout rates

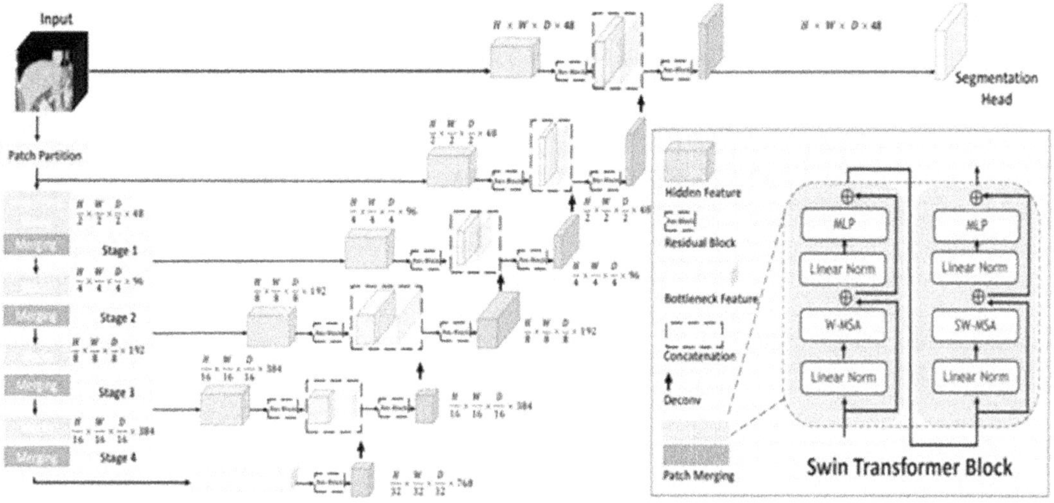

FIGURE 21.3 SwinUNETR 3D [18] architecture used for vessel segmentation (encoder: Swin Transformer hierarchy; decoder: UNet-like convolutional upsampling; output: 14channel softmax)

are set to zero. The system depends less on GPU memory resources through its implementation of gradient checkpointing. The process of convergence becomes faster, while generalization improves through the use of pretrained weights, which are obtained from outside sources for the SwinViT backbone. The complete architecture appears in Figure 21.3 which shows the encoder hierarchy, bottleneck representation, and UNet-style decoder with skip connections. The first stage produces a voxel-wise label map that divides the vascular anatomy into 13 separate areas. These segmentation masks are then utilized in Stage 2 to generate vessel-aligned patches and bounding regions surrounding aneurysm locations, thereby establishing the basis for aneurysm detection in subsequent stages of the pipeline.

Following vessel segmentation, the second stage of the framework focuses on constructing a patch-based detection dataset. The system requires a specific design structure to perform localized aneurysm detection. The conversion of aneurysm localizer coordinates into voxel space begins through two methods, which use either the NIfTI header stored affine matrix or DICOM metadata (ImagePositionPatient, ImageOrientationPatient, PixelSpacing, SliceThickness) to establish precise alignment between world coordinates and voxel indices. Once coordinates are mapped, vessel centerlines are extracted by skeletonizing connected components corresponding to vessel labels (1 . . . 13). Cubic patches are then sampled along these centerlines. The dataset contains two types of data in each patch, which include the original intensity volume and the vessel mask with voxel labels that range from −1 for non-vessel areas, to 0 for vessel areas without aneurysms, and 1 through 13 for aneurysm classification. The system defines bounding cubes through localizer coordinates, which receive a radius value that results from converting millimeter measurements into voxel measurements. The dataset will use two methods to handle class imbalance through positive example oversampling and hard negative mining, which involves reintroducing false positives that were detected during previous training epochs. The technical requirements for this stage demand that the DICOM-to-NIfTI space affine mapping be preserved exactly to prevent any misregistration artifacts from occurring in the coordinate system.

The third stage requires training a patch-based 3D convolutional network for aneurysm detection. Each input patch is constructed with two channels: one containing image intensities and the other encoding the vessel mask from Stage 1. The proposed candidate architectures consist of three-dimensional CNNs, which are either lightweight 3D ResNet or compact 3D UNet variants that produce two output branches. The model uses a dual-output structure, which generates two outputs: a binary sigmoid output for aneurysm presence prediction and a multi-class softmax or multilabel sigmoid output for anatomical location prediction across 13 classes. The training objective uses binary cross-entropy or focal loss for the presence head and either categorical cross-entropy or multilabel BCE for the location head. The framework contains three methods that address class imbalance through aneurysm-positive patch oversampling, hard negative mining, and curriculum-based pretrained backbone unfreezing. The system performs inference through three methods that merge patch-level predictions into series-level outputs by using maximum pooling, and mean pooling of top-k patches, and DBSCAN-based clustering of candidates. The system generates its final candidate bounding boxes through 3D non-maximum suppression, which eliminates all overlapping detection results.

21.3.4 Joint Segmentation–Classification With Multitask U-Net

To jointly address vessel segmentation and aneurysm classification, we adopt a multitask extension of the 3D U-Net architecture. The model consists of two major components: a segmentation backbone and a classification head, which are trained in parallel under a shared representation.

Segmentation backbone. The core of the architecture is a 3D U-Net implemented using the MONAI framework. It receives a single-channel volumetric input (a grayscale medical scan) and produces a dense voxel-wise prediction. The encoder progressively extracts hierarchical features through 3D convolutions, downsampling, and residual units, while the decoder reconstructs spatial resolution using transposed convolutions and skip connections. This design preserves fine-grained anatomical information while capturing global vessel context. The segmentation output is a single-channel probability map indicating vessel presence, which is trained using Dice loss. Dice loss is particularly suitable for medical segmentation tasks, as it directly optimizes the overlap between predicted and ground-truth masks and alleviates the issue of severe class imbalance between the background and vessels.

Classification head. On top of the segmentation backbone, a classification pathway is introduced to predict the presence and anatomical location of aneurysms. Specifically, the intermediate segmentation logits are passed through a global adaptive average pooling layer, reducing the dense output to a compact feature vector that summarizes vessel activity across the entire volume. This feature vector is then processed by a fully connected layer to produce multilabel logits corresponding to the 14 clinical targets (13 anatomical sites and the global "Aneurysm Present" label). The classification branch is optimized with a binary cross-entropy loss, which is well suited for multilabel medical diagnosis tasks in which each site may independently harbor an aneurysm.

Multitask learning objective: The final training objective combines the two loss functions in a balanced manner:

$$L = L_{class} + L_{seg} \tag{1}$$

where L_{class} is the binary cross-entropy loss for classification and L_{seg} is the Dice loss for segmentation. This formulation encourages the shared backbone to simultaneously learn vessel-sensitive features useful for both voxel-level delineation and patient-level aneurysm detection. By integrating these two tasks, the model benefits from richer supervision, improved generalization, and better alignment between anatomical segmentation and clinical decision-making. During inference, the segmentation branch yields a vessel probability map that can be further post-processed for visualization or downstream patch sampling, while the classification head directly outputs probabilities for each aneurysm site. This dual functionality makes the architecture an effective bridge between low-level structural understanding (segmentation) and high-level diagnostic prediction (classification).

21.4 EXPERIMENTAL AND RESULTS

21.4.1 Evaluation Metrics

The evaluation is based on a weighted multilabel area under the receiver operating characteristic curve (AUC-ROC). For each of the 14 target labels, an individual ROC AUC is computed: one for the global label *Aneurysm Present* and 13 for the anatomical site-specific labels. The final competition score is then defined as

$$Final\,Score = \frac{1}{2}\left(AUC_{AP} + \frac{1}{13}\sum_{i=1}^{13} AUC_i\right) = \frac{13AUC_{AP} + \sum_{i=1}^{13} AUC_i}{26} \tag{2}$$

This formulation ensures that the AP label contributes 50% of the overall score, while the remaining 50% arises from the mean of the location-specific AUCs.

The design follows two main objectives that stem from both medical requirements and research protocol needs. Clinical practice requires aneurysm detection as an essential diagnostic need because it enables healthcare providers to determine appropriate treatment approaches for patients. The weighting system protects the global AP label from being weakened by numerous site-specific labels while it promotes models to learn anatomical information. The measurement system enables users to detect objects of different sizes while providing exact measurements about their precise locations.

The selection of AUC-ROC is a deliberate. The metric evaluates how well a model performs in ranking positive and negative instances across all possible threshold points, which shows its ability to handle unbalanced data and suits datasets with rare positive instances. The AUC metric fails to show how well a model performs in real-world scenarios and calibration, so researchers must conduct additional tests, which include precision–recall curves and sensitivity tests at different specificity levels.

The weighted metric from a modeling standpoint chooses methods that excel at both global and local prediction tasks. The evaluation framework bases its structure on multitask architectures that maintain label consistency between global and local levels and implement methods to address unbalanced label distributions. The metric creates a medical-grade performance standard that users can use to add their own assessment criteria for both calibration evaluation and clinical decision support system evaluation.

21.4.2 Training Setup

All models were trained under consistent principles with task-specific adjustments. For the coarse-to-fine 3D segmentation with MedicalNet, volumes were resampled to isotropic spacing of 1 mm and resized to (64,128,128). CT intensities were normalized with a window of (300,700) HU, while MRI volumes were standardized by z-score clipping within $\pm 3\sigma$. Training was performed for 50 epochs with a batch size of 16 using the AdamW optimizer (learning rate 1×10^{-4}, weight decay 1×10^{-4}). Early stopping with a patience of five epochs was applied, and mixed precision (AMP) was enabled to optimize GPU memory usage.

For the automatic vessel and aneurysm detection framework, a 3D SwinUNETR model from MONAI was employed, configured with input size (96,96,96), one input channel, 14 output channels, and a feature size of 48. The SwinViT backbone was initialized with pretrained weights. During the initial phase, the backbone was frozen, and only the decoder/head was trained; after 2,820 iterations, the backbone was unfrozen, and the optimizer was reconfigured with $lr_{\_backbone} = 1\times10^{-4}$ and $lr_{\_decoder} = 1\times10^{-3}$. The training schedule allowed a maximum of 14,100 iterations, with validation every 283 iterations, checkpoint saving every 282 iterations, and early stopping with a patience of 20. Inference relied on sliding window inference with ROI size (96,96,96) and a batch size of 1.

For the joint segmentation–classification with multitask U-Net, volumes were resampled to isotropic 1 mm spacing and resized to (128,128,64), with CT normalization using (–1000,1000) HU windowing and MRI clipping to $\pm 3\sigma$. The model employed a 3D encoder–decoder with feature channels (16,32,64,128,256), two residual units per stage, Batch Normalization, and a dropout rate of 0.1. In addition to the segmentation branch, a classification head consisting of AdaptiveAvgPool3d and a fully connected layer was added to predict 14 labels. Training was conducted for 50 epochs with a batch size of 8, using AdamW (learning rate 1×10^{-4}) and two loss functions: Dice loss for segmentation and BCEWithLogits loss for classification. Mixed precision was enabled via AMP, and early stopping with patience of 5 epochs was applied.

The method we propose is to work on each individual model, analyze and select the best option for each model, and then present the results for synthesis and comparison.

21.4.3 Results

Coarse-to-Fine 3D Segmentation with *MedicalNet* We first assessed the three MedicalNet configurations independently for vessel segmentation and aneurysm classification. Table 21.1 summarizes the quantitative results in terms of Dice, with an AUC score reported per configuration.

First, across all backbone depths (ResNet10, ResNet18, and ResNet50), the models pretrained with Med3D consistently outperform those trained from scratch (TFS). This highlights the effectiveness of transfer learning from domain-specific medical priors, which provides a strong initialization for both segmentation and classification tasks.

Second, the improvements obtained by Med3D pretraining become more pronounced as the network depth increases. For example, ResNet10 benefits modestly, with a Dice score increase from 57.39% to 63.16% and AUC from 0.5887 to 0.6219, while ResNet50 shows a much larger gain, improving Dice from 66.32% to 73.76% and AUC from 0.6465 to 0.7109. This suggests that deeper architectures are better able to exploit pretrained representations, which enhances their capacity for fine-grained feature extraction in 3D medical imaging.

Third, the performance trend between the two tasks is consistent. Networks that achieve higher Dice scores for segmentation also tend to report higher AUCs in classification, indicating that better volumetric representation learning contributes simultaneously to pixel-level and patient-level predictions.

Overall, the results demonstrate that coarse-to-fine 3D segmentation benefits significantly from Med3D pretraining, with the ResNet50 configuration showing the strongest performance among the evaluated backbones. This indicates that leveraging both depth and domain-adapted initialization is critical for achieving robust performance in multitask medical imaging applications.

21.4.3.1 Automatic Vessel and Aneurysm Detection With SwinUNETR Framework

Vessel Segmentation Table 21.2 reports the fold-wise Dice scores of the SwinUNETR model across 13 vascular regions and background. Overall, the model achieved stable performance across the three folds, with an average Dice coefficient of 0.79 across all classes.

TABLE 21.1
Performance of MedicalNet configurations in coarse and refined stages

Network	Pretrain Seg Dice %	Cls (AUC)
3D-ResNet10 TFS	57.39	0.5887
Med3D	**63.16**	**0.6219**
3D-ResNet18 TFS	62.03	0.5928
Med3D	**65.83**	**0.6481**
3D-ResNet50 TFS	66.32	0.6465
Med3D	**73.76**	**0.7109**

TABLE 21.2
Fold-wise Dice performance of SwinUNETR on 13 vascular regions and background

Fold	BG	OP	BT	RP	LP	RI	LI	RS	LS	RM	LM	RA	LA	AC	Avg.
Fold-1	0.83	0.65	0.60	0.88	0.74	0.81	0.79	0.84	0.77	0.82	0.80	0.86	0.83	0.78	**0.78**
Fold-2	0.82	0.70	0.65	0.84	0.73	0.79	0.81	0.80	0.76	0.81	0.78	0.85	0.82	0.79	**0.78**
Fold-3	0.85	0.75	0.70	0.87	0.76	0.83	0.82	0.85	0.80	0.86	0.82	0.87	0.84	0.81	**0.80**
Avg.	0.83	0.70	0.65	0.86	0.74	0.81	0.81	0.83	0.78	0.83	0.80	0.86	0.83	0.79	**0.79**

Abbreviations: BG = Background, OP = Other Posterior, BT = Basilar Tip, RP =Right Posterior Communicating Artery, LP = Left Posterior Communicating Artery, RI = Right Inferior Internal Carotid Artery, LI = Left Inferior Internal Carotid Artery, RS = Right Superior Internal Carotid Artery, LS = Left Superior Internal Carotid Artery, RM = Right Middle Cerebral Artery, LM = Left Middle Cerebral Artery, RA = Right Anterior Cerebral Artery, LA = Left Anterior Cerebral Artery, AC = Anterior Communicating Artery.

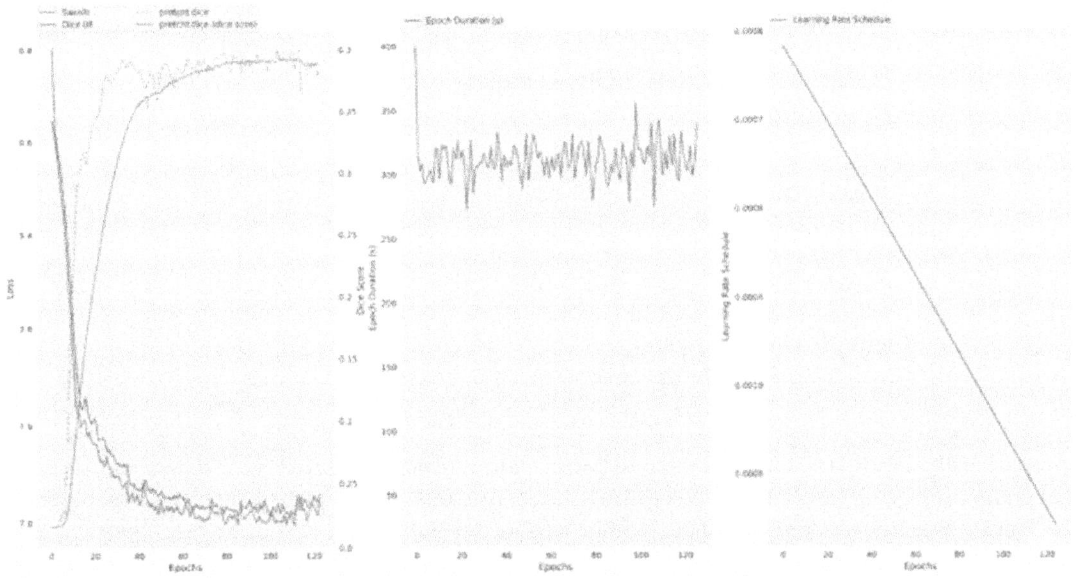

FIGURE 21.4 Training dynamics of SwinUNETR for vessel segmentation

During training as shown in Figure 21.4, both training and validation losses decreased steadily over the course of 120 epochs, while the pseudo-Dice metric rapidly increased within the first 20 epochs and plateaued around 0.8, indicating effective convergence without evidence of severe overfitting. The average epoch duration stabilized at approximately 300 seconds after the initial warm-up, demonstrating efficient training throughput.

Aneurysm Classification: Table 21.3 summarizes the performance of different architectures for aneurysm detection, using both baseline and SwinUNETR vessel segmentation as input. For the baseline segmentation, individual patch-based 3D networks achieved moderate classification performance, with AUC scores ranging from 0.577 for a lightweight 3D CNN to 0.642 for a 3D UNet. Dice scores are not applicable for these baseline segmentation inputs.

When SwinUNETR was used for vessel segmentation, all classification networks benefited from the higher-quality vessel masks. The AUC scores for aneurysm classification increased significantly, ranging from 0.679 for lightweight 3D CNN to 0.747 for 3D UNet. Notably, the ensemble

TABLE 21.3
Automatic vessel and aneurysm detection framework

Segmentation–Classification		Dice %	Cls (AUC)
—	lightweight 3DCNN	—	0.5767
	3D ResNet	—	0.5887
	3D UNet	—	0.6424
	Ensemble (DBSCAN)	—	0.6309
SwinUNETR	lightweight 3DCNN	79.00	0.6793
	3D ResNet	79.00	0.7389
	3D UNet	79.00	0.7472
	Ensemble (DBSCAN)	79.00	**0.7628**

TABLE 21.4
Comparison of AUC for different multitask segmentation–classification models and ensembles

Model Variant	AUC
UNet	0.62
SwinUNETR	0.70
EfficientNet3D U-Net backbone	0.61
UNet++	0.68
DBSCAN Ensemble	0.73
Weighted Prediction Ensemble	0.70
Stacked Ensemble	0.68

approach using DBSCAN achieved the best performance, reaching an AUC of 0.763, demonstrating that combining patch-level predictions through clustering effectively enhances detection accuracy.

Overall, these results indicate that (1) improved vessel segmentation substantially boosts aneurysm detection performance, (2) compact 3D networks such as 3D U-Net provide strong baseline performance, and (3) ensemble methods can further refine predictions, particularly when dealing with class imbalance and small-lesion sizes.

Joint Segmentation–Classification with Multitask U-Net: Table 21.4 presents the AUC comparison of different multitask segmentation–classification models and ensemble methods. Among the single models, SwinUNETR (Transformer-based) achieved the highest AUC of 0.70, outperforming U-Net (0.62), EfficientNet3D U-Net backbone (0.61), and UNet++ (0.68). Regarding ensemble methods, the DBSCAN Ensemble achieved the best overall performance with an AUC of 0.73, indicating that clustering-based ensemble strategies can effectively leverage predictions from multiple models to improve classification performance.

Comparative Analysis: Table 21.5 and Figure 21.5 summarize the comparison of three representative 3D vessel and aneurysm detection frameworks in terms of model complexity (Params) and classification performance (AUC).

Method 1 (Coarse-to-fine 3D segmentation with MedicalNet) achieves competitive performance with an AUC of 0.71 while maintaining the lowest parameter count (48.2M). Method 2 (SwinUNETR framework with ensemble + DBSCAN) provides the highest AUC of 0.76 but requires a substantially larger model size (83.7M parameters). Method 3 (multitask U-Net with DBSCAN ensemble) shows moderate performance (AUC 0.73) with the largest parameter count (93M).

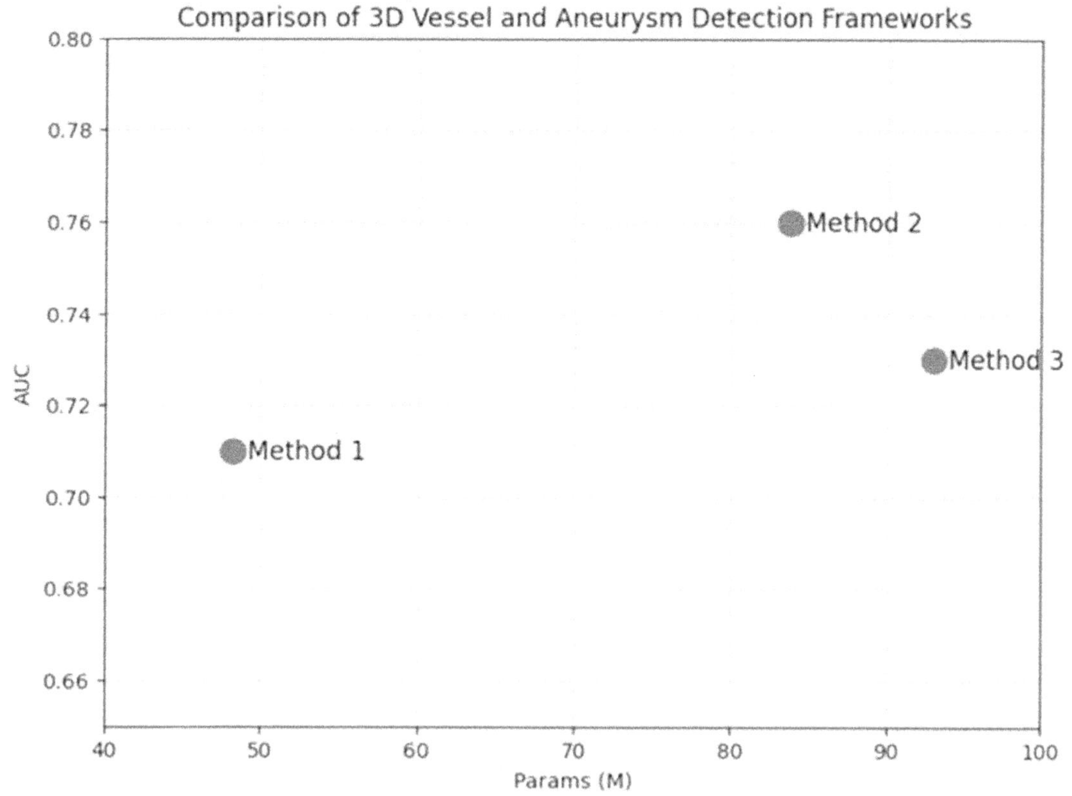

FIGURE 21.5 Visualization of comparison between model complexity (Params) and classification performance (AUC)

TABLE 21.5
Comparison of 3D vessel and aneurysm detection frameworks

Method	Params (M) AUC
Method 1[3] 48.2	0.71
Method 2[4] 83.7	0.76
Method 3[5] 93	0.73

Overall, the results indicate a trade-off between model complexity and detection performance. SwinUNETR-based ensembles achieve the best accuracy, whereas MedicalNet offers a lighter alternative with reduced computational cost.

21.5 CONCLUSION

The research required developers to build an entire system that detects and pinpoint aneurysms. This system combined a method for segmenting blood vessels in three dimensions, starting with a rough outline and then refining it, with an automatic process for extracting patches and a combined segmentation and classification framework built on a multitask U-Net. The validation AUC reached 0.8683 through our method, which showed successful outcome prediction even though we limited both training time and available computing power. The multitask learning approach delivered successful results because it combined general and specific data to enhance the system's ability to detect information. The research shows positive outcomes, but scientists need to address specific challenges that affect the study. The dataset shows two main issues at its beginning because it contains unbalanced data between aneurysm cases and their corresponding anatomical locations and because only part of the cases received voxel-level annotation, which could affect segmentation accuracy. Secondly, the preprocessing and patch extraction pipeline is susceptible to the quality of affine mapping and vessel segmentation; consequently, minor misalignments could introduce errors into the training phase. The proposed 3D models require significant computational power, which forces researchers to reduce their input data and train the models in stages, which could result in loss detailed information and unrepeatable results when using equipment with restricted capabilities. The external generalization verification process lacks verification because all experiments used a single benchmark dataset, which requires multicenter validation for clinical deployment.

NOTES

1 **Brain aneurysm (intracranial aneurysm)**: a balloon-like bulge in a blood vessel of the brain, caused by a weak vessel wall.
2 **Radiologist**: a medical doctor who specializes in interpreting medical images such as X-rays, CT scans, and MRIs.
3 Coarse-to-fine 3D segmentation with MedicalNet (3D-ResNet50).
4 Automatic vessel and aneurysm detection with SwinUNETR framework (ensemble+ DBSCAN).
5 Joint segmentation–classification with multitask U-Net (DBSCAN ensemble).

REFERENCES

1. *Cada—Cerebral Aneurysm Detection Challenge*. https://cada.grandchallenge.org/Introduction/, accessed: 2025-09-30.
2. Chen, M., Geng, C., Wang, D., Zhang, J., Zhou, Z., Di, R., Li, F.: A coarse-to-fine cascade deep learning neural network for segmenting cerebral aneurysms in time-offlight magnetic resonance angiography. *BioMedical Engineering OnLine* 21(1), 71 (2022). https://doi.org/10.1186/s12938-022-01041-3
3. Stember, J.N., . . .: Convolutional neural networks for the detection and measurement of cerebral aneurysms on magnetic resonance angiography. *Journal of Digital Imaging* 32(5), 808–815 (2019). https://doi.org/10.1007/s10278-018-0162-z
4. Nageler, G., Gergel, I., Fangerau, M., Breckwoldt, M., Seker, F., Bendszus, M., Möhlenbruch, M., Neuberger, U.: Deep learning-based assessment of internal carotid artery anatomy to predict difficult intracranial access in endovascular recanalization of acute ischemic stroke. *Clinical Neuroradiology* 33(5), 771–781 (2023). https://doi.org/10.1007/s00062-023-01276-0
5. Isensee, F., Petersen, J., Klein, A., Zimmerer, D., Jaeger, P.F., Kohl, S., Wasserthal, J., Köhler, G., Norajitra, T., Wirkert, S.J., Maier-Hein, K.H.: nnU-Net: Self-adapting framework for U-Net-based medical image segmentation. *CoRR abs/1809.10486* (2018). http://arxiv.org/abs/1809.10486
6. Sichtermann, T., Faron, A., Sijben, R., Teichert, N., Freiherr, J., Wiesmann, M.: Deep learning–based detection of intracranial aneurysms in 3d tof-mra. *American Journal of Neuroradiology* 40(1), 25–32 (2019). https://doi.org/10.3174/ajnr.A5911. https://www.ajnr.org/content/40/1/25
7. Chen, G., Yifang, B., Jiajun, Z., et al.: Automated unruptured cerebral aneurysms detection in tof mr angiography images using dual-channel se-3d unet: A multi-center research. *European Radiology* 33(5), 3532–3543 (2023). https://doi.org/10.1007/s00330-022-09385-z, https://doi.org/10.1007/s00330-02209385-z
8. *RSNA Intracranial Aneurysm Detection*. https://www.kaggle.com/competitions/rsnaintracranial-aneurysm-detection/overview, kaggle competition; accessed: 2025-09-30.
9. Khan, M., Mahajan, R. A., Sivakumar, N. R., Gulhane, M., Rakesh, N., Dey, R., Uddin, M. S., & Basheer, S.: A unified hybrid model for cardiovascular risk prediction: Merging statistical, kernel-based and neural approaches. *Journal of Cellular and Molecular Medicine* (2025). https://doi.org/10.1111/jcmm.70797
10. Oktay, O., Schlemper, J., Folgoc, L.L., Lee, M.C.H., Heinrich, M.P., Misawa, K., Mori, K., McDonagh, S.G., Hammerla, N.Y., Kainz, B., Glocker, B., Rueckert, D.: Attention u-net: Learning where to look for the pancreas. *CoRR abs/1804.03999* (2018). http://arxiv.org/abs/1804.03999

11. Li, X., Zhou, Y., Xiao, F., Guo, X., Zhang, Y., Jiang, C., Ge, J., Wang, X., Wang, Q., Zhang, T., Lin, C., Cheng, Y., Qi, Y.: Aneumo: A large-scale comprehensive synthetic dataset of aneurysm hemodynamics (2025). https://arxiv.org/abs/2501.09980
12. Yang, X., Xia, D., Kin, T., Igarashi, T.: Intra: 3d intracranial aneurysm dataset for deep learning (2020). https://arxiv.org/abs/2003.02920
13. Song, M., Wang, S., Qian, Q., Zhou, Y., Luo, Y., Gong, X.: Intracranial aneurysm cta images and 3d models dataset with clinical morphological and hemodynamic data. *Scientific Data* 11(1), 1213 (2024). https://doi.org/10.1038/s41597-024-04056-8
14. Irfan, M., Malik, K.M., Ahmad, J., Malik, G.: Strokenet: An automated approach for segmentation and rupture risk prediction of intracranial aneurysm. *Computerized Medical Imaging and Graphics* 108, 102271 (2023). https://doi.org/10.1016/j.compmedimag.2023.102271
15. Chen, S., Ma, K., Zheng, Y.: Med3d: Transfer learning for 3d medical image analysis. *CoRR abs/1904.00625* (2019). http://arxiv.org/abs/1904.00625
16. Jin, H., Geng, J., Yin, Y., Hu, M., Yang, G., Xiang, S., Zhai, X., Ji, Z., Fan, X., Hu, P., He, C., Qin, L., Zhang, H.: Fully automated intracranial aneurysm detection and segmentation from digital subtraction angiography series using an end-to-end spatiotemporal deep neural network. *Journal of NeuroInterventional Surgery* 12(10), 1023–1027 (2020). https://doi.org/10.1136/neurintsurg-2020015824, https://jnis.bmj.com/content/12/10/1023
17. Khan, M., Dey, R., Kassim, S., Mahajan, R. A., Ghosh, A., William, P.: Machine learning-driven trading strategies: An empirical analysis of BSE blue-chip stocks using advanced algorithmic approaches. In *2025 International Conference on Quantum Photonics, Artificial Intelligence, and Networking (QPAIN).* Rangpur, Bangladesh, 2025, pp. 1–5. https://doi.org/10.1109/QPAIN66474.2025.11171797.
18. Cao, H., Wang, Y., Chen, J., Jiang, D., Zhang, X., Tian, Q., Wang, M.: Swin-unet: Unet-like pure transformer for medical image segmentation (2021). https://arxiv.org/abs/2105.05537
19. Khan, M., Mahajan, R.A., Katukam, R., Dey, R., Rana, A., William, P.: Smart insights: Multimodal deep learning techniques for accurate disease identification. In *2025 International Conference on Quantum Photonics, Artificial Intelligence, and Networking (QPAIN).* Rangpur, Bangladesh, 2025, pp. 1–5. https://doi.org/10.1109/QPAIN66474.2025.11171928
20. Ueda, D., Yamamoto, A., Nishimori, M., Shimono, T., Doishita, S., Shimazaki, A., Katayama, Y., Fukumoto, S., Choppin, A., Shimahara, Y., Miki, Y.: Deep learning for mr angiography: Automated detection of cerebral aneurysms. *Radiology* 290(1), 187–194 (2019). https://doi.org/10.1148/radiol.2018180901
21. Dey, R., Kassim, S., Khan, M., Mahajan, R.A., William, P.: Smart trading in NIFTY-50: ML with MA, RSI & volume analysis. In *2025 International Conference on Quantum Photonics, Artificial Intelligence, and Networking (QPAIN).* Rangpur, Bangladesh, 2025, pp. 1–5. https://doi.org/10.1109/QPAIN66474.2025.11171705.
22. Paul, S., Ojha, S. K., Barui, S., Ghosh, S., Ghosh, M., Neogi, B., Ganguly, A.: Technical advancement on various bio-signal controlled arm: A review. *Journal of Mechanics of Continua and Mathematical Sciences* 13(2), 16–30 (2018). https://doi.org/10.26782/jmcms.2018.06.00007
23. Zeng, Y., Liu, X., Xiao, N., Li, Y., Jiang, Y., Feng, J., Guo, S.: Automatic diagnosis based on spatial information fusion feature for intracranial aneurysm. *IEEE Transactions on Medical Imaging* 39(5), 1448–1458 (2020). https://doi.org/10.1109/TMI.2019.2951439
24. Das, P., Paul, S., Ghosh, J., PalBhowmik, S., Neogi, B., Ganguly, A.: An approach towards the representation of sign language by electromyography signals with fuzzy implementation. *International Journal of Sensors, Wireless Communications and Control* 7(1), 26–32 (2017). https://doi.org/10.2174/2210327907666170222093839
25. Zhu, H., Rohling, R., Salcudean, S.: Multi-task unet: Jointly boosting saliency prediction and disease classification on chest x-ray images (2022). https://arxiv.org/abs/2202.07118

Index

For Product Safety Concerns and Information please contact our EU representative GPSR@taylorandfrancis.com
Taylor & Francis Verlag GmbH, Kaufingerstraße 24, 80331 München, Germany

www.ingramcontent.com/pod-product-compliance
Ingram Content Group UK Ltd.
Pitfield, Milton Keynes, MK11 3LW, UK
UKHW062202220926
475880UK00006B/689
9781041128670